The Care of the Uninsured in America

T0214434

Nancy J. Johnson • Lane P. Johnson
Editors

The Care of the Uninsured in America

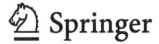 Springer

Editors
Nancy J. Johnson
El Rio Community Health Center
Tucson, AZ
USA
nancyj@elrio.org

Lane P. Johnson
Arizona Health Science Center
Tucson, AZ
USA
oneherbal@msn.com

ISBN 978-1-4899-8350-3   ISBN 978-0-387-78309-3 (eBook)
DOI 10.1007/978-0-387-78309-3
Springer New York Dordrecht Heidelberg London

© Springer Science+Business Media, LLC 2010
Softcover re-print of the Hardcover 1st edition 2010
All rights reserved. This work may not be translated or copied in whole or in part without the written permission of the publisher (Springer Science+Business Media, LLC, 233 Spring Street, New York, NY 10013, USA), except for brief excerpts in connection with reviews or scholarly analysis. Use in connection with any form of information storage and retrieval, electronic adaptation, computer software, or by similar or dissimilar methodology now known or hereafter developed is forbidden.
The use in this publication of trade names, trademarks, service marks, and similar terms, even if they are not identified as such, is not to be taken as an expression of opinion as to whether or not they are subject to proprietary rights.

Printed on acid-free paper

Springer is part of Springer Science+Business Media (www.springer.com)

To Our Patients

Preface

As the director of a Faith Based Community Health Center, I daily find myself interacting with medically uninsured patients and their families. At our clinic, we are blessed with wonderful staff and volunteers. We make a significant difference in the lives of the people we serve, and I have learned that the effort also makes a significant difference in the lives of our staff and volunteers.

As I interact each day with our patients and their families, I come away recognizing that there is no individual face of poverty. Having lived my adult life relatively well off financially, I am struck with how many of our patients look like my friends and neighbors; that there is no particular ethnicity or age. Our patients look pretty much like the rest of us.

The sobering fact is how close to the truth that may be. The difficulty of being medically uninsured is only the tip of the iceberg. Many Americans are only a few paychecks away from homelessness, and less than that to lose (if they ever had) their medical insurance. For most of our patients, it is not about choice, it is about circumstance. Joblessness, homelessness, accident or illness, advancing age, disability, and mental illness are all merely predisposing factors. Every day at our clinic, we count our blessings and realize how fortunate we are to be able to provide health services, and that it is a fine line to cross and find one's self in need of health services.

The least we can provide is respect and caring, and we strive for that with every interaction. It is not always easy, but respect and compassion are the real foundation of a medical home.

As we have come to work with other organizations in our communities to address the larger problems of the medically uninsured, we recognized that there were few resources to help us figure out what the issues are, and how we might go about trying to resolve them. Practically every community in the United States has to address these issues. Rather than continuing to reinvent the wheel, we have compiled this book as a collection of thoughts and ideas that may help get you started.

Bless you for your compassion and caring. Let us all move forward together.

Nancy J. Johnson, RN, PhD(c)
Executive Director
El Rio Community Health Center
Tucson, AZ, USA

Preface

As a physician, I have been trained to take care of each person's medical issues as I see them, and consider the ethnic, cultural, economic, and demographic issues primarily as they relate to the medical concerns. Even though my career has been focused on the medically underserved. Even though I have a degree in public health, and despite what I teach my students.

What the editing of this book has reminded me is how important it is to consider our patients collectively if we are going to be effective in the long run. We can take care of patients through our days, our years, our entire careers, and still not affect the system that helps to perpetuate the conditions in which our patients find themselves.

As a physician, one learns to compartmentalize, and at times this is a useful strategy in taking care of patients. But it allows us to too easily separate ourselves from our patients and their conditions, to think of them and us.

There are very few of us in the United States who are far away from the possibility of no medical coverage. That we are the only developed country that is in this position, and over 25% of our residents are without any medical coverage insurance, is shameful. It is about us, and we all must do more to correct these inequities. There are sufficient resources in this country to accomplish the goal of health care for everyone. What we lack as a country is sufficient political will.

Some other lessons I have learned or been reminded of in this editing process:

What we have written is a snapshot in time. The past influences the future, but we cannot dwell on it. We have to consider what the most effective means are to provide care to the medically uninsured, and move forward.

Among medically uninsured populations, the diversity is as significant as the commonalities. There is no single fix.

Regardless of a patient's background, the single most important tool we have in taking care of the medically uninsured is the development of a medical "home" which patients can identify as the place they can come to get care. What is a medical home? Nancy said it best. Where you are respected and cared for as the person you are, not the circumstances that have placed you in the position you are in. I am convinced it is from this concept that a viable system can be developed.

As Dr. Cullen's chapter on information technology points out, what is required is not just a new electronic system that follows the patients, but a new language that creates and defines a system that can appropriately care for the patient. What we design for the complexities of caring for the medically underserved can serve as model for caring for everyone in this country.

Many innovative, bold, and wonderful solutions have been developed as local/ regional models. As communities and states we can learn from, and support, each other. But the local models are not, by and large, self-sustaining. Ultimately, solutions to the lack of medical insurance in this country will require a national perspective, and federal funding. That is part of the work we all must do, and Dr. Dalen's chapter points out some of the possibilities and pitfalls other countries have experienced.

When I wonder how the system we have hasn't already collapsed from its own weight, I just need to look at the people working within it. Healthcare is a service industry, and we have been blessed with professionals who understand and live the concept of service in their daily lives, who go the extra mile for the patient despite the vagaries, the barriers, and the sometimes mean spiritedness of the organizational infrastructure. At times I look at the ascending generation and wonder if they have the heart, the vision, the courage, the resolve, and the tenacity to even continue to try to weave new thread in this patchwork quilt of a healthcare system. But then I look at the young workers at Nancy's clinic, or my own students, and my heart is filled again with hope.

Lane P. Johnson, MD, MPH
Associate Professor, Clinical Family and Community Medicine
Associate Clinical, Professor, Mel and Enid Zuckerman
Arizona College of Public Health
Arizona Health Sciences Center
Tucson, AZ, USA

Contents

Contributors

Fran (Reina) Bartholomeaux, RN, MS, CCRN Fran Bartholomeaux is currently an Assistant Professor at Grand Canyon University. She has a Master of Science from the University of Arizona. She has had an extensive nursing career in hospital nursing including, ICU, CCU, and Emergency Nursing. She has been a staff nurse, clinical leader, manager, and director in her career. She graduated with her BSN in 1977 from the University of Arizona.

Fran has a special place in her heart for special need populations and communities in need. She has worked with domestic violence prevention and disaster preparedness for the community and schools. She has been a school nurse in an underserved community in Tucson, AZ. She is a firm believer in blending the art, heart, and science of nursing.

Judy Clinco, RN Judy Clinco, a former New Yorker, has lived in Tucson for 28 years. After completing RN training, she worked in different New York hospitals gaining valuable surgical, critical care, and administrative experience. In 1980, shortly after relocating to Tucson, Ms. Clinco founded Catalina In-Home Services, Inc. and continues as Catalina's CEO.

Her innovations in caregiver training, service quality, and employee compensation and retention have earned many local, regional, and national awards. Ms. Clinco is widely recognized as a leader in the private duty home care industry, publishes articles in the lay and professional press, and is a popular speaker at industry conferences. In 2000, she created a model training program called the Direct Care Giver Association. This program has brought unprecedented cooperation to Tucson's long-term care providers in addressing the common goal of assuring a sufficient number of highly trained, qualified Direct Caregivers for a rapidly increasing elder population.

Terry Cullen, MD, MS Terry Cullen is a Rear Admiral in the United States Public Health Service (USPHS), currently serving as the Chief Information Officer and Director of the Office of Information Technology for Indian Health Service (IHS). She previously worked as the senior medical informatics consultant for IHS, Clinical Director at the Sells Indian Health Service Hospital, and a General Medical Officer in Sells and San Carlos, AZ. The Indian Health Service Clinical Reporting

System received the Davies Award for Public Health Informatics in 2006. Dr. Cullen was recognized with the Fed 100 award for information technology in 2006 as well as a meritorious service medal from the USPHS. She continues to maintain a clinical practice.

Dr. Cullen is Board Certified in Family Practice with an additional certification in Addiction Medicine. She attended the University of Arizona College of Medicine, interned at Cook County Hospital in Chicago, and completed her residency in Family Practice at the University of Arizona. She received a Masters in Science in administrative medicine from the University of Wisconsin. Her professional interests include Medical Informatics, cross-cultural issues in medicine, rural medicine, addiction medicine, prevention, and women in medicine.

James E. Dalen, MD, MPH   James Dalen is the former Vice President for Health Sciences and Dean of the University of Arizona College of Medicine, and is currently Professor Emeritus of medicine and public health. During his tenure at the Arizona Health Sciences Center, he established the Mel and Enid Zuckerman College of Public Heath.

Dr. Dalen is the former editor of the *Archives in Internal Medicine* and was a member of the editorial board of the *Journal of the American Medical Association*. He is Board Certified in Cardiology. He is a Master Fellow of the American College of Chest Physicians (ACCP) and is past president of that organization. He received his BS in 1955 from Washington State University, his MA in 1956 from the University of Michigan, his MD in 1961 from the University of Washington, and his MPH in1972 from the Harvard School of Public Health.

Howard J. Eng, MS, DrPH, RPh   Howard Eng is Assistant Professor in the Division of Community, Environment and Policy and Rural Health Office at the University of Arizona, Mel and Enid Zuckerman College of Public Health. Educated as a pharmacist, public health professional, and health services researcher, he holds BS in Pharmacy and MS in Hospital Pharmacy Administration degrees from the University of Arizona, and DrPH in Community Health from the University of Texas. He has more than 30 years of experience in health care and has been a faculty member in the Colleges of Pharmacy (2), Medicine, and Public Health.

Dr. Eng's expertise includes health services and policy research, health economics, epidemiology, public health, border health, rural health, and pharmacy. He was the recipient of the 1990 SAGE's Outstanding University of Florida Faculty Award for Excellence in Research on Aging and the 1998–1999 University of Arizona Health Sciences Center Deans' Teaching Scholars, and selected to the 2003–04 National Rural Health Leadership Development Program sponsored by the Office of Rural Health Policy.

Dr. Eng has conducted rural health research for more than 15 years in which more than 10 of those years in border health. His research interests are (1) to identify the best methods/practices that will enhance the delivery of health services that will lead to the improvement of rural, border, and/or tribal health, (2) to study factors that impact the community health services delivery system (e.g., access to health services, health services financing, barriers to health services utilization, workforce trends, health services quality improvement, and diffusion/adaptation of new technology), (3) to identify effective strategies that will reduce health disparities among minority populations, and (4) to study methods that will improve pharmaceutical usage patterns that will improve community therapeutic outcomes.

Sara Heron, MD   Originally from San Diego, CA, Dr. Heron completed her undergraduate training at Yale University where she received a bachelor of arts in psychology. She attended medical school at Case Western Reserve University where she received the Evans-Machlup award, given to a fourth year medical student who demonstrates excellence in understanding the psychological development of children and the relationship between mental and physical well-being. During that period, she was also awarded the Jeanne Spurlock Minority Fellowship, by the American Academy of Child and Adolescent Psychiatry, which afforded her the opportunity to participate in both clinical and research experiences in the child psychiatry department at University Hospitals of Cleveland. She completed a clerkship in Child Advocacy and Protection, during which she assisted with organizing an SCHIP (State Children's Health Insurance Program) rally in the greater Cleveland area.

Dr. Heron will be completing her internship year in psychiatry at the University of Arizona College of Medicine in 2009. Her particular interests within psychiatry include working with socioeconomically and racially underserved populations. She is also interested in pursuing a fellowship in child and adolescent psychiatry.

Lane P. Johnson, MD, MPH   Lane Johnson is Director of the MD–MPH Dual Degree Program at the University of Arizona College of Medicine. He is an Associate Professor of Clinical Family and Community Medicine, and a Clinical Associate Professor in the Mel and Enid Zuckerman Arizona College of Public Health. He is Board Certified in Family Practice. He is clinically active in Family Practice at University Physicians Hospital and Healthcare on Kino campus.

Dr. Johnson's areas of special interest and research include public health, clinical prevention, medically underserved populations, medical education, rural health, and alternative therapies. His practice has included the use of herbal treatments and acupuncture. He authored a book about herbs for clinicians in 2001, *Pocket Guide to Herbal Remedies*, and received a Health Education Multi-Media Yearly (HEMMY) award in 2005 for his work with herbs used by Hispanic women with diabetes.

Dr. Johnson is a graduate of the University of Arizona College of Medicine (1983), where he was a founding member of the Commitment to Underserved People (CUP) Program. He also completed his residency in Family Practice at the University of Arizona. After a year at the Campus Health Center at the University of Michigan, he returned to southern Arizona, where for 6 years he was Medical Director for United Community Health Center, a consortium of clinics in rural Southern Arizona. He was a physician and Medical Director at Broadway Family Health Center, a University of Arizona Family Practice Clinic. He is also a volunteer physician for the Commitment to Underserved People (CUP) Clinic, and at St. Elizabeth of Hungary Clinic.

Nancy J. Johnson RN, PhD(c)   Nancy Johnson comes from a family of health-care professionals. She completed her undergraduate nursing education at Illinois Wesleyan University with a BSN. And went on to work at the University of Illinois Hospital in Chicago in medical nursing and later, critical care nursing. Upon completing her Masters in Nursing with a specialty in Teaching and Administration from the University of Illinois, she began teaching at Illinois Wesleyan University while maintaining clinical practice at Mennonite Hospital in Bloomington, IL. She relocated to Tucson in 1982 to teach at the University of Arizona College of Nursing. The following year she was recruited by Tucson Medical Center to work in their Nursing Education and Research Department where she initiated and developed the Community Health Center for Tucson Medical Center developing their community education, employee wellness program, and corporate wellness services for the business community. She completed a second Masters Degree in Marketing and Business from the University of Arizona in 1988 and became involved in Tucson Medical Center's development of their managed care organization. In 1992, she was selected as a National Healthier Communities Fellow through the Healthcare Forum. Ms. Johnson is the Chief Operating Officer for El Rio Neighborhood Health Center, and the former Executive Director for St. Elizabeth of Hungary Clinic, a faith-based organization which provides medical, dental, and health services for the uninsured and underserved in Tucson and Southern Arizona. She serves as a Board Member for the Arizona Association of Community Health Centers as well as on their Legislative Committee. She is also an adjunct faculty in Nursing at the University of Arizona, Grand Canyon College, and the University of Phoenix, where she has received the Teaching Excellence Award twice in the past two decades. She is currently finishing her doctoral dissertation for her PhD in Health Services with research interests in innovative care management for high-risk populations and those with chronic diseases.

Francisco A. Moreno, MD   Dr. Moreno is an Associate Professor of Psychiatry at the University of Arizona College of Medicine. He has been conducting research in biology and treatment of mood and anxiety disorders, geared to improve our understanding of the brain basis for mental illness and the underlying mechanism of action of antidepressants/antianxiety drugs, and treatment resistance. He is originally from Mexico where he obtained his MD at the University of Baja California, then completed his psychiatry residency and research training in Neuropsychopharmacology at The University of Arizona Health Sciences.

Dr. Moreno, through his research collaborations, utilizes various research methodologies such as molecular, biochemical, electrophysiological, pharmacological, and behavioral correlates of depression and anxiety disorders. His work is funded by grants from the National Institutes of Health, Private Foundations, and Collaborations with Industry. He has supervised and mentored a number of interdisciplinary students, psychiatry residents, research fellows, and junior faculty. His clinical interest and expertise include treatment resistant mood and anxiety disorders, and work with underserved Hispanic patients. Dr. Moreno serves often as a psychopharmacology consultant to government institutions, health insurances, and pharmaceutical/device industry.

Lynne Tomasa, PhD, MSW   Lynne Tomasa is a gerontologist and medical educator. She is an assistant professor at the University of Arizona, College of
Medicine, in the Department of Family and Community Medicine. For the past 20
years, she has worked in various capacities and projects, most of them related to
supporting the quality of life for older adults. Dr. Tomasa has taught family practice
residents and medical students about aging and care of the older adult; designed
competency-based curriculum and interprofessional activities; and is currently
working on transitional care issues in the lives of older persons and individuals with
disabilities. She also continues to work as a court investigator.

Jennifer Vanderleest, MD, MSPH   Jennifer Vanderleest trained in Family
Medicine at the University of California San Francisco, San Francisco General
Hospital. She has worked in a clinic for sex workers and a Health Care for the
Homeless clinic, and as the Medical Director of the Pima County HIV/STD
Program. She is currently a Clinical Assistant Professor in Family and Community
Medicine, and is core faculty in the Arizona AIDS Education and Training Center
and the Institute for LGBT Studies at the University of Arizona. She is committed
to working with medically underserved people including people living with HIV,
sex workers, the incarcerated, homeless, and LGBT communities.

Who Are the Uninsured?

Howard Eng

The Andersons are a family of four. Jim Anderson is 35 years old and works for a local taxi company. The company offers health insurance only to full-time employees (minimum of 40 hours per week), but Jim could not afford the 40% employee premium contribution, so he decided not to purchase the company's health insurance plan. Liz Anderson is 33 years old and works part time (20 hours per week) for a local gift shop that does not offer health insurance benefits to their employees. Jim and Liz have two children; Sally, 13 years old, and Bud, 10 years old. The Andersons are an uninsured family who are not eligible for the Medicaid program because their family income is too high. Although the children would be eligible for the State Children's Health Insurance Program, Jim and Liz decided not to enroll the children because of the costly monthly premiums.

The Andersons do not have a personal family physician, but use the local Community Health Center once in a while. Although the Community Health Center offers a sliding scale for the Andersons, they rarely use it unless there is an urgent health issue or something is required for work or school.

Last year, Jim was sick with a respiratory infection in mid February. He delayed seeing a medical provider due to the cost. After missing several days of work, Jim decided to go to the Emergency Room (ER) at the local community hospital. The ER physician wrote two prescriptions, an antibiotic and a cough medicine. The antibiotic was written for 14 days of an expensive brand name product; Jim decided to fill and take only half of the prescription. His infection became much worse and he was admitted to the hospital for 10 days of treatment. The cost of hospitalization was more than $5,000 since the Andersons did not have health insurance and had to pay the full amount out-of-pocket. They had to use their entire savings account to pay one-third of the hospital bill, and agreed to pay the remainder over the next 24 months. In addition, Jim lost 2 weeks of pay as a result of his hospitalization. This single medical event, along with being medically uninsured, has put the Andersons on the brink of bankruptcy for the intermediate future, and fearful of any other medical problems.

H. Eng
Division of Community, Environment and Policy and Rural Health Office, University of Arizona, Mel and Enid Zuckerman College of Public Health, Tucson, AZ, USA

N.J. Johnson and L.P. Johnson (eds.), *The Care of the Uninsured in America*,
DOI 10.1007/978-0-387-78309-3_1, © Springer Science+Business Media, LLC 2010

Introduction

The U.S. Census Bureau reported in 2007 that 45.3 million (15.3%) people living in the United States (US) did not have health insurance (U.S. Census Bureau 2007a). There was a decrease in the medically uninsured of about 2 million from the previous year as 3 million more people received medical coverage under government programs (U.S. Census Bureau 2007a). The number of medically uninsured native-born people decreased, while the number of foreign-born people stayed the same. The percentage of people covered by private insurance decreased marginally from 67.9 to 67.5% during the same year, while the percentage of people covered by employment-based insurance also decreased, from 59.7% in 2006 to 59.3% in 2007 (U.S. Census Bureau 2007a). Between 2001 and 2006, the US uninsured population increased by 7.2 million (18.2%), an average increase of the uninsured population of 1.2 million per year (3.0%). Figure 1 shows the 7-year uninsured trend.

In addition to the large number of medically uninsured people in the US, the economic impact of this population is even more staggering. Nationally, those who are medically uninsured for any part of 2008 will spend a total of $30 billion out-of-pocket for healthcare services; they also receive about $56 billion in uncompensated care. Included in this number are the resources provided by philanthropic foundations and organizations along with many health professional volunteers (Hadley et al. 2004).

This chapter will define *key terms* related to the medically uninsured, consider the various methodologies used to count the medically uninsured population, discuss

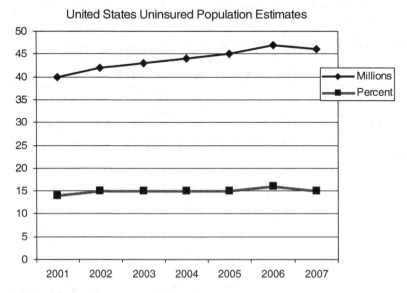

Fig. 1 United States uninsured population estimates

the impact of the number of medically uninsured individuals including the economic consequences for community, state, and national programs, as well as provide a picture of medically uninsured populations in the US.

Medically Uninsured: Definitions

Many definitions are possible in considering medically uninsured populations; the most straightforward definition is that of residents of the US who do not have health insurance coverage. The complicating factors of assessing the problem of lack of health insurance begins when we consider those who are uninsured for a short period of time, those who are children, those who are adults and do not qualify for governmental programs, those who are pregnant – and the list continues with the variety that comprises our nation. As discussion continues, the uninsured will be the diverse large number of residents in our country who do not have health insurance coverage. This is a different frame of reference from access to healthcare. Other definitions needed to fully understand the issues include: federal poverty guidelines, healthcare "safety net," health disparities and medical homes.

The federal poverty guidelines are established and published annually in the Federal Register by the Department of Health and Human Services (2005). These are the guidelines utilized to determine if uninsured individuals are eligible for state and federal programs.

The *healthcare "safety net"* was defined by the Institute of Medicine (2000) as:

"…those providers who organize and deliver a significant level of healthcare and other health-related services to uninsured, Medicaid and other vulnerable patients." The Institute of Medicine also took it a step further by identifying the concept of core safety net providers as having two distinguishing characteristics. These are: "…by legal mandate or explicitly adopted mission, they maintain an "open door" offering access to services to patients regardless of their inability to pay; and secondly, a substantial share of their patient mix is uninsured, Medicaid, and other vulnerable patients (Institute of Medicine 2000)."

As the uninsured are further described, *health disparities* are frequently referenced in terms of their existence in a population and potential methods in which they may be reduced. The Agency for Healthcare Research and Quality U.S. DHHS (2008) defines health disparity populations as "populations in which there is significant disparity in the overall rate of disease incidence, prevalence, morbidity, mortality, or survival rates as compared to the health status of the general population (U.S. DHHS 2008)."

Lastly, the concept of a *medical home* is newly popular in addressing the challenges in caring for the uninsured. The term medical home was first used in the 1960s to define the care coordinated for special needs children. A medical home, according to the American College of Physicians (2004) ,is identified as a patient-centered, provider-guided, cost-effective, longitudinal relationship for care which strives to avoid episodic, emergent and expensive healthcare utilization. In regards to the medically uninsured population, this definition of medical home applies the added features of coordinating an interdisciplinary team to manage needed care, more focus on health promotion and disease prevention and utilizing various staff members and models to further engage this frequently vulnerable population.

Counting the Medically Uninsured

The national and state uninsured figures reported in the literature vary depending on the results of the different health surveys and the definition used for medically uninsured. There are many *different* definitions used by health policy researchers, dependent on the data sources. A review of seven national surveys that include health insurance coverage questions showed differences in sampling methods used, the sampling numbers used, the over sampling of minority populations, the pooling of multiple years of survey data, types of healthcare coverage included in the survey, time period of being uninsured, and the release date of findings (refer to Fig. 2 for comparison summary). The surveys reviewed include: (1) Behavior Risk Factor Surveillance Survey – BRFSS, (2) Current Population Survey (CPS), (3) Community Track Survey – CTS, (4) National Health Interview Survey – NHIS, (5) National Survey of American Family – NSAF, and (6–7) Survey of Income and Program Participation #1 and #2 – SIPP #1 and #2.

As a result of these differences, each survey will report its *own* estimates. In 2005, the uninsured percentages for those below 65 years of age reported from four surveys ranged from 14.5 to 19.5 (Fig. 3). The CPS reported the uninsured percentage as 17.2, while the BRFSS reported as 14.5, MEPS reported as 19.5, and NHIS reported as 16.4 (U.S. Census Bureau 2007a; U.S. Census Bureau 2007b; Centers for Disease Control and Prevention 2007a, b; Rhoades 2006). However, the primary characteristics of the uninsured reported are fairly consistent.

The CPS data that is used by the U.S. Census Bureau is the most common used data source by health policy researchers (e.g., The Access Project, Center for Risk Management and Insurance Research, Commonwealth Fund, Employee Benefit Research Institute, The Henry J. Kaiser Family Foundation, The Urban Institute, and Institute of Medicine, and William M. Mercer, Incorporated) to estimate uninsured rates at the federal and state levels. The estimates can be used to determine the state level estimated uninsured rate trends over time and to compare the states' uninsured rates for the 50 states. CPS estimates are consistent, available on an annual basis, and are useful for examining health insurance trends.

The primary purpose is to collect labor force data on the civilian non-institutional population 16 years of age and older. In participating housing units, respondents are asked about both their and other household member enrollment in any of multiple private or public health insurance programs in the previous calendar year. The data are collected every March. The CPS collects data about employment-based health insurance, individually purchased health insurance, Medicare, Medicaid, Military,

Veterans Administration, Indian Health Service, and state-specific health programs. It is currently being used to allocate federal funding for the State Children's Health Insurance Program (SCHIP) to states, and to evaluate the effectiveness of SCHIP in reducing the number of uninsured children (Eng et al. 2002).

The CPS is the *only* ongoing survey that provides an annual estimate of health insurance coverage that can be used for national as well as cross-state comparisons. However, states using the CPS data should understand the type of information it can provide and how best to present estimates given that the data this survey provides are limited due to sample size and questionnaire design (e.g., overestimate the uninsured by including those who were uninsured during a short period of time, does not capture gaps or overlaps of coverage during the calendar year, may underestimate public program coverage such as Medicaid, and does not capture publicly funded health programs of state).

National Surveys	Year	Uninsured	Sample Size	Time Frame of Uninsured Estimate	State Estimates	Other Limitations
BRFSS	1998	22 millions	120,000	Uninsured at the time of interview.	All	Children and other members of household not included in survey.
CPS	March 1999	44 millions	116,000	Uninsured throughout calendar year.	All	Some states have small sample sizes.
CTS	July 1996- July 1997	35 millions	60,000	Uninsured at time of interview.	Not Possible	
MEPS	March- June 1996	44 millions	24,000	Uninsured throughout 3-6 month period.	Possibly Some	Data must be accessed thru NCHS Data

Fig. 2 Seven national health insurance coverage surveys comparison on counting the uninsured

						Center.
NHIS	1997	41 millions	103,47 7	Uninsured at time of interview.	All	Some states have small sample size.
NSAF	Feb.- Nov. 1997	36 millions	110,00 0	Uninsured at time of interview.	13	Only thirteen states are included.
SIPP #1	1994	19 millions	47,000	Uninsured throughout calendar year.	41 and DC	Many states have small sample size.
SIPP #2	Oct. 1994 - Sept. 1995	31 millions	47,000	Average monthly uninsured	41 and DC	Many states have small sample size.

Source: Paul Fronstin, May 5, 2000, Health Insurance Coverage Survey Matrix Comparison.

BRFSS   =   Behavior Risk Factor Surveillance Survey

CPS   =   Current Population Survey

CTS   =   Community Track Study

MEPS   =   Medical Expenditure Panel Survey

NHIS   =   National Health Insurance Survey

NSAF   =   National Survey of American Family

SIPP   =   Survey of Income and Program Participation

Fig. 2 (continued)

Depending on state, the CPS may or may not be used to make precise within state estimates of insurance coverage. Because of small sample sizes and the fact that the CPS sample does not include all Primary Sampling Units (a unit composed of a metropolitan area, a large county, or a group of neighboring smaller counties)

United States Uninsured Population Estimates for
Four Surveys: Under 65 Years of Age for 2005

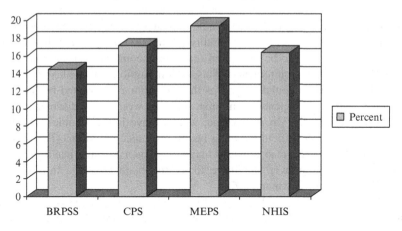

Source: BRFSS, CPS, MEPS, and NHIS

Fig. 3 United States uninsured population estimates for four surveys: Under 65 years of age for 2005

or counties within each state, analysis may have an unacceptable amount of error. For example, it is often *not* possible to make uninsured population estimates for each county within a state because not all counties are included in the sample. In addition, small sample size may make precise estimates for specific population groups defined by age, race, or county of origin difficult.

Because of sample size limitations, it has been suggested that researchers use 3-year rolling averages of CPS estimates when reporting health insurance coverage rates within states. Pooling 3 years of sample from a specific state *can* reduce the amount of sampling errors associated with specific state coverage and allows more precise estimates of coverage for a specific state to be made. Even with its limitations, the CPS is the most commonly used data source in reporting and monitoring the US' uninsured rates and figures.

In this book, we will use the most recent Current Population Reports of the US Census Bureau (U.S. Census Bureau 2008) as the primary data source.

Pictures of Medically Uninsured Populations

The medically uninsured population in the US is not a single, homogeneous population which can easily be identified; it also consists of a number of smaller subpopulations. In this section, a brief overview of the medically uninsured population by gender, age, race/ethnicity, citizenship, income, employment, geography, and rural/urban residency will be provided.

Gender: The CPS, BRFSS, NIHS, and MEPS reported that men are more likely to be uninsured than women (U.S. Census Bureau 2007a; U.S. Census Bureau 2007b; Centers for Disease Control and Prevention 2007a, b; Rhoades 2006). Figure 4 below shows the male and female uninsured percentages for 2006 (U.S. Census Bureau 2007a). The Kaiser Commission in 2000 reported that low-income men are the most likely to be uninsured than low-income women because of the Medicaid's eligibility requirements (Kaiser Commission on Medicaid and the Uninsured 2001). The population groups that are primarily targeted by Medicaid are children, parents of dependent children, pregnant women, the disabled, and the medical indigent elderly. On an average, women have lower incomes than men; thus, they have greater difficulty paying health insurance premiums (Patchias and Waxman 2007). Women also are less likely than men to have health coverage through their own employer and more likely to obtain coverage through their spouses (Patchias and Waxman 2007).

Age: In 2006, the uninsured are more likely to be young (DeNavas et al. 2007). Figure 5 shows that 67.9% of those under age 35 are uninsured. Young adults in the age group of 18–25 are more likely to be uninsured (29.3%) than the other five age groups. The primary reasons for the high risk of uninsured in this group are: (1) having low paying jobs that do not provide for employer-sponsored health insurance or employee cost-sharing, health-sharing portion is not affordable, (2) seeing themselves as indestructible ("Superman effect") with no need for health insurance, (3) determining health insurance is not a high priority need, and (4) losing Medicaid and SCHIP children eligibility at age 19 and may not qualify as an adult under Medicaid. A 2004 Commonwealth Fund study found that employers who offer health coverage, nearly 60% do not insure dependent children over age 18 or 19 if they do not attend college (Patchias and Waxman 2007). Those in 25–34 age group are the next highest uninsured group (26.9%).

U.S. Percentage of Medically Uninsured by Gender: 2006

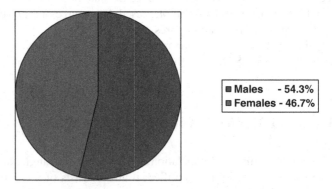

Source: U. S. Census Bureau: Health Insurance Historical Table HI10

Fig. 4 U.S. Percentage of medically uninsured by gender: 2006

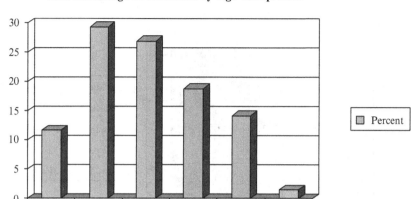

Source: U. S. Census Bureau: Health Insurance Historical Table HI10

Fig. 5 U.S. Percentage of uninsured by age group: 2006

Most elderly are covered by Medicare. Only a small percentage of elderly are uninsured (1.5%). There are several reasons for not qualifying under Medicare: (1) may not have accumulated the requisite 10 years of Medicare-qualifying employment, (2) certain job positions are ineligible for Medicare such as domestics or farm laborers, (3) household income too low to buy into Medicare, and (4) ineligible because of citizen status (Okoro et al. 2005). Medically uninsured elderly populations will be further addressed in a later chapter.

The percent of uninsured increased by 2.2 million in 2006, largely due to a decline in employer-sponsored insurance (DeNavas et al. 2007). Of the 2.2 million, 2.1 million were non-elderly (1.4 million were adults and 710,000 were children – under 18 of age) and 100,000 newly uninsured elderly (Holahan and Cook 2007). Although Medicaid and Children Health Insurance Programs are available to many children, 11.7% of their age group are still uninsured. Of the 710,000 newly uninsured children, 70% were in families with incomes at 200% or more of the federal poverty level (FPL) (Holahan and Cook 2007). The largest growth of uninsured children occurred between 200 and 399% of the FPL.

Race/Ethnicity: In 2005, the uninsured are more likely to be Whites than other races or ethnicities, comprising about half of the uninsured US population (48%) (DHHS 2005). However, minorities (Hispanics, American Indians, Blacks, Asian-Pacific Islanders) are more disproportionately uninsured than Whites (*see* Fig. 6 for details). The highest minority with disproportionately uninsured rates are the Hispanics (32.7%) followed by the American Indian population (31.4%). Even though most American Indians have access to the Indian Health Service they still have high uninsured rates.

Hispanics represented 14% of US residents, but comprised 30% of the uninsured in 2005 (DHHS 2005). Nearly two-third (62%) of Hispanics adults – an estimated 15 million people – were uninsured (Doty and Holmgren 2006). Hispanics had the

U.S. Percentage of Uninsured by Race/Ethnicity:
3 Year Average 2004 - 2006

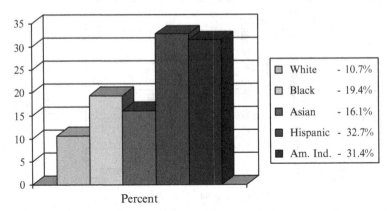

Source: U. S. Census Bureau Report - Income, Poverty, and
Health Insurance Coverage in the United States: 2006, August 2007

Fig. 6 U.S. Percentage of uninsured by race/ethnicity: 3 year average 2004–2006

highest uninsured rate of all working-age adults (Doty and Holmgren 2006). The higher uninsured rate for Hispanics is primarily associated with type of jobs they are employed in,such as construction and agriculture that do not offer employer-sponsored health insurance (DHHS 2005).

In 2005, immigrants made up 16% of all nonelderly adults in the US among whom about 18 million of the total 29 million adult were non-citizens (Schwartz 2007a). Non-citizens include legal permanent residents (immigrants with green cards), refugees, temporary immigrants, and undocumented immigrants. The majority of the non-citizens were: Hispanics (61%), Asian/Pacific Islanders(18%), Whites (15%), and Blacks (6%)(Schwartz 2007a). Non-citizens form a high dispro-portionate percentage of the uninsured; especially, those who are low-income (below 200% of the poverty level). Low-income non-citizens who have been in the US for less than 5 years are the least likely to have health coverage (67%) (Schwartz 2007a). More than three-quarter (78.2%) of the uninsured are citizens in 2006 (U.S. Census Bureau 2007a). It is 3.4 times more likely for a non-citizen to be uninsured than a native (*see* Fig. 7).

In 2005, the uninsured rates for minorities below the 200% of FPL are *not* the same as those at the 200% or greater of FPL in 2005. The uninsured minority rates are (1) Hispanics (<200% of FPL=44% and 200%≥of FPL=21%), (2) American Indians (<200% of FPL=44% and 200%≥of FPL=16%), (3) Asian Americans (<200% of FPL=37% and 200%≥of FPL=11%), and (4) Blacks (<200% of FPL=29% and 200%≥of FPL=12%) (Kaiser Commission 2006). Medically uninsured immigrant and refugee populations will be further addressed in a later chapter.

U.S. Percentage of Uninsured by Citizenship: 2006

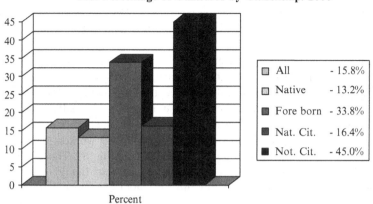

□ All	- 15.8%
□ Native	- 13.2%
■ Fore born	- 33.8%
■ Nat. Cit.	- 16.4%
■ Not. Cit.	- 45.0%

Percent

Source: U. S. Census Bureau: Health Insurance Historical Table HI-7

Fig. 7 U.S. Percentage of uninsured by Citizenship: 2006

Federal Poverty Level: Based on the March 2006 CPS data, the Kaiser Commission on Medicaid and the Uninsured reported that low-income Americans, those who earn less than 200% of the FPL or $39,942 for a family of four were more likely to be uninsured than those who earn 200% greater than or equal of the FPL in 2005 (Kaiser Commission 2006). Thirty-six percent of the poor those <100% of the FPL and the near-poor those 100–199% of FPL (29%) make up nearly two-thirds the uninsured population. Over 8 in 10 uninsured came from working families – almost 70% from families with 1 or more full-time workers and 11 from families with part-time workers (Kaiser Commission 2006). Low-wage workers, unskilled laborers, service workers, and those employees in small business are the most likely of being uninsured.

Employment: The primary source of health insurance in the US is employer-sponsored health benefits. In 2006, 59.7% of the US population had employer-sponsored health insurance (U.S. Census Bureau 2007a). This was a 523,000 decrease in employer-sponsored health benefit from the year before (60.2%) (U.S. Census Bureau 2007a). There had been a steady decrease of employer-sponsored coverage during 2001–2006 (63.2–59.7%). Most of the decline in employer-sponsored health insurance can be attributed to *rising* cost of health insurance premiums in which the employers had discontinued offering health insurance to their employees because of cost or employees' premium cost sharing had become so high that they cannot afford to purchase the health insurance.

Although the premium cost increases were less in 2006 than 2005, the growth in health insurance costs still *outpaced* the rate of inflation and the growth in workers' wages (Kaiser Family Foundation 2006). In 2006, the annual premium for employer-sponsored health insurance was $4,242 for single coverage in which the employer contributes an average of $627, and $11,480 for family coverage in which the employee contributes an average of $2,973 (Kaiser Family Foundation 2006). There were increases of $218 for single coverage ($2,024 in 2005) and $600 for family coverage ($10,880 in 2005) between 2005 and 2006 (Kaiser Family Foundation 2005).

Small employers including self-employed individuals face higher costs (e.g., administrative and premium costs) than larger employers for providing the same benefits (economies of scale); thus, the smaller firms are less likely to offer health insurance. In addition, small firms because of employee size usually paid a higher premium cost because of the increased probability of having higher users of health services. There is twice the likelihood that a firm with 3–9 workers will *not* offer health insurance than a firm with 50–199 workers (*see* Fig. 8). Those who work part-time or part-year, usually seasonal workers, are less likely to be offered employer-sponsored health coverage than full-time and full-year workers. Part-time or part-year workers accounted for 30.2% of the employed population in 2005, but accounted for 41.4% of the uninsured workers (Fronstin 2006). The number of uninsured varies among occupations. The service-sector occupations or blue-collar jobs have a higher disproportionality of uninsured. In 2005, 24.1% of the US work-force was blue-collar-type jobs (e.g., farming, fishing, forestry, construction, extraction, maintenance, production, transportation, and material moving), and of these, 36.1% of the workers were uninsured (Fronstin 2006). Other employment-related reasons for becoming uninsured include: (1) losing a job that provided for health insurance (e.g., employer going out of business or being laid off) and (2) divorce or death of a spouse who provided the health insurance through his/her employer (Institute of Medicine 2001).

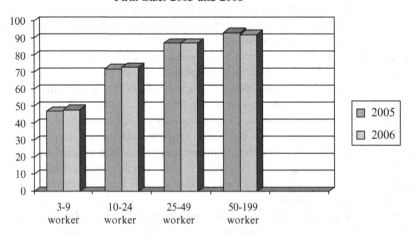

Percentage of Firms Offering Health Benefits, by Firm Size: 2005 and 2006

Source: The Kaiser Family Foundation and Health Research and Education
Trust: Employer Health Benefits 2006 Summary of Findings

Fig. 8 Percentage of firms offering health benefits, by firm size: 2005 and 2006

Geography: The highest percentages of the uninsured occur in the four U.S.-Mexico border states (California, Arizona, New Mexico, and Texas) and some southern states (Arkansas, Georgia, Florida, Mississippi, Louisiana, South Carolina, and Texas). These states appeared at least once in the top 10 uninsured states during 2004 to 2006 (*see* Fig. 9). However, all four U.S.-Mexico border states appeared in the top 10 uninsured states in all 3 years. The top 5 uninsured states – those with fewer than 10% uninsured in 2006 were: (1) Vermont, (2) Rhode Island, (3) Wisconsin, (4) Hawaii, and (5) Minnesota.

The 2008 edition of *Income, Poverty and Health Insurance Coverage in the United States; 2007* from the US Census Bureau shows 3- year averages of the percentage of people without health insurance by state from 2005 to 2007. Massachusetts, which has implemented a bold plan to provide medical insurance to a broader range of residents in the State, has jumped to the first place with the lowest percentage of people without health insurance coverage. Other state standings remain consistent with figures presented above (U.S. Census Bureau 2007a).

Top Ten Uninsured States for 2004 to 2006

Rank	2004		2005		2006	
1	*Texas*	*24.2*	*Texas*	*23.6*	*Texas*	*24.5*
2	**New Mexico**		**New Mexico**	20.3	**New Mexico**	22.9
3	*Florida*	*19.4*	*Florida*	*20.2*	*Louisiana*	*21.9*
4			**Arizona**	**19.6**	*Florida*	*21.2*
5			**California**	**18.8**	**Arizona**	**20.9**
6			*Georgia*	*18.3*	*Mississippi*	*20.8*
7	**California**	**18.0**				
8			*Louisiana*	*17.7*	*Arkansas*	*18.9*
9	**Arizona**	**16.7**	*Arkansas*	*17.5*		
10	*Mississippi*	*16.7*	*South Carolina*	*17.3*	**California**	**18.8**

Source: U. S. Census Bureau: Health Insurance Historical Table HI-4
Bold = Four U.S.-Mexico Border States
Italics =Southern States

Fig. 9 Top ten uninsured states for 2004–2006

Local and state programs to increase health insurance coverage will be reviewed in a later chapter.

Rural versus Urban: The demographics of the rural population are older, poorer, and less healthy compared to people living in urban areas. Among the 42 million non-elderly uninsured in the US based on March 2000 CPS data, 18% live in rural areas in 1999. Persons living in sparsely populated counties or counties not bordering a metropolitan area are less likely to be employer-sponsored. For example, the Kaiser Family Foundation reported that 70% of urban residents had employer-sponsored coverage in 1997, while only 66% of those living in counties next to metropolitan areas and 55% of residents in non-adjacent counties had health insurance through their employers (Kaiser Commission 2001). The probability of being uninsured of those in counties not bordering large cities were 50% higher than urban residents (22% versus 14%).

More than three-quarter (84%) of the rural uninsured are working or have workers in their families, and with 73% from families with at least one full-time worker. Among the uninsured who are poor, 47% of those in rural areas are from families with full-time workers compared to 38% of the poor urban uninsured. Rural residents (24%) between the ages of 45 and 64 are more likely to be uninsured than urban residents (19%).

Medical Care Research and Review reported that when health insurance offered, enrollment rates were similar for rural and urban workers at 68% (Kaiser Commission 2001). However, rural residents are less likely to have job-based coverage because their employers are less likely to offer them health insurance. This is primarily due to the *types* of business/industry employer located in rural areas. Small businesses that do not offer health insurance are very common in rural areas, such as farming, general labor, service, and repair work. One-third of rural workers are employed in firms with less than 25 employees and a third of these workers are self-employed. These combinations of small size businesses with lower wages are the major factors that contributed to the lower levels of job-based coverage. The rural medically uninsured will be further addressed in a later chapter.

Who are the most likely to be uninsured in the US: Although there is not a single group that is uninsured in the US, there are population characteristics that increase the likelihood that one will be uninsured. The more characteristics one has, greater is the probability that one will become uninsured. Those characteristics include:

- Younger adult males, especially those 18–25 years of age, are more likely to be uninsured than older adult males.
- Younger adult males are more likely to be uninsured than young adult females due to Medicaid eligibility requirements.
- Minorities are more likely to be uninsured than Whites.
- Hispanics are more likely to be uninsured than other minority groups.
- Even though most American Indians have the availability of Indian Health Service their rating is still higher-than-average of uninsured.
- Lower income persons, especially those below the 200% of FPL, are more likely to be uninsured than higher income persons.

- Unemployed persons are more likely to be uninsured than employed persons.
- Part-time and seasonal employees are more likely to be uninsured than full-time employees.
- Employees of small firms are more likely to be uninsured than employees of large firms.
- Residents living in US -Border and some southern states are more likely to be uninsured than other parts of the country.
- Rural residents are more likely to be uninsured than urban residents.

Health Consequences of the Medically Uninsured

One of the major barriers to the access of healthcare is being uninsured – not having the means to pay for health services. The uninsured do not have a medical home or a regular source of care that provides the full spectrum and needed continuity for the prevention of disease and maintenance of optimal health status. Thus, many uninsured seek care through healthcare safety net providers such as community health centers, free clinics, public health facilities, school-based health centers, and ERs. Most of these safety-net providers do not provide a full continuum of care for the uninsured, but provide immediate relief or treatment for the problem at hand. Community health centers for example, provide ambulatory services, but not hospital services.

There are many health consequences as a result of not receiving preventive and ongoing health services as well as services in a timely manner. Many of the uninsured will forego preventive services; the uninsured are less likely to be screened for serious illnesses. The uninsured are more likely to postpone or fail to receive needed medical care. Not receiving care in a timely manner may result in entering the healthcare system in poorer health or at a more advanced disease stage. This leads to the uninsured frequently having worse health outcomes, and requiring more intensive and expensive care (e.g., longer hospitalization) than those with private health insurance or publicly financed health coverage programs (e.g., Medicaid) as a result of seeking care with more serious symptoms or illnesses. Even if the uninsured receive care, they may not be able to follow-up with treatment such as prescription drugs or surgery. The uninsured may not fill their prescription drugs because they cannot afford it. Thus, there is no improvement in their health conditions, chronic or acute, and conditions may even become worse. In addition, there may be a delay with follow-up physician visits or diagnostic tests such as laboratory tests or X-rays.

Studies have shown that the uninsured who cannot afford to pay for health services frequently do not have a personal physician or healthcare provider, and receive fewer needed medical visits. Preventive visits in the uninsured population also rank less than in the insured population. Adults who have been uninsured for more than 1 year are three to four times more likely to not have had their blood pressure checked or any cancer screenings completed. This lack of access to timely preventive care causes more than 20,000 uninsured adults to die prematurely each year (Kaiser Family Foundation 2008).

The State Health Access Data Assistance Center (SHADAC 2006) reported: 56.8% of the uninsured adults (18–64 years) did not have a personal physician or healthcare provider compared to 15.5% of the insured adults. In addition, 41.1% of the uninsured adults were unable to see a physician when needed due to the *cost*; whereas, only 9.2% of the insured adults reported the same circumstance in the past 12 months. SHADAC also reported the uninsured adults were less likely to have received recommended cancer screenings than insured adults. For example, uninsured adult women ages 40–64 who did not receive a mammogram in the past 2 years was reported as 50.8%; whereas, insured adult women who did not receive a mammogram for the same time frame was only 22.8%. The review of other preventive cancer screening tests such as Pap smears, PSA tests, and sigmoidoscopies or colonoscopies yield the same findings. Uninsured adult women who had not had a pap smear in the past 3 years were 24.6% with insured women reporting 12.2%. Nearly 75% of uninsured men ages 40–64 had not had a PSA in the past 2 years compared to 52.2% in their insured counterparts. The uninsured adult population had lower sigmoidoscopies or colonoscopies than the insured population with 74.2% never having had one. The insured population reported 50.5% not having either diagnostic screening (SHADAC 2006). In addition to these illustrated cancer screenings, other health screenings are also lower in the uninsured population. For example, uninsured adults not receiving hypertensive screening were reported at 19.5%, with the insured adults at 5.6%. Lastly, uninsured adults reported no cholesterol screening at 40.5%, compared to the insured rate of 18% (Hadley 2006).

The Urban Institute examined the medical care sought after and obtained by uninsured and insured non-elderly individuals following an unintended injury or onset of a chronic condition. The uninsured were less likely to obtain any medical care than the insured individuals for either of the health problem. However, regardless of healthcare coverage, there was a greater likelihood that medical care would be obtained for onset of a chronic condition than unintended injury (Hadley 2007).

Uninsured adults with chronic health conditions are more likely than the insured adults to have substantially higher unmet health needs. A Robert Wood Johnson Study in 2005 reported that 49% of uninsured adults with chronic conditions reported foregoing needed medical care or prescription drugs due to the cost. Thirty-four percent of the uninsured reported unmet needs for medical care as well as unmet needs for prescription drugs (Davidoff and Kenny 2005). This same study showed that more than half of the uninsured adults with arthritis-related conditions (59%), diabetes (57%), heart disease (56%), and asthma (52%) had an unmet need for either medical care or prescription drugs (Davidoff and Kenny 2005). For these four health conditions, the unmet need for prescription drugs was also far higher than the average of 34% for arthritis-related conditions (47%), diabetes (43%), heart disease (42%), and asthma (42%). The impact of unmet medical and prescription needs in the uninsured population has huge implications for health outcomes.

Lastly, this impact on individual health outcomes in the uninsured can have a significant impact on the US population life expectancy. Premature death can be attributed to the inability to access the needed medical care due to the lack of health insurance. The Kaiser Commission on Medicaid and the Uninsured (2002) estimates that the effect of extending insurance coverage to all US residents would reduce mortality rates of the uninsured by 10–15%. The Institute of Medicine (Health Care Leadership Council 2007) estimates the number of unnecessary deaths in the uninsured population to be 18,000 each year.

Economic Cost of the Medically Uninsured

The economic cost of lacking health insurance extends beyond the uninsured individuals and their families. The Institute of Medicine (IOM 2003) reported that the financial, physical, and emotional well-being of all members of the uninsured family may be in jeopardy if any individual becomes ill or injured and incurs substantial medical bills (Democratic Policy Committee 2003). The uninsured or "self-pay" individuals are usually penalized for not having insurance by being charged higher fee-for-service rates for healthcare services and *not* given the discounts afforded to insured patients (Robert Wood Johnson Foundation 2006). A study published in *Health Affairs* (Himmelstein et al. 2005) found that an uninsured patient paid up to twice as much as an insured patient for care. To pay for the accrued medical bills, families may have to cut back on basic living expenses such as food, heat, or rent, may have to use up or close saving accounts, borrow from other family members and friends, obtain loans or a second mortgage on their home, or declare bankruptcy (IOM 2003; Long 2003; Schwartz and Artiga 2007b).

High uninsured rates have negative economic impacts on society and the healthcare system. The society costs include: (1) lost health and reduced length of life, (2) higher costs for publicly supported health programs such as Medicaid and Medicare, (3) increased financial risks and anxiety in families, and (4) financial stresses for – and instability of – healthcare providers in communities with high uninsured rates (IOM 2003; Kellermann 2003). By default, the many state, county, and municipal health facilities serve as providers for their uninsured populations (Kellermann 2003). Public funding for the safety-net may be considerable depending on the community uninsured rate. Using 2004 dollars, the Kaiser Commission on Medicaid and the Uninsured Report found that federal, state, and local governments covered as much as 85% of the estimated $41 billion spent on uncompensated care (Hadley et al. 2004). This cost was paid mostly by the taxpayers.

The impact on the healthcare system reported by the IOM include: (1) the uninsured use fewer services and are less able to pay the full cost of care, which creates financial pressures and lowers revenues for healthcare providers in high-uninsured areas, (2) to avoid the burden of uncompensated care, physicians and hospitals in high-uninsured areas may reduce services, scale-back staffing, limit hours, relocate or close, (3) hospitals with high uninsured rates offer fewer services, and (4) public health departments in high-uninsured areas may have to divert resources away from public health activities that benefit the entire community it order to provide care to the uninsured (Democratic Policy Committee 2003; Public Health Reports 2003).

High uninsured rates have *significant* impacts on the business community and the nation's economic productivity. To make up for financial losses due to extensive uncompensated care of the uninsured, health providers have to charge more for health services, and these are reflected in health insurance company contracts. Thus, the health insurers have to increase their premium costs to compensate for the higher health provider charges. This cost is passed on to the employers who provide health insurance to their employees. A USA Families study in 2005 reported that health insurance premiums for families who have insurance through their private employers paid on an average $922 higher in 2005 due to the cost of healthcare for the uninsured that was not paid for by the uninsured themselves or by other sources of reimbursement (Family USA 2005). Employers also bear the costs of uninsurance through workers who miss work, leave their jobs, or retire early for health reasons. A 2005 study from the Commonwealth Fund found that 69 million workers reported missing days due to illness for a total of 407 million days of lost time at work (IOM 2003).

Providing universal health care coverage for the US population could have a significant impact on the nation's economy. The IOM (2003) estimated that the potential economic value gained from providing health insurance for all Americans (leading to improved health and longer life spans) would be between $65 billion and $130 billion a year (Democratic Policy Committee 2003). The estimate was based on higher expected lifetime earnings due to improved productivity and educational and developmental outcomes (Robert Wood Johnson Foundation 2006).

Later chapters will discuss how other developed countries have provided universal healthcare coverage to their populations, and how community, state, regional and other programs are attempting to provide health coverage to a broader base of their populations in the US.

References

American College of Physicians (2004) Patient-centered, physician-guided care for the chronically III: The American College of Physicians Prescription for Change, Oct 2004. Available at: http://www.worldcongress.com/events/nw600/pdf/luminarySeriesPDF/Tooker_1.pdf. Accessed 28 Sept 2009

U.S. Census Bureau (2007a) Health Insurance Historical Tables 4, 6 and 7. Available at http://www.census.gov/hhes/www/hlthins/historic/hihistt4.html. Accessed 9 July 2007

U.S. Census Bureau (2007b) Annual Social Economic (ASEC) Supplement Table HI10. Available at http://pubdb3.census.gov/macro/032007/health/h01001.htm. Accessed 30 Sept 2007

U.S. Census Bureau (2008) Income, Poverty, and Health Insurance Coverage in the United States: 2007. Available at http://www.census.gov/prod/2008pubs/p60-235.pdf. Accessed 28 Sept 2009

Centers for Disease Control and Prevention (2007a) Behavioral risk factor surveillance system: Prevalent data nationwide 2005. Available at: http://apps/need.cdc.gov/brfss/display.asp?cat=HC&yr=2005&qkey=868&state=UB. Accessed 1 Oct 2007

Centers for Disease Control and Prevention (2007b) Summary of health statistics for the U.S. population: National Health Interview Survey 2005. Series 10, Number 233

Davidoff A, Kenny G (2005) Uninsured Americans with chronic health conditions: Key findings from the National Health Interview Survey. Robert Wood Johnson Foundation, pp 1–22. Available at: http://www.urban.org/UploadedPDF/411161_uninsured_americans.pdf. Accessed 28 Sept 2009

Democratic Policy Committee (2003) The uninsured in America: Expert panel spotlights Consequences of not having health insurance. Available at: http://democrats.senate.gov/dpc/dpc-new.cfm?docname=fs-108-1-355. Accessed 1 Oct 2007

DeNavas C, Proctor B, Smith J (2007) Income, poverty, and health insurance coverage in the United States: 2006. U.S. Census Bureau, Current Population Reports: Consumer Income. pp 1–78

Department of Health and Human Services, Office of the Assistant Secretary for Planning and Evaluation (2005) Overview of the uninsured in the United States: An analysis of the 2005 Current Population Survey. Issue Brief, pp 1–11

U.S. DHHS (2008) 2007 National Healthcare Disparities Report. U.S. Agency for Healthcare Research and Quality, Rockville, MD

Doty MM, Holmgren AL (2006) Health care disconnect: Gaps in coverage and care for minority adults. Commonwealth Fund. Issue Brief, pp 1–11

Eng HJ, Resnick C, Yordy K, DuVal M, Vogel R, Brill J, Paz-Ono E, Parces M, Voloudakis M, Khandokar I, Clarihew B, Jacobs J (2002) Health care coverage in Arizona: Full Assessment. Southwest Border Rural Health Research Center, pp 1–55

Family USA (2005) Paying a premium: The added cost of care for the uninsured. A Report by Family USA, pp 1–17

Fronstin P (2006) Sources of health insurance and characteristics of the uninsured: Analysis of the March 2006 Current Population Survey. Employee Benefit Research Institute. Issue Brief, pp 1–30

Hadley J (2006) Cover Missouri project report: Consequences of lack of health insurance on health and earnings. Missouri Foundation for Health, pp 1–21. Available at: http://www.urban.org/UploadedPDF/1001001_CoverMo1.pdf. Accessed 28 Sept 2009

Hadley J (2007) Insurance coverage, medical care use, and short-term health changes following an unintended injury or onset of a chronic condition. J Am Med Assoc 297(10):1073–1084

Hadley J, Holahan J, Cook A (2004) The cost of care for the uninsured: What do we spend, who pays, and what would full coverage add to medical spending? Kaiser Commission on Medicaid and Uninsured: Issue Paper, pp 1–14

Healthcare Leadership Council (2007) The uninsured. Available at: http://www.hlc.org/html/uninsured.html. Accessed 1 Oct 2007

Himmelstein DU, Warren E, Thorne D, Woolhander S (2005) Market watch:Illness and injury as contributors to bankruptcy. Health Aff 10:63–73. Available at: http://content.healthaffairs.org/cgi/reprint/hlthaff.w5.63v1. Accessed 28 Sept 2009

Holahan J, Cook A (2007) What happened to the insurance coverage of children and adults in 2006? The Kaiser Commission on Medicaid and Uninsured. Issue Paper, pp 1–10

Institute of Medicine (2000) America's Health Care Safety Net: Intact but Endangered. National Academies Press. Available at http://books.nap.edu/openbook.php?record_id=9612&page=47. Accessed 28 Nov 2008

Institute of Medicine (2001) Coverage matters: Insurance and health care. National Academy Press, Washington, DC, pp 1–8

Institute of Medicine (2003) Hidden costs, value lost: Uninsured in America. pp 1–196

Kaiser Commission on Medicaid and the Uninsured (2002) Sicker and poorer: The consequences of being uninsured, pp 1–24

Kaiser Commission on Medicaid and the Uninsured (2006) Fast facts. Henry Kaiser Family Foundation

Kaiser Commission on Medicaid and the Uninsured (2006) The uninsured: A primer – key facts about Americans without health insurance, pp 1–45

Kaiser Family Foundation (2008) Five basic facts on the uninsured. Available at: http://www.kff. org. Accessed 29 Nov 2008

Kaiser Family Foundation and Health Research and Educational Trust (2005) Employer health benefits 2005 summary of findings, pp 1–8

Kaiser Family Foundation and Health Research and Educational Trust (2006) Employer health benefits 2006 summary of findings, pp 1–8

Kellermann A (2003) A shared destiny: Effects of uninsurance on individuals, families, and communities. Testimony before Subcommittee on Labor, Health and Human Services, and Education Committee on Appropriations, U.S. Senate. Available at: http://www7.nationalacademies.org/ocga/testimony/healthcareaccessaffordability.asp. Accessed 1 Oct 2007

Long S (2003) Hardship among the uninsured: Choosing among food, housing, and health insurance. The Urban Institute, pp 1–7

Okoro CA, Young SL, Strine TW, Balluz LS, Mokdad AH (2005) Uninsured adults aged 65 years and older: Is their health at risk? J Health Care Poor Underserved 16(3):453–463

Patchias EM, Waxman J (2007) Women and health coverage: The affordability gap. Commonwealth Fund. Issue Brief, pp 1–11

Public Health Reports (2003) Community consequences of lack of health insurance. Public Health Reports: News and Notes 118:382–383

Rhoades JA (2006) The uninsured in America: First half of 2005: Estimates for the civilian noninstitutional population under age 65. Agency for Healthcare Research and Quality, MEPS Statistical Brief #129

Robert Wood Johnson Foundation (2006) The consequences of uninsurance. Available at http:// statecoverage.net/coverage/consequences.htm. Accessed 1 Oct 2007

Schwartz K (2007a) Spotlight on uninsured parents: How a lack of coverage affects parents and their families. Kaiser Commission on Medicaid and Uninsured, pp 1–7

Schwartz K, Artiga S (2007b) Health insurance coverage and access to care for low income noncitizen adults. Commonwealth Fund, Issue Brief, pp 1–11

State Health Access Data Assistance Center (SHADAC) (2006) The coverage gap: A state by state report on access to care, pp 1–25

Why Are People Uninsured?

Nancy J. Johnson

Lisa and Gary are responsible parents and follow the advice of their pediatrician in raising their two young children. They do not have access to employer group insurance in that Gary is self-employed as a music production supervisor and Lisa is at home with the children. However, as careful healthcare consumers, they purchased individual premiums for each of them as well as each of the children. Then last spring, they received a rejection notice from their insurance company for the youngest child. The reason was a congenital hip misalignment of their 18- month daughter, which the pediatrician had determined 'minor' and most likely 'temporary'. However, the insurance company determined the baby 'uninsurable' due to the need for monitoring and radiology services. Since then, they have not been able to replace the insurance coverage for their young daughter and she is ineligible for government-funded health programs due to the family's income.

Introduction

In the late 1990s, there was a brief period of time in which the number of Americans without health insurance was *not* increasing annually. Since 2001, the number increased from about 42 million to approximately 46.5 million in 2005 (US Census Bureau 2006). However, the number of uninsured Americans under age 65 fell by 1.5 million between 2006 and 2007 (US Census Bureau 2008). The primary reason for this decline was the growth in public health insurance coverage from Medicaid and Medicare, as well as the growth in military programs such as the Veterans Administration and the TRICARE military insurance plan. This represents the first decline in the number of uninsured in over a decade. However, 45 million is still a large number of uninsured individuals in the United States, representing the gaps

N.J. Johnson
El Rio Community Health Center, Tucson, AZ, USA
e-mail: NancyJ@elrio.org

N.J. Johnson and L.P. Johnson (eds.), *The Care of the Uninsured in America,*
DOI 10.1007/978-0-387-78309-3_2, © Springer Science+Business Media, LLC 2010

between private and public health insurance coverage. Over 80% of the uninsured under age 65 are members of working families (Institute of Medicine 2003).

So, why are so many Americans uninsured at any point in time? This chapter will explore many of the causes for people in the United States (US) being medically uninsured, the forces that allow this situation to continue, and preview some of the options and alternatives that may change this situation.

Medical Insurance in the US

Many believe that the challenges faced from the increased cost of health insurance as well as the number of Americans without insurance is primarily due to *how* insurance is acquired in the US. The government currently, actually, pays for health insurance for over 50% of Americans. Medicare provides public insurance for all those over age 65 and the disabled in the US. The government provides Medicaid for the very poor and low-income pregnant women as well as the state children's health insurance programs (SCHIPS) for low-income children. Medicare is funded through payroll taxes, federal general revenues and beneficiary premiums; while Medicaid is funded through federal and state taxes. Veterans may receive much of their healthcare through the Veterans Health Administration.

The growth of these three programs was the primary reason for a decline in the uninsured in the most recent reported data from 2007. However, this description of sources for healthcare insurance does not address the issues of the various governmental programs or the the amount of money utilized to identify who is eligible and who is not eligible, as well as to enforce the benefit limits to which individuals are entitled. There are also many uninsured who may qualify for these programs, but are *not* enrolled as well. Other groups of Americans who receive their health insurance through private insurance usually do so through employers, but that also presents the challenges of benefit limits, pre-existing conditions, non-covered services, and waiting periods. This can lead to starts and stops in coverage, disruption in treatment, and continually influences the numbers of uninsured at any point in time.

Employer health coverage is also subsidized through the federal tax system because workers do not need to pay taxes on compensation received as employer provided healthcare benefits, and premiums paid by employers that are part of an employee's compensation are exempt from payroll tax, as well as income taxes. Finally, there is also the working poor, a group which doesn't have access to employer-offered insurance, or cannot afford their portion of the employer premium, and have too much income to qualify for governmental health insurance programs. Investigation of the American structure of options for healthcare coverage illustrates the complexity, both financially and programmatically, and provides some indications as to why so many people are uninsured (Fig. 1).

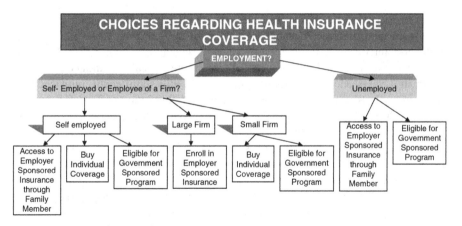

Fig. 1 Choices regarding health insurance coverage

Causes of Being Uninsured

Medical Insurance Is Not Affordable

The most commonly cited reason for being uninsured is the cost of health insurance. This is heard from employers as well as from employees and individuals who choose not to enroll. Employers continue to see increasing costs in offering insurance to their employees and consequently, employees do not enroll when it is offered, due to their share of the cost. The Robert Wood Johnson Foundation (2005) reported that the average health insurance premium for single coverage in 2004 was $308 per month and family coverage was $829 per month. On average historically (St. Luke's Health Initiative 2007), the employee has paid approximately 16% of single coverage premium, whereas, the average percent paid for family coverage was 28%. In 2008, the average percentage paid by the employee for their portion of family coverage has risen to 40% in some markets (HealthNet of Arizona 2008).

For industries that tend to pay lower wages, the cost for health insurance is greater for the employee. In addition, the out-of-pocket costs such as co-payments and deductibles have continued to rise significantly since 2001 (RWJ 2005). Lastly, in the past 25 years, except for a short period of time in the mid-1990s, the rise in health insurance costs has been substantially greater than increases in worker wages. If these rates of increases continue, health insurance will cost a family upwards of $36,000 per year by the year 2014. In 2004 (St. Luke's Health Initiative 2007), Out-of-pocket expenses were estimated at 17% and currently, they are greater than 35% with some health insurance plans. A glance at the recent data supports this with an annual increase in Medicaid enrollment of 5.8% in 2003 while the employer plans decreased by 4.8% (Kaiser Family Foundation 2006). However,

60% of the population continues to access health insurance through their employer and, for the first time in a decade, the data from 2007 did not show a decline in employer-offered health insurance coverage (Holahan and Cook 2008). National employer surveys in 2007 did indicate the lowest rate of health insurance premium growth in 4 years. However, this growth of 6.1%, still significantly outpaced the growth in workers' wages which was 3.7% and overall inflation of 2.6% (St. Luke's Initiatives 2007). The continuance of the trend would depend upon the economy and efforts for healthcare reform in the future.

Employers continue to work with strategies designed to control costs such as disease management programs, closed provider networks and higher employee deductibles and co-payments. A survey of employers (EBRI 2007) identified various perceptions as to why healthcare insurance premiums continue to rise. These included: higher insurance company profits, higher spending for hospital care, higher spending for physician services, higher spending for prescription drugs and an aging population.

A comprehensive study by Cunningham (2007) investigating the problem of paying medical bills for American families documenting that about 57 million individuals were in families with problems paying medical bills in 2007. This represents an increase of about 14 million since 2003 (Cunningham 2007). Although the uninsured had more challenges in affording healthcare, most people with medical debt (42.5 million) had insurance coverage.

Fewer Employers Offer Medical Insurance

There are various characteristics of employers that indicate the likelihood of health insurance that will be offered in the future. These include the size of the business, the number of part-time employees employed, the nature or type of business, and whether the business is unionized or not. Regardless of these characteristics, there has been a decline in the number of employers that offer health insurance to their employees as mentioned above. Small employers comprise most of the decline. Currently, less than 43% of employers with less than 50 employees offer health insurance benefits (RWJ 2005). The greater the number of part-time employees and the greater number of low-wage positions existing in the business results in a greater likelihood that insurance benefits will not be offered. Industries which tend to offer lower or no health benefits or none at all include service, wholesale/retail, construction, agriculture, and the forestry service.

The RWJ Foundation (2005) reports that nearly 50% of low-wage workers are not offered any type of health insurance benefit currently. The Kaiser/HRET (2006) survey of small employers with size ranging from 3 to 199 employees indicated that 79% of small employers cited cost as the major issue to not offering a health insurance benefit, found that benefits were variable each year in terms of cost and covered services (e.g., mental health, cost for families). Some employers simply pass on market premium increases directly to the employee that impacts re-enrollment by the employee and their dependents. For the past decade, there has been an average of a 10% annual increase in healthcare premiums (Kaiser Foundation 2008).

Insurance Plans Offer Different and Confusing Benefits and Costs

In addition to the challenges for employers to provide affordable health insurance plans for their employees and their families, various designs of insurance plans are confusing for many employees. The differing features of plan designs and the restrictions have many unknowns that can lead to insured individuals and their families avoiding access to the healthcare system and not receiving regular preventive care. Surprises of co-payments for outpatient screening procedures such as colonoscopies and emergency room visits as well as the varying co-payments for differing tiers of pharmaceuticals can incent insured individuals to avoid utilization of needed services and decrease adherence to recommended treatment plans. Providers of healthcare are frequently just as uncertain as to what various insurance plans may or may not cover. This places the providers such as hospitals, clinics, and physicians in an uncomfortable position in terms of managing care and service delivery. There is a notable *absence* of tools or lists of desirable characteristics for health insurance policies that would enable health care consumers to make wise choices about options for healthcare insurance.

Workers Are Not Eligible to Enroll, or Choose Not to Enroll

Although employers may offer insurance, some workers are not insured due to being part-time workers or having a waiting period before eligibility begins. However, for workers who are eligible, approximately 13% choose not to enroll (Kaiser Foundation 2006). There is a relationship with declining income and choosing not to enroll in employer-offered health insurance as well. As health insurance premiums increase, some choose to take the risk of *not* having health care coverage. Some insured families lose coverage due to the worker changing jobs or getting laid off in poor economic times. Divorce and death can also cause families to lose insurance coverage.

Individuals Are Not Able to Find a Medical Insurance Plan Due to Cost or Pre-Existing Medical Conditions

Individuals and families who do not have access to employer health insurance benefits, or who do not work, or who are self-employed, may try to purchase health insurance in the individual market. Some states offer small group coverage for the self-employed and nationally; this is about 6% of the non-elderly Americans (RWJ 2005). As a result, most self-employed Americans or small businesses find their health insurance premiums determined primarily on age and health status. Insurance companies in some states must insure all individuals who apply for coverage, yet can charge whatever premiums they choose for those they expect to have high medical utilization and costs.

Individuals who have been employed full time and insured by an employer with greater than 20 employees, they may be eligible to continue coverage through the Consolidated Omnibus Reconciliation Act (COBRA) after employment has been terminated. However, this is also a much more expensive option that can only be used for up to 36 months post-employment.

Another barrier to being insured is the existence of previous medical conditions, commonly called "pre-existing conditions," which can result in expensive premiums. Some states, *allow* insurance companies to simply deny coverage for an individual perceived as being high risk. Individuals with pre-existing medical conditions, at times, cannot purchase any sort of insurance for any amount of money in the marketplace. The best strategy for these individuals is to affiliate themselves with an employer who offers insurance in order to gain medical insurance since no one can be selected out or denied in the group insured model.

Diabetes, for example, is a chronic disease in which individuals struggle to acquire and keep healthcare coverage. The American Diabetes Association has identified the inability for many Americans with diabetes to find healthcare coverage to be a primary issue for advocacy (http://www.diabetes.org, 2008). Nearly, 21 million American children and adults have diabetes and many are uninsured and unable to access the necessary supplies, medications and education needed to self-manage their disease and prevent expensive and life-threatening complications such as heart disease, retinopathy, kidney failure, and vascular disease. Health insurance problems make it harder for people to manage their diabetes, and uninsured adults with diabetes are less likely to receive needed care and effectively manage their disease. Even those with insurance struggle to obtain needed care when the insurance is inadequate. People with diabetes need health insurance that is available, affordable, and adequate to provide care for their chronic illness (http://www.diabetes.org, 2008)

In 2004, a team of researchers at Georgetown University Health Policy Institute (2005), studied the experiences of 851 individuals who had diabetes and the role of health insurance. These individuals were all under 65 years of age and either were uninsured, about to lose their insurance, or insured with problems. They echoed the problems that many face who have a chronic health condition. Despite having some sort of insurance, they struggled with medical debt, trying to find less expensive test strips and medications on E-Bay, or from Canada, and some had serious expensive complications from lack of management of their diabetes. Essentially, when people have a chronic health condition and their insurance coverage breaks down, they frequently lose their jobs and struggle with financial resources as well as healthcare status.

Another scenario illustrates a family in which one parent suffered from asthma and the other from hypertension. Based upon the continued increases in their employer-based health insurance and out-of-pocket costs, they both sought employment for less compensation but improved healthcare benefit plans.

There Are Limited Medical Insurance Programs for Low-Income Adults Without Children

Although Medicaid helps provide health insurance coverage for low-income individuals, the financial eligibility requirements are very limited and differ from state to state depending on the local economy, the number of families who are low-income, and the design of the state's Medicaid program. Most State guidelines for childless adults are very restrictive and even the poorest are often not eligible. In addition, the process of enrolling and staying enrolled is challenging for this low-income population. Convenience of enrolling in Medicaid programs is seen as one of the most effective methods to improve enrollment for those eligible for Medicaid (RWJ 2005). For other subgroups of Americans, such as immigrants and refugee populations, this assistance with enrollment is an essential strategy. Flores et al. (2005) found that the barriers to insuring eligible children in Latino families included lack of knowledge about the application process, language barriers, family mobility, and system problems such as lost paperwork and excessive waits.

Another recent study released by the National Institute for Health Care Management (2008) reported that one in four are eligible for Medicaid and the State Children's Health Insurance Program (SCHIP) but are not enrolled. The study cited reasons that included not being aware of the programs, not knowing how to enroll, fear of being linked to a publicly financed program and the challenge of staying enrolled.

Most of the 12 million eligible in the US are low-income families which include 6.1 million children (64% of the uninsured children in the US). The study was based upon the 2006 data from the 2007 Current Population Study and also reported that of the 10 million uninsured non-US citizens, 5.6 million are undocumented immigrants, and 4.4 million are legal residents (NIHCM Foundation 2008). These numbers illustrate that an additional 25% of the uninsured would be insured if outreach programs addressing some of the barriers to eligibility completion were addressed. Fortunately, governmental health insurance programs tend to include children; however, children frequently lose eligibility around age 19, creating a gap in coverage. Young adults frequently face challenges in finding employment, which provides health insurance benefits.

Changes in Income or Eligibility; Job Change, Move, Layoff, Marital Status

Approximately, *two million Americans* lose their health insurance each month. Health insurance transitions can happen when there is a job change, layoffs, a move, change in marital status, or a change in income status. Individuals purchasing coverage from the marketplace or their employers could potentially be uninsured at any point in time. For example, a large stable employer in the southwest experienced an employee strike which lasted for approximately 2½ months. After 30 days, as prescribed in the employee medical insurance benefit, the striking employees and their families did not have health insurance. Suddenly, these seemingly stable families were struggling with paying out-of-pocket for health and medical care. Regularly taken prescription medications were the key stumbling point for individuals who suddenly discovered that the cost of purchasing their regular medications for chronic illnesses totaled over $800–$1,000 per month. Needless to say, anyone could become uninsured or experience a transition in insurance coverage and be at risk for a period of time.

Some people transition directly from one health insurance plan to another, but many are uninsured for a month or longer. Research shows that people in poor health are twice as likely to encounter a lengthy spell without health insurance compared to people in good health (Kaiser Foundation 2006). About 80% of the diabetics studied in the Georgetown study had problems arise directly related to health insurance transitions (NIHCM Foundation 2008).

What Do These Causes for Being Medically Uninsured Tell Us?

With healthcare insurance being a "choice," rather than a mandate in the US, there is great variability in what research-identified barriers tell us about why people are uninsured. While some individuals may have many options for securing health insurance, it is still a *choice*. Some individuals simply choose to not purchase and/ or participate in health insurance options, while others will pay whatever the cost to assure health insurance coverage. Some individuals choose not to enroll in public health insurance programs, even when the cost is zero, and will seek healthcare on an as-needed basis. These differences and the diversity in the population create a challenge in attempting to insure as many as possible in a complex "patchwork quilt" of methodologies by which to enroll or purchase health insurance.

Today, most of the uninsured are the "working poor." As discussed above, they usually make too much money to qualify for Medicaid, yet have too little income to be able to purchase private health insurance. For example, in 2008, a family of four at 200% of the federal poverty level would be earning $42,400 and therefore, not qualifying for Medicaid, but finding local prices for healthcare insurance ranging anywhere from $900 to $1,500 per month for family coverage. Purchasing health insurance for a family in this income range can exceed 10% of the family's income. Only 59% of persons with household incomes less than 150% of the federal poverty level are able to cover the entire family. As the household income increases to 200% of the federal poverty level, 90% of families have all household members insured (Institute of Medicine 2003).

Insurance Mandates and High Risk Pools

As mentioned previously, in many states, insurance companies can charge more because someone is sick or simply deny coverage. Individuals with chronic conditions such as diabetes may not be able to purchase insurance. Some states such as Illinois and Indiana, however, mandate that insurance be sold with comprehensive benefits to all residents regardless of health status. In addition, they may *not* charge these individuals more than they could charge healthy individuals in the community (http://www.naschip.org, 2008). Again, the Georgetown University study reports in that 395 people with diabetes needed to purchase individual health insurance and only 15 were successful (NIHCM Foundation 2008). The federal legislation of COBRA, mentioned earlier, allows certain people who would lose their insurance when their employment ends to purchase the existing employer-based plan for, anywhere from, 18 to 36 months. However, the individual must pay the entire premium and this is frequently cost prohibitive. When COBRA expires, another federal law passed in 2003, HIPAA (Health Information and Affordability Act) requires individuals to be offered non-group coverage. Again, there are no specific regulations for the type of insurance, so the actual insurance policy can be weak and expensive to purchase as well.

Thirty-three states in the United States have now created high-risk pools for individuals who have been turned down by private insurers and do not qualify for Medicaid assistance. The first of these high risk pools was established in 2002 and insures about 6% of its individually insured population. A few other states that focus on consumer outreach insure about 2–3% of the states' individually insured population (http://www.insure.com, 2008). These high risk pools for the uninsured are also expensive, require much paperwork, and have some caps on how much a benefit will pay for the individual. To begin with, a high-risk insurance pool is the last resort for those with pre-existing conditions, whose employers do not provide coverage and have individually been denied coverage because of their health status. The high risk pool coverage generally insures the middle class who do not qualify for Medicaid. Legislators created these pools as a safety net; each state operates differently depending on how much is funded by the state.

Essentially, the state government contracts with private insurers to administer the program, collect the premiums, and pay the claims. Although the benefits vary, most mirror basic health insurance coverage. However, these pools are allowed to charge up to 130–200% of the market cost for an individual premium. According to Families USA (2008), most states cap the premium at 150% of the market value and risk pools are ineligible for federal grants if they are not at 200% or below in pricing premiums. Those individuals in high risk pools have their choice of deductibles usually ranging from $500 to $10,000 depending on the state and choices offered. High risk pool policy holders can open tax-free Health Savings Accounts (HSAs) to save for deductibles, co-pays, and other out-of-pocket expenses.

Individuals must demonstrate proof of denial, as well as not being eligible for Medicaid or Cobra benefits. Lastly, there is generally a 6–12-month waiting period for individuals to have active coverage. High risk pools are continuing to expand as an option for uninsured individuals.

As mentioned above, high risk pools are quite expensive and are not feasible for the working poor who do not qualify for governmental healthcare programs. Cunningham (2007) investigated whether uninsured people paid full or reduced costs when they received healthcare services and if they were aware of providers in their communities who did charge less for uninsured individuals. Their research found that less than half of the uninsured in their sample population (47.5%) used or were aware of lower-priced providers. Promoting lower-priced providers in communities may also be another method for improving access to needed healthcare for the working poor.

What's Driving Risking Healthcare Costs?

All Americans recognize the continuing increases in medical insurance as well as the out-of-pocket expenditures. There are many factors driving these rising costs that include an aging population, increased utilization of healthcare services, new and more prescription medications available, cost-shifting from federal programs to state programs, new and better technology for diagnosis and treatment, corporate profits, medical liability, and the uncompensated care of the uninsured and underserved.

It is also evident that the healthcare system focuses on managing the care of those who are ill. In any given year, close to 50% of all healthcare spending pays for the care received by only 5% of the population (Kaiser Foundation 2006). In 2004, almost half the people in the US had a chronic condition that ranged from mild to serious. Healthcare for those with chronic conditions accounts for 75% of total healthcare costs (US DHHS 2002). As the population ages, healthcare spending begins to increase at around age 55 and healthcare costs for patients between the ages of 76 and 84 are nearly eight times as much as for the care of children ages 1–5 years of age (US DHHS 2002). The CDC Report on Aging and Health in America (2007) predicts that by 2030, 20% of the US population will be over 65 years of age and healthcare expenditures will increase by 25% without factoring in the cost of new technology and inflation. The majority of healthcare services are also utilized by the older population.

The uninsured and underserved traditionally receive little preventive and primary care, and frequently may not follow up on initial care; this can result in more acute episodes of illness. Community outreach and the current work to help the uninsured establish a low-cost medical home may help to minimize more expensive utilization of tertiary care services.

Results of No Health Insurance

The results of having no health insurance can lead not only to adverse health consequences, but also adverse financial consequences. For example, uninsured women with breast cancer are less likely than insured women to receive breast-conserving surgery. The uninsured are also less likely to receive care even when they have serious symptoms and uninsured children are 70% more likely to go without care for ear infections, asthma, and sore throats. Uninsured children are five times more likely not to have a needed prescription filled. Reviewing the potential financial consequences, 27% of families reported they struggled to pay for expenses, such as food, rent, and heat. Almost 44% reported they were forced to use most or all of their savings to pay medical bills and one out of five said they had run up a large credit card debt or had to take out a loan against their home to pay medical expenses (Commonwealth Fund 2004). In a 2007 Health Confidence Survey (EBRI 2007), 63% of the respondents reported an increase in the costs they are responsible for, and the negative impact of those increases on their financial health of their household. Fifty-two percent reported a decrease in their savings overall due to healthcare expenditures.

What Tradeoffs and Options Exist for the Medically Uninsured?

Most Americans are concerned about the continually rising cost of healthcare and what might happen to their coverage in the future as well as their ability to afford medical care. The challenge in determining what can be done revolves around three issues: cost, access, and quality. Many options are possible that stretch from expanding governmental coverage, offering Americans financial incentives or tax credits for health coverage, allowing the free market to set access and price, expanding primary prevention and primary care access, or developing clinical information systems to save money, along with other alternatives. However, due to the complex nature, potential consequences, and sheer size of the healthcare industry, local communities and states may do better to improve cost, access, and quality than the federal government.

Critical Thinking Case Studies

Sheila's husband works for a small restaurant chain that offers health benefits. However, the coverage is about $1,200 per month for the family and also requires an additional policy for prescription drugs. Sheila has diabetes and her children require asthma medications monthly which result in a monthly prescription bill of about $400. When money is tight, Sheila buys the children's medications, but foregoes her own.

She also tests her blood sugar only occasionally to save test strips. The last time she saw her physician, her blood sugar was *elevated*.

What assistance might be available for Sheila?

What options are there for her family?

Charlie lost his health insurance when he was laid off about a year ago. He was offered COBRA but could *not* afford it and was without insurance for 3 months paying for his high blood pressure and cholesterol medications on his credit card. He then was able to qualify for a new policy at $400 per month. However, his medications and physician visits were not covered. He elected to continue to use his credit card, but recently ended up in the hospital with chest pain. He has been discharged with a $16,000 hospital bill and no insurance. The hospital has coordinated a payment plan for him.

What might be the options for Charlie as his employer does not offer medical or dental benefits?

What would be the initial considerations in terms of his level of income and pre-existing conditions?

References

Center for Communicable Disease (2007) The state of aging and health in America. Center of Disease Control and Prevention, Atlanta, pp 1–46

Commonwealth Fund (2004) Affordability crisis in healthcare. Issue Brief

Cunningham PJ (2007) Identifying affordable sources of medical care among uninsured persons. Available at http://www.hschange.com/content/912/?topic=topic06. Accessed 29 Nov 2008

Employee Benefit Research Institute (2007) 2007 Health confidence survey: rising costs are changing the ways Americans use the healthcare system. Available at http://www.ebri.org/pdf/notespdf/EBRI_Notes_11a-20071.pdf. Accessed 23 Nov 2008

Families USA (2008) Failing Grades: State Consumer Protection in the Individual Health Insurance Market. Families USA. Available at: http://www.familiesusa.org/assets/pdfs/failing-grades.pdf. Accessed 28 Sept 2009

Flores G, Abreu M, Brown V, Tomany-Korman SC (2005) How Medicaid and the State Children's Health Insurance Program can do a better job of insuring uninsured children: the perspectives of parents of uninsured Latino children. Ambul Pediatr 5(6):332–340

Georgetown University Health Policy Institute (2005) Falling through the cracks: Stories of how health insurance can fail people with diabetes, pp 1–48

HealthNet of Arizona (2008) Interview re: employer provided plans with Provider Network Representative, July 8, 2008

Holahan J, Cook A (2008) Changes in economic conditions and health insurance coverage, 2000–2004. *Health Affairs*, Available at http://content.healthaffairs.org/cgi/reprint/hlthaff.w5.498v1. Accessed 12 Oct 2008

Holahan J, Cook A (2008) The decline in the uninsured in 2007: why did it happen and can it last? Kaiser Family Foundation, Washington, DC, pp 1–19

http://www.covertheuninsured.org (2008) Accessed 1 April 2008

http://www.diabetes.org (2008) Accessed 12 April 2008

http://www.insure.com (2008) Accessed 28 Nov 2008

Institute of Medicine (2003) Uninsurance facts and figures: the uninsured are sicker and die sooner

Kaiser Family Foundation (2006) The uninsured: a primer key facts about Americans without health insurance. The Kaiser Commission on Medicaid and the Uninsured

Kaiser Family Foundation (2008) Few low-income uninsured buy non-group coverage. Available at http://www.ahanews.com/ahanews_app/jsp/display.jsp?dcrpath=AHANEWS/AHANews. Accessed 12 Oct 2008

National Association for State Comprehensive Health Insurance Plans (2008) Available at http://www.naschip.org/. Accessed 30 Nov 2008

National Institute for Health Care Management Foundation (2008) Available at http://www.nihcm.org. Accessed 6 July 2008

Robert Wood Johnson Foundation (2005) Why are people uninsured? Available at http://www.statecoverage.net. Accesssed 16 Oct 2008

St. Luke's Health Initiatives (2007) Arizona health futures: employer-sponsored health insurance coverage, pp 1–7

US Census Bureau (2006) Health insurance statistics. Available at http://www.census.gov/hhes/www/hthins/hthin06.html. Accessed 15 Oct 2008

US Census Bureau (2008) Health insurance statistics. Available at http://www.census.gov/hhes/www/hthins/hthins07.html. Accessed 21 Nov 2008

US Department of Health and Human Services (2002) Medical expenditure panel survey. Available at http://www.hhs.gov. Accessed 17 March 2008

The Culture of Poverty and the Uninsured

Nancy Johnson

Living in Poverty-Episodic, Cyclical or Chronically?

Lisa was employed part-time and lived with her husband and three children.

Her husband left and she was left without *medical insurance as well as a* decrease *in family income. Financially, she was unable to make ends meet and struggled to find afford-able day care as well as move to a full-time job, which might offer insurance for her and her children. Lisa ended up losing her home but was able to qualify for Medicaid for medical coverage. Upon finding a job with higher wages, she then was unable to qualify for Medicaid and was* uninsured *again.*

Joe was 53 years old, employed at a stable but minimum wage job that did not *provide health insurance. Then he was involved in a serious automobile accident. Due to his accident, he lost his job and all his funds were going to make payments for medical bills and expenses. He soon was unable to pay the rent on his apartment and was evicted. However, at this point in time, he was able to enroll in Medicaid for his medical expenses. Joe stayed with a friend for three months before he was able to get a new job and begin to save for his own apartment again. So far, he is still enrolled in Medicaid for medical coverage.*

Cecilia is 20 years old, single, never married and has a five-year-old son. She lives with her grandmother and works to help the family. She did not *graduate from high school and always found school difficult. Her son has asthma and Cecilia is continually anxious about her ability to afford his inhaler. Cecilia would like to go back to school and try to improve her position in life and ability to support her family, but doesn't know what steps she would need to take and how she would make ends meet.*

In each of these situations, what sort of poverty is illustrated? What are the assets each individual has to work with and what are the barriers to getting out of poverty?

N. Johnson (✉)
El Rio Community Health Center, Tucson, AZ, USA;
College of Nursing, Grand Canyon University, 3300 W. Camelback Road, Phoenix,
AZ, 85017, USA

N.J. Johnson and L.P. Johnson (eds.), *The Care of the Uninsured in America*,
DOI 10.1007/978-0-387-78309-3_3, © Springer Science+Business Media, LLC 2010

Introduction

Despite the fact that the US is a very prosperous nation with the resources, experience and knowledge to virtually eliminate poverty, many Americans continue to *live in* poverty. According to the most recent governmental data in 2005, nearly 37 million people or approximately 12.6% of the American population have incomes below the federal government's poverty line (US Census 2007). From the year 2000 to the most current data collected in 2007, poverty has worsened with an increase of 5.3 million more Americans living in poverty. These figures represent an all-time high for the US and are growing faster than the general population. Although the US is a much wealthier country than other industrialized nations, it has more people living in long-term poverty than many other countries. Poverty level is far higher with the US ranked 24th among 25 countries for the number of individuals living below 50% of the median income level (CAP 2007). This is not because of individuals working less than workers in other countries, but is more about US policies and infrastructures failing to assure that workers have sufficient resources to withstand the fall to poverty (Oswald 2007).

When the definition of poverty is considered, it is, at times, *subjective*. The current official definition of poverty was established originally in the 1960s. Although many other economic measures have changed over the years, the definition of poverty has *not* changed. According to the definition of poverty, a family of four is considered poor in the year 2009 if it has an annual income of less than $22,050. However, if other Americans and governmental officials were to be interviewed, most would believe that a family of four at a much higher annual income would be classified as poor. In fact, a recent survey of Americans identified a minimum annual income of $40,000 necessary to simply support basic necessities of life for a family of four to survive (http://www.sixstrategies.org/about/about.cfm 2006). Upon review of the 2009 United States Health and Human Services Poverty Guidelines (http://aspe.hhs.gov/poverty/08poverty.shtml), two slightly different versions are presented of the federal poverty measure. The first is the poverty thresholds, which represent the original measure of poverty as described. They are updated by the Census Bureau annually and used for statistical purposes. However, the poverty guidelines, frequently referred to as the "federal poverty level" are issued annually in the federal register by the Department of Health and Human Services. They are used for administrative purposes such as defining eligibility for certain state and federal programs (Table 1).

These guidelines are frequently used in percentage multiples, such as 125% of the federal guidelines, to determine eligibility for programs such as Head Start and Food Stamps. However, these guidelines are not used for cash public assistance programs such as Temporary Assistance for Needy Families or supplemental Security Income.

Most other developed nations use a poverty measure that is generally set at about 50% of the income of the median family. By contrast, the US' definition of poverty represents about 28% of the income of the median family. Lastly, as the definition

Table 1 2009 HHS poverty guidelines

Persons in family or household	48 Contiguous states and D.C.	Alaska	Hawaii
1	$10,830	$13,530	$12,460
2	$14,570	$18,210	$16,760
3	$18,310	$22,890	$21,060
4	$22,050	$27,570	$25,360
5	$25,790	$32,250	$29,660
6	$29,530	$36,930	$33,960
7	$33,270	$41,610	$38,260
8	$37,010	$46,290	$42,560
For each additional person, add	$3,740	$4,680	$4,300

Source: Federal Register (2009) 74(14), 23 Jan 2009, pp 4199–4201

of poverty is looked at, it defines poverty from a one-dimensional perspective. Poverty is *not* simply about income, but should also include the *lack of* other resources such as access to *healthcare, assets*, and the *ability* to manage and direct one's life. These other attributes define human poverty.

There are many myths about poverty in the US and some of them include that poor people choose not to work and rely on governmental assistance programs for their source of income and healthcare. Many believe that poverty *happens* to poor people and that they represent a different segment of the communities. However, the reality about poverty in the US is a different picture. Some of the facts about poverty include:

- Poverty affects many Americans. Nearly one-half of Americans will experience poverty for a year or more at some time in their lives before they reach age 60. Of this group, another half will have lived in poverty at some time in their life for over 4 years or more.
- Over 40% of the poor work full-time. Nearly, two-out-of-three working families with incomes below the federal poverty level include one or more workers. These individuals and families are frequently uninsured as their incomes are too high to qualify for Medicaid; they do not have access to employer-paid insurance and cannot afford to purchase it in the marketplace too. Only about 3% of those classified as poor receive more-than-half their annual income from Food Stamps, Supplemental Social Security and Temporary Assistance for Needy Families.
- Most poor Americans are Whites rather than the common myth that they are of ethnic minorities. About 47.0% are White and non-Hispanic. However, for various ethnicities, in 2007, 24.5% of blacks and 21.5% of Hispanics were poor (University of Michigan).
- Involuntary reduction in work hours caused 48% to become poor.
- 18% became poor due to loss of employment.
- 10% became poor due to loss of the *breadwinner* through divorce. Poverty rates are the highest for families headed by single women.
- 16.5% of foreign-born residents lived in poverty, compared to 11.9% of residents born in the US.

(US Census 2007)

These myths and realities of poverty in the US illustrate why there are so many misconceptions about poverty and Americans. Another common belief is that poverty is due to individual problems and failures, rather than the problems and failures of the *structures* that society has created through the political and economic choices (Buck 2003). While most believe that individual choices and behaviors can influence the risk of living in poverty, the structures and policies developed are much more powerful in their relationships to people living in poverty.

The results of poverty are many and frequently include the lack of education, safe housing, inadequate nutrition, and reliable transportation along with a lack of access to medical, dental and healthcare. Poverty can result in a lifetime of reduced opportunities for individuals and families. Poverty is also detrimental to the American family. When parents have to work two or three jobs in order to support their families, the stress negatively impacts relationships and family life.

Aspects of Poverty

Although this discussion started with the income definitions of poverty, that information is *not* of particular use when attempt is made to strategize on policy and programs to help reduce the level of poverty and improve health status. Historically, the World Bank's World Development Report (1980) identified poverty as "a condition of life so characterized by malnutrition, illiteracy, and disease as to be beneath any reasonable definition of human decency." This speaks to what living in poverty is like, rather than identifying income as a feature of poverty. So, human poverty may be about having a lack of food, lack of education and little or no access to healthcare. In addition, the definition of human poverty is perceptual, based upon how rich a community or country is , so the definition of what human poverty looks like varies greatly between developed and developing countries.

There are two frameworks for understanding poverty in the US. The first that is frequently cited is poverty as a *personal* problem or the "culture of poverty" (Lewis 1966). The second viewpoint is that poverty is a *social* problem and results from failures in societal structure (Iceland 2006).

The culture of poverty is described as resignation, dependence, present-time orientation, lack of impulse control, weak ego structure, sexual confusion and the inevitable inability to defer gratification (Lewis 1966). Payne (1998) comments that generational poverty is often conveyed in the attitude that society owes one a living. This framework assumes that the pathway out of poverty is there for those who make an effort and the rest exhibit the characteristics in some part described by Lewis. This upward mobility belief is an American myth in that most economists believe the US to be one of the least upwardly mobile societies among industrialized nations. People who are born poor are likely to die poor, despite working to travel the pathway out of poverty.

The opposite framework of societal failures as described by Iceland (2006) presents the conceptual view that economic inequities result from economic systems and infrastructure that foster the accumulation of money and assets in one segment of society, often at the expense of another, or from broad economic shifts that produce instability and disruption in the labor market. Basically, the belief that upwardly mobile economic pathways are either non-existent or blocked for members of our society is the premise.

Many others also view poverty from a structural approach, rather than an individual approach (Oswald 2007). This means there is a structural vulnerability in that some people have a *greater* chance of experiencing poverty than others. Some factors that increase this chance include lack of income and resources, isolation, physical weakness, powerlessness and vulnerability. In contrast, the development of assets or resources and education are the two criteria that improve the opportunities to rise above poverty. Buck (2003) originally classified poverty in three differing levels consisting of episodic, cyclical and extreme/chronic poverty. These three levels were based upon access to employment rather than the length of time spent in poverty. Buck also supports that poverty is continually seen as a personal problem rather than one present and belonging to today's society. Buck believes that poverty will persist until it is recognized as a societal challenge, a failure of structural systems, and not that of the individual. Oswald proposes a "maze of poverty" that is based upon the presence of resources. The fewer the resources, the less likely the person will reach economic stability and more sporadic the "maze." These resources are defined as employment, housing, access to medical and healthcare, education and others. This model assumes that poverty is *structurally* created rather than the direct consequences of individual choices.

The episodic poor as defined by Buck are those who have at least one significant episode of poverty due to loss of employment, layoff, death, divorce or other uncontrollable life events. This category represents approximately 13% of those living in poverty at any point in time. The cyclical poor are those who move in and out of poverty on a regular basis, which represents about 20% of those living in poverty and about 18% of the general population (US Census 2007). Lastly, the chronically poor are living in poverty greater than 80% of the time and for more than 5 years. It is important to acknowledge that these three kinds of poverty "categories" need different strategies for interventions and assistance. In addition, all three "categories" result in various and sporadic, and ineffective access to the healthcare system.

In summary, poverty is best addressed as an issue of income and assets, not character. The current system of governmental programs and infrastructure does not promote escape from poverty or provide the needed resources on a regular basis. Twice in recent history, the US has significantly reduced the poverty level. First, during "The New Deal" from the 1930s to 1940s, the 60–80% poverty rate was reduced to 25%. In addition, during the 1960–1970s with the "War on Poverty", the poverty rate was reduced from 25% to 12–15% (Iceland 2006).

These are the only two times in history when poverty was treated as a structural problem rather than an individual problem. Although there is no single or simple solution to helping individuals escape the poverty trap, antipoverty policy that has been most effective includes education and training, cash assistance, child care/early childhood education, affordable housing and access to healthcare (Iceland 2006).

Poverty and Lack of Healthcare

A common belief in the US is that the poor are receiving their medical, dental and other healthcare through governmental programs designed to serve those living in poverty. Although many Americans do receive emergency medical and dental care through Medicaid or state-funded sliding scale healthcare programs, many fall into the "notch" group. This group constitutes the working poor in the US whose income knocks them out of eligibility for most governmental funded health insurance programs. However, the cost of insurance may be too expensive or they may have a pre-existing condition such as hypertension or diabetes which influences the cost of insurance. Many employers do *not* offer their employees insurance and for those employers who do offer medical insurance, the employee portion of the premium may be *cost prohibitive*.

Poverty and the resulting lack of medical insurance results in basically no or minimum preventive care and screenings for these individuals and families, as well as the lack of exposure to much needed health education and health information. The CDC (Woolf 2006) reports that as salaries drop, uninsured individuals also tend to lead less-healthy lifestyles and seek even less healthcare services. In addition, individuals living in poverty seek urgent care facilities as well as emergency rooms for their urgent or emergent medical and dental care needs. This results in the delivery of episodic care as well as high costs and expenses for individuals and families who cannot afford the fees. An additional adverse outcome of the lack of healthcare for those living in poverty is the lack of early detection of chronic and serious illnesses such as diabetes, high blood pressure and cancer. These individuals present at times with advanced disease, resulting in expensive surgeries, treatments and medications, and sometimes death or disability occurring with what may have been a *manageable* health condition or disease if diagnosed earlier. A recent scenario of an uninsured woman in her mid-fifties illustrates the concern. She was brought to a community health center by her son, who felt she may have broken her hip when she fell. An X-ray did indicate a broken hip and additional blood work and diagnostics were completed. This woman was suffering from untreated lymphoma of which the broken hip was a secondary symptom due to loss of calcium in the bones. She survived for only 4 months with medical bills totaling over $85,000 for her care and treatment. Would access to affordable healthcare have improved her outcome or enhanced her quality of life?

Poverty and disease go hand-in-hand as aspects of public health are considered. Most infectious diseases and injuries which are prevalent among the poor are a result of a lack of income, clean water, sanitation, safe housing, education and access to healthcare. In addition, when the poor become ill, they are unable to work; therefore, further adding to the loss of assets and resources with less hours worked or the loss of employment. A recent study funded by the Agency for Healthcare Research and Quality (Fiscella and Holt 2007) investigated health disparities and the use of preventive services such as influenza vaccinations, colorectal screenings, mammography and pap smears. They discovered that poverty-related factors such as low income, and low education were more significant in the lack of completing preventive screenings, rather than the lack of access to primary care. Fiscella and Holt (2007) make the point that longer office visits need to be scheduled with patients dealing with poverty to confirm their understanding of the need for preventive screenings as well as address and overcome the financial barriers which may play a role in completing and following up on preventive screenings.

Strategies for Building Health with Individuals Living in Poverty

Individuals living in episodic, cyclical or chronic poverty frequently are dealing with the crisis "du jour" which many times reflect the base of Maslow's hierarchal pyramid of safety, food and security. Preventive healthcare and the management of chronic diseases do not factor into this paradigm when individuals and families are addressing paying rent, putting food on the table and possibly dealing with basic safety issues. However, healthcare professionals and healthcare systems have the opportunity to thoughtfully work with individuals to develop their assets and resources, which may hopefully lead to ongoing and preventive use of the healthcare system. Initially, healthcare professionals must have the community knowledge to leverage existing resources for those living in poverty and lacking medical and dental insurance. Some of the existing resources for healthcare professionals and organizations to collect include the services available from the county health department, volunteer-based healthcare clinics, eligibility for Medicaid and other state or federally funded programs and programs for discounted prescriptions. However, the reality of caring for the uninsured and poor is initially about establishing the relationship that will position the healthcare professional as a resource for the individual or family no matter what the medical needs.

For individuals and families living in poverty, there are barriers to using healthcare even when it is available and affordable, that poverty has created. These may include crisis living, involving basic needs such as safety and food. Other barriers may include lack of resources, distrust of governmental entities, lack of planning skills, coexisting problems, transportation and not knowing the rules of the various economic classes. Healthcare professionals must assess these basic issues prior to addressing ongoing healthcare and preventive care that may be needed. These barriers greatly influence the ability to adhere to treatment recommendations. Although many times, healthcare professionals assist the uninsured and underserved with directions regarding completion of treatment and receipt of services, the goal is to build planning and self-management skills about one's own health status with the patient population rather than building enabling patterns of behavior.

The recognition that relationships are the key to change and learning is critical in working with people who are uninsured and have low income. Healthcare professionals should offer non-judgmental, caring environments that focus on solving the concrete problems first. People living in poverty must first address the shelter, food and safety needs for themselves and their families. Healthcare systems can assist with this by providing the healthcare-provider with access to an interdisciplinary team to help the individual resolve barriers in the way of healthcare and eventually, learn some planning and goal-setting skills. An illustration of this effective team has been documented frequently in the community health worker literature working with underserved individuals and families seeking prenatal care, asthma management and other chronic care services (Metzger 2005). Community health workers can, many times, address culture, language and literacy barriers that may be interfering with access to needed healthcare.

The establishment of the "medical home" for those living in poverty has been documented frequently in the past 3 years. The "medical home" is identified as the resource for individuals to access their healthcare needs, to go to rather than the hospital emergency room and to receive the needed continuity of care (AAFP 2008). To begin the establishment of a medical home, education must start with the individual who has viewed his or her healthcare as an acute need rather than an ongoing process, which necessitates management. Uninsured individuals can be referred from emergency rooms to local community health centers to establish medical homes, but the community health center must follow up and work to rehearse and cement those relationships. Community Health Centers are also able to provide sliding scale affordable healthcare and can advocate and guide individuals through the community network of primary, secondary and tertiary care. Other avenues to identify those who would benefit from a "medical home" are community outreach efforts such as fairs at community food banks, WIC clinics, neighborhood centers and volunteer clinics held in schools and churches. Currently, St. Elizabeth's Health Center, a faith-based community health center in Tucson, Arizona collaborates with St. Mary's Hospital Emergency Room in striving to create "medical homes" for uninsured and underserved patients. Daily, all patients seen in the emergency room for non-emergent conditions, who do not have a primary care provider or insurance, are referred to St. Elizabeth's Health Center to establish sliding scale medical and/or dental care. These names, after patient consent is obtained, are sent to St. Elizabeth's Outreach staff, for followup daily. Generally, there are 12–15 referrals per day for the community health workers to contact from simply one community emergency room setting. Of the total number of referrals, approximately 20% provide erroneous names, addresses and telephone numbers to the emergency room fearing a large medical bill they *cannot* afford to pay. From the resulting patients who are reached by the community health worker, they are invited to visit St. Elizabeth's Health Center and to learn about services which are available and hopefully, establish care. The ability to engage the individual in this initial encounter begins the relationship, which hopefully leads to the establishment of a "medical home." Currently, 18 months of data show that approximately 19% of the patients establish "a medical home" as measured by the completion of the initial new patient visit (Johnson 2008). The long-term question is whether simply establishing medical homes for those without insurance will improve health status for those living in poverty.

A Nation Without Poverty?

Initiatives and policy efforts are continually generated by various groups in the hope of reducing poverty in US with all the various benefits touted with improved health status being one of them. As noted previously, declines in the nation's poverty rates have only been seen twice, with the New Deal era and the War on Poverty in the 1970s. Both these initiatives focused on structural changes in programs as well as a multifaceted approach. Today's initiatives stress the importance of listening to stakeholders from low-income families, government officials, neighborhood coalitions, healthcare professionals and others about what possibilities and partnerships may make a difference. Components of current initiatives comprise many structural and financial incentives, which may help to move some individuals and families out of poverty. Some of these include access to basic healthcare for all, access to safe and affordable child care, more affordable housing and the creation of better job opportunities. As policy and structural changes are attempted, an improvement in health indicators and a decrease in health disparities for those living in poverty may be hoped.

Most recently, the Center for American Progress convened a Task Force on Poverty (2007) to examine the causes and consequences of poverty in the US and prepare an action plan. This initiative came about in response to the increase of approximately 5 million more Americans living in poverty with more than 1 in 20 being poor for 10 or more years (CAP 2007). The Task Force advocates for the US to adopt the following four guiding principles to help reduce poverty in the country. They include:

1. Promote decent work to pay enough that families can pay for basic needs and save for the future.
2. Provide opportunity for all through available jobs, educational resources and good neighborhoods.
3. Ensure economic security through stable job opportunities with livable wages.
4. Help people build wealth through education and savings.

The Task Force has identified a 12-step program to cut poverty in half over the next decade. They suggest:

- Raise minimum wage to half the average hourly wage, which would be approximately $8.40/h.
- Expand the Earned Income Tax Credit and Child Tax Credit
- Promote unionization by enacting the Employee Free Choice Act.
- Guarantee child-care assistance to low-income families and promote early education for all.
- Create 2 million new opportunity housing vouchers and promote equitable development in and around central cities.
- Connect disadvantaged and disconnected youth with school and work.
- Simplify and expand Pell Grants and make higher education accessible to residents of all states.

- Help former prisoners find stable employment and re-integrate into their communities.
- Ensure equity for low-wage workers in the Unemployment Insurance system.
- Modernize means-tested benefits programs to develop a coordinated system that helps workers and families.
- Reduce the high cost of being poor and increase access to financial services.
- Expand and simplify the Saver's Credit to encourage saving for education, homeownership and retirement.

These 12 steps are estimated to cost approximately $90 billion per year, but the Task Force recommends a fairer tax system in which to accomplish the 50% cut in poverty over the next 10 years. The recognition that poverty is a result of a variety of societal and governmental structures including housing, wages, tax policies, education and welfare policy is essential for our communities in order to reduce poverty and improve health status.

References

American Academy of Family Physicians (2008) Medical homes. Available at http://www.aafp. org. Accessed 1 Apr 2008

Buck RE (2003) The causes of poverty. An unpublished manuscript

Center for American Progress (2007) Task force on poverty in the United States. Available at www.americanprogress.org. Accessed 1 Feb 2009

Federal Register (2009) 74(14). 23 Jan 2009, pp 4199–4201

Fiscella K, Holt K (2007) Impact of primary care patient visits on racial and ethnic disparities in preventive care in the United States. J Am Board Fam Med 20(6):587–597

Iceland J (2006) Poverty in America: a handbook, 2nd edn. University of California Press, Los Angeles

Johnson N (2008) Turning emergency room visits in medical homes with the uninsured. An Unpublished Article

Lewis O (1966) The culture of poverty. In: Gmelch G, Zenner W (eds) Urban life. Waveland Press, Long Grove, IL

Metzger N (2005) Community health workers and diabetes. In: Handbook of diabetes management. Springer, New York

Oswald WT (2007) Understanding poverty: a critical look at who is poor and why?. Springfield College, San Diego

Payne R (1998) A framework for understanding poverty. Aha Process, Highland, TX

Six Strategies (2007) Six strategies for low income families project. Available at http://www. sixstrategies.org. Accessed 31 Mar 2008

U.S. Bureau of the Census (2007) Income, poverty and health insurance coverage in the United States: Report, P60, n. 235, p53. U.S. Bureau of the Census, Washington, DC

Woolf SH, Johnson RE, Geiger JH (2006) The Rising Prevalence of Severe Poverty in America: A Growing Threat to Public Health. Amer J of Prev Med 31(4):332–421

World Bank (1980) World Development Report 1980. Available at: http://www-wds.worldbank. org/external/default/WDSContentServer/WDSP/IB/2000/12/13/000178830_98101911111283/ Rendered/PDF/multi_page.pdf. Accessed 28 Sept 1009

Health Disparities and the Uninsured

Nancy J. Johnson

Florence is a 61-year-old African American woman with six grown children and very little money. She was widowed 4 years ago and has been uninsured ever since. When she thought she might be sick because of changes in her bowel habits, she put off going to the doctor for a year because she knew she could not afford the medical bills. By the time she did see a doctor, her cancer had spread from her colon to her liver. Although she had surgery, she declined to have chemotherapy due to the costs. She decided to put her faith in God and died within the year. If Florence had had health insurance, preventive screenings via a colonoscopy might have discovered the cancer earlier and saved her life. Being uninsured is a disparity by itself limiting the access of timely care as well as receiving the current standard of care.

Introduction

Despite the many improvements in the overall health of our nation, health disparities continue to be widespread among Americans as they relate to race, ethnicity, age, socioeconomic status and education. In healthcare, the term health disparity refers to the unequal treatment of patients on the basis of race, ethnicity, gender, age, or other characteristics – such as being uninsured (McGuire et al. 2006). Many believe these disparities have their roots in American society, which has been characterized by poverty, discrimination and unequal opportunities. The Institute of Medicine's Report, "Unequal Treatment: Confronting Racial and Ethnic Disparities in Healthcare," describes disparities as "complex, … rooted in historic and contemporary inequities, and involve many participants at several levels, including health systems, their administrative and bureaucratic processes, utilization managers, healthcare professionals, and patients" (2002). In addition to the complex challenge of reducing health disparities, is the issue of patients being uninsured – a disparity all on its own. The disparity of being uninsured will not be eliminated until access to healthcare is available for everyone.

N.J. Johnson
El Rio Community Health Center, Tucson, AZ, USA
e-mail: njohnson@ccs-soaz.org

N.J. Johnson and L.P. Johnson (eds.), *The Care of the Uninsured in America*,
DOI 10.1007/978-0-387-78309-3_4, © Springer Science+Business Media, LLC 2010

Ayanian (2008) discusses the disparity of being uninsured as an additional overriding barrier to the poor, racial and ethnic minorities, and disenfranchised Americans. He identified that all Americans must overcome seven potential barriers in order to receive healthcare. These include: (1) having health insurance, (2) getting enrolled in insurance, (3) having coverage for effective providers and needed services, (4) becoming well informed about the treatment options, (5) having a regular source for primary care, (6) getting referred for needed specialty care, and (7) having providers deliver high quality care (Ayanian 2008). These seven challenges are important factors in looking at health disparities in the US. Even for those with health insurance, issues related to low literacy, minimal education, culture and language represent health disparities. Healthcare providers lacking insight and culturally sensitive communication skills can add to the problem. The overall healthcare system and its providers have the challenge of addressing many variables that cause disparities and lead to their persistence.

These various categories of disparities are a challenge in that they are interrelated without evidence as to the strength of each alone. Many correlations can be identified between ethnicity and lack of insurance, age and lack of preventive screenings, and employment and access to care to name a few, but the power of various factors on the presence of disparities is not known. Zuvekas and Taliaferro (2003) identified that we can examine the influence that the healthcare system, insurance coverage and access to care have on disparities, but many other equally important factors influence disparities including age, employment, and gender. While lacking health insurance is a disparity in itself, other disparities such as education, age, ethnicity, culture, literacy, and employment continue to influence the existence of health disparities in Americans.

In the US, racial and ethnic groups have significant differences in health status when compared to the white population. In 2005, the US Census (2008) reported that people of color make up nearly one third of the US population. Hispanics are the largest ethnic minority group. By the year 2050, the US Census (2005) estimates that nearly half of the US population will be Hispanic, African American or Asian. The proportion of Hispanics and Asians are expected to *double* in the next 50 years.

Much of the US' ethnic diversity is geographical. For example, states such as Arizona, Hawaii and California have some of the highest percentages of minorities ranging from 55 to 81%; whereas, the northeast states such as Maine and Vermont range from 1 to 5% minorities. People of color are also reported by the census to be more likely to have family incomes less than 200% of the federal poverty level. The proportion of children who are poor or near-poor is also higher in families of color. Elderly non-whites are far more likely to have incomes less than 200% of the federal poverty level. Nearly 70% of elderly Hispanics, nearly 2/3 of elderly African Americans, and 50% of elderly Pacific Islanders and American Indian/ Alaska Natives are poor or nearly poor. Elderly whites who are poor represent about 38% of the population (U.S. Census 2005). These changing demographics of the US, along with the data on poverty illustrate health status as a trait influenced by many variables. As discussed above, lack of health insurance is a major disparity and impacts the ability of an individual to seek and receive preventive services, as well as medical care and treatment, placing these identified populations at risk for poor health status.

Populations at Risk for Health Disparities

In 2000, the Kaiser Commission on Medicaid and the Uninsured collaborated with the UCLA Center for Health Policy to assess health insurance and access to care by various minority populations. The study identified that 37% of non-elderly Hispanics were uninsured, is nearly double the number of White uninsured. This is primarily due to the fact that 43% of Hispanics receiving health insurance from their employers, with 76% of Whites reporting employer-sponsored insurance coverage (www.kff.org, 2009). The high percentages of Hispanics who are uninsured are reflected in low numbers of those receiving care; however, even for Hispanics with insurance, access to care is less than White populations. Some of these disparities may be due to cultural, linguistic and literacy barriers. However, when Hispanic children are covered by Medicaid, the disparity in access to care disappears completely and utilization of healthcare services is the same between Hispanic and White children (www.kff.org, 2009). The study also examined African Americans and their insurance status and access to care. African Americans represent about 13% of the US population and their health indicators are worse than Whites in the US. African Americans have double the infant mortality and three times as many die from diabetes than the White population (www.kff.org, 2009). Between private health insurance and Medicaid, about 77% of African Americans have insurance. However, African Americans are three times as likely to live in poverty, compared to the White population. Upon assessment of American Indians/Alaska Natives, this group represents 2.4 million individuals with many disparities for health indicators. For example, American Indian/Alaska Native infant mortality rate is 1½ times greater than White populations; they have a higher incidence of diabetes. Native Americans also present with lower incomes, less access to healthcare and limited health insurance. Lastly, Pacific Islanders/Asian Americans, although counted by the census data as one minority group, are a very diverse population. These groups have different languages, socioeconomic status and citizenship status. Some subsets of this group match Whites in terms of being uninsured, while others have uninsured rates matching those of other minority groups living in the US. However, most of the Pacific Islanders/Asian Americans are reported to have about 20% of uninsured population (www.kff.org, 2009).

Racial and ethnic minorities of all groups except the Pacific Islanders/Asian Americans reported their overall health status as worse than that of Whites. All low-income groups report their health status worse than those with higher incomes. Poorer reports of health status are also linked to higher rates of mortality among racial and ethnic minorities (www.kff.org, 2003).

The use of preventive care among racial and ethnic groups is also less than that of non-Hispanic whites. The National Commission on Preventive Priorities (2007) reported that Hispanic Americans have lower utilization to non-Hispanic Whites and African Americans for various preventive services. Hispanic smokers were 55% less likely to seek assistance with smoking cessation, 39% less likely to be current on colorectal cancer screening, and 55% less likely to have received a pneumococcal vaccine at age 65 or older. However, regardless of insurance status, Asian adults had the lowest utilization for breast, cervical and colorectal cancer screening, (NCPP 2007). African Americans had higher screening percentages for colorectal cancer and breast cancer; however, they also have the *highest* mortality rates for these two cancers. Access to insurance would increase preventive screenings in these racial and minority populations.

Although much research on health disparities is organized around racial and ethnic populations, disparities are also apparent with other classifications. Specifically, the lack of insurance is a powerful influence on the presence of disparities. Shen and Washington (2007) compared insured and uninsured patients who had suffered a cerebral vascular accident or stroke. They identified that the uninsured group had a higher level of neurologic impairment, a longer average hospital stay and higher mortality risk. The researchers felt that the uninsured population lacked access to outpatient and preventive care that would detect and provide early treatment for hypertension in the asymptomatic stages. An additional study completed by DeLia and Belloff (2006) in New Jersey supported *income* as the most important factor in differences between both the rural and urban insured and uninsured populations. A third study (Shone et al. 2005) reviewed the changes in health disparities among children after enrollment in the State Children's Health Insurance Plan. Prior to enrollment in the insurance program, White childrens' parents reported the lowest unmet healthcare needs percentage compared to both African American and Hispanic parents' reports. After insurance enrollment, all the three racial and ethnic groups reported the same percentage of unmet healthcare needs; eliminating the disparities between the groups. Without health insurance for all Americans, elimination of health disparities seems unlikely.

National Disparity Improvement Projects

The data collected from The National Healthcare Disparities Report (NHDR) (AHRQ 2007) is being used for tracking changes in healthcare disparities among racial, ethnic, and socioeconomic groups. This annual report describes the quality of and access to care for multiple subgroups across the US. The data show significant disparities continue to exist since the first report in 2000, compared to the 2005 data. Significant improvements have been made in childhood immunizations for most populations, due to the Vaccines for Children program, outreach to schools, pediatric practices, community health centers, community locations and a concentrated effort to reach all children. With this effort, the disparity of being uninsured was eliminated for children needing immunizations. Some of the biggest disparities in this most recent report include:

- Blacks had a rate of new AIDS cases ten times higher than Whites.
- Hispanics had a rate of new AIDS cases over 3.5 times higher than that of Whites.
- Asian adults age 65 and over were 50% less likely than Whites to have a pneumonia vaccine.
- American Indians/Alaska Natives were twice as likely to lack prenatal care in the first trimester compared to Whites.
- Poor children were over 28% more likely than high-income children to experience poor communication with their healthcare provider (NHDR 2007).

As mentioned previously, the interrelatedness between access to care and quality of care is complex, but this report also supports the challenges that the uninsured have in getting access to high quality care. The report also identifies that based upon their core set of measures, being uninsured is the key factor to a lack of better quality care (NHDR 2007). The possibility of reducing disparities is hampered due to so many Americans lacking health insurance.

The NHDR (2007) also compared uninsured individuals with individuals who had insurance with core quality, and access to care study measures. The data illustrated that uninsured individuals measured worse on almost 90% of the quality measures and did worse on 100% of the access measures than the insured individuals. The uninsured were six times as likely to lack a usual source of care and four times as likely to be without a source of care for financial reasons. Uninsured individuals were nearly three times as likely to not get care when needed for illness or injury. They were also twice as likely not have a screening mammogram after age 40. A subset of the NHDR core indicators is illustrated in Fig. 1. However, despite the strength of the correlations between uninsured status and quality and access indicators, it is still important to remember the other factors influencing disparities, including poverty, race, ethnicity, age, education, and gender.

Other governmental programs continue to study and address health disparities. These include the Federal Collaboration on Health Disparities Research (FCHDR), which has been developed by the Centers for Communicable Disease (CDC), and the Office of Public Health and Science's Office on Minority Health. This collaborative is focusing on disparities around obesity, building environments which includes schools, houses, parks, and other systems, mental healthcare, and co-morbidities. A second collaborative group is the Health Disparities Roundtable which is sponsored by the Office of Minority Health and the Agency for Healthcare Policy and Research. This group is partnering with the Institute of Medicine to reduce health disparities by engaging sciencepolicy makers, educators, healthcare professionals, and government and industry leaders.

The Centers for Disease Control and Prevention (2007) has also created the REACH Program (Racial and Ethnic Approaches to Community Health). This is a program specifically targeting health disparities and health inequities across the life span through integration of programs in communities, schools, churches, worksites,

National Healthcare Disparities Report 2007
Core Measures with the Largest Disparities
Between Uninsured and Insured Individuals

ACCESS

- Persons who have a specific source of ongoing care
- Persons without a usual source of care who indicate a financial or insurance reason for not having a source of care
- Persons who have a usual primary care provider.

QUALITY

- Adults who can sometimes or never get care for illness or injury as soon as wanted
- Women age 40 and over who reported they did not have a mammogram within the past two years
- Children whose parents reported poor communication with their health providers

National Healthcare Disparities Report, 2007.

Fig. 1 National Healthcare Disparities Report (2007) Core measures with the largest disparities between uninsured and insured individuals

and neighborhoods. The REACH program uses community-based participatory approaches and strives to identify the root causes of health disparities. An example of a REACH program is "The Access Community Health Network" (ACCESS), which is a partnership with the University of Illinois in Chicago. This collaborative program works with faith leaders in the community to recruit low-income earning and uninsured women of color to be screened for breast and cervical cancers. Breast cancer is the second leading cause of cancer deaths among African American women and the leading cause of death among Hispanic women in the US. African American women are more than twice as likely to die from cervical cancer than White women, with Hispanic women about 1.5 times more likely to die when compared to White women. Lastly, women without insurance are 28% less likely to have a routine mammogram and 12% less likely to have a routine Pap test than women with insurance. Uninsured women are 2–3 times more likely to have breast cancer diagnosed at a later stage. This REACH project reaches women by getting support from faith leaders, recruiting lay health workers, and holding educational groups in the various churches in the community. The REACH project also collaborates with various primary care providers to serve the uninsured in the Chicago area. Since they began their program more than 5 years ago, they have reached over 10,000 African American and Hispanic women with education on breast and cervical cancers and have screened over 5,200 women with mammograms and Pap tests.

African American women aged 40 and over who received even one piece of educational information about mammography are 80% more likely to get a mammogram (CDC 2009). REACH funds more than 40 different projects across the US with specific programs and progress information available at http://www.cdc.gov/reach/about.htm.

Skills and Strategies for Addressing Health Disparities

Although lack of insurance remains a powerful determinant for health disparities, all healthcare providers can develop skills to address other factors contributing to disparities. Over the past 20 years, much has been written and developed to address health disparities which stem from racial and ethnic factors. In addition, all the sliding fee scale programs, community health centers, Medicaid, other forms of low cost healthcare and health-reform efforts have been targeting, and continue to target, lack of insurance as a key disparity.

To begin to address healthcare disparities, one can start with the exploration of culture and *how* to effectively care for all patients. Many definitions of culture can be pulled from the literature which includes the words values, beliefs, language, religion, color, behavior, and norms. For healthcare professionals however, culture is best defined by what the patient tells us it is. Every individual we encounter presents his own world view; and our recommendations and guidance for care need to be the ones the patient can integrate into their culture, lifestyle and belief system. If not, the health provider has fewer opportunities and chances to improve health status (and decrease disparities) for that individual. Being aware of patients who lack medical, dental and health insurance provides insight into their world view before conversation begins. Providing care for an individual or family without insurance requires thoughtful consideration of resources available such as money, transportation, childcare, caregivers, shelter, as well as other factors considered with all patients which include language, literacy, beliefs and values, family support, and education.

For the uninsured patient, a priority will most likely be managing their illness, surgery, or chronic condition on a budget. In addition, as data are collected about health history, family health, and social health, behaviors and current concerns, more of the individual's culture emerges. All this data allow the healthcare provider to plan and execute what is referred to as "culturally competent" care. Cultural competence is defined as a set of congruent behaviors, attitudes, and policies that come together in a system, agency or among healthcare providers to enable them to work effectively in cross-cultural situations (Cross 2000). However, at times, healthcare providers equate cultural competency with ethnicity and language. It is agreed that language and knowledge of an individual's ethnicity is helpful, but never a surety for achieving cultural competency. Cultural humility as proposed by Tervalon and Murray-Garcia (1998) provides that clinicians and healthcare providers make a lifelong commitment to self-evaluation and critique, pay close attention to the relationship between the individual and the provider and to develop mutually beneficial partnerships. For example, in caring for two Chinese-speaking patients, who have both lived in the US for 10 years, the care could be drastically different. One individual has married an American and is much acculturated into American ways, whereas the second individual lives with her elderly Chinese parents and continues to practice many of the customs and beliefs of her home country and her parents. Clinical discussion about diet, exercise, medications, and many other health issues would or could result in very different conversations and clinical interventions.

Upon reviewing some of the commonalities of many of our uninsured patients, they may have challenges with literacy and health literacy issues, confusion over utilization of the healthcare system, and possibly English as not the primary spoken language of choice. Tools and skills to address these needs are essential for clinicians and organizations serving diverse uninsured populations.

Cultural Caring for the Uninsured

Although each individual will present with their own worldview for exploration by the healthcare provider, some guidelines for beginning assessment include:

- Consider all patients as individuals of their own unique culture.
- Never assume that age, insured status, ethnicity or race tells you anything about an individual.
- Turn your "facts" into questions regarding each individual.
- Identify strengths in an individual's culture that can be used to improve their health.
- Know your own attitudes about various cultural groups, attributes, and lifestyles. Suspend them.
- Let your patient tell you what cultural attributes are useful in their care.
- Never forget that caring, empathy, and compassion cross all cultures and worldviews.

In addition, there are many indicators of culture that can be observed and assessed in forming relationships with patients and crossing cultures. Some of them include family structure, important family events, role of the family members, rules of interpersonal interactions, communication and linguistic rules, rules of decorum and discipline, religious beliefs, standards for health and hygiene, food preferences, dress and personal appearance, holiday and celebrations, and many others as they relate to time, work, and play. Establishing medical homes for patients without insurance is a strategy that enables this knowledge of their unique culture and crossing boundaries to occur over time to enhance health outcomes. Chapter Seven discusses the concept of medical homes in greater detail.

Creating Culturally Caring Healthcare Organizations

From the healthcare organization point of view, developing a healthcare delivery site that is culturally appropriate involves leadership to create the desired environment for patients. Office of Minority Health, US Department of Health and Human Services (2000). National Standards for Culturally and Linguistically Appropriate Services (CLAS) in Healthcare with the intent to increase healthcare provider's awareness of how attitudes, beliefs, biases, and behaviors can impact clinical care (Fig. 2).

National Standards for Culturally and Linguistically Appropriate Services (CLAS) in Health Care

Culturally Competent Care:

1. Health care organizations should ensure that patients/consumers receive from all staff members effective, understandable, and respectful care that is provided in a manner compatible with their cultural health beliefs and practices and preferred language.
2. Health care organizations should implement strategies to recruit, retain, and promote at all levels of the organization a diverse staff and leadership that are representative of the demographic characteristics of the service area.
3. Health care organizations should ensure that staff at all levels and across all disciplines receive ongoing education and training in culturally and linguistically appropriate service delivery.

Language Access Services:

4. Health care organizations must offer and provide language assistance services, including bilingual staff and interpreter services, at no cost to each patient/consumer with limited English proficiency at all points of contact, in a timely manner during all hours of operation.

5. Health care organizations must provide to patients/consumers in their preferred language both verbal offers and written notices informing them of their right to receive language assistance services.

6. Health care organizations must assure the competence of language assistance provided to limited English proficient patients/consumers by interpreters and bilingual staff. Family and friends should not be used to provide interpretation services (except on request by the patient/consumer).

7. Health care organizations must make available easily understood patient-related materials and Post signage in the languages of the commonly encountered groups and/or groups represented in the service area.

Organizational Supports:

8. Health care organizations should develop, implement, and promote a written strategic plan that outlines clear goals, policies, operational plans, and management accountability/oversight mechanisms to provide culturally and linguistically appropriate services.
9. Health care organizations should conduct initial and ongoing organizational self-assessments of CLAS-related activities and are encouraged to integrate cultural and linguistic competence-related measures into their internal audits, performance improvement programs, patient satisfaction assessments, and outcomes-based evaluations.
10. Health care organizations should ensure that data on the individual patient's/consumer's race, ethnicity and spoken and written language are collected in health records, integrated into the organization's management information systems, and periodically updated.
11. Health care organizations should maintain a current demographic, cultural, and epidemiological profile of the community as well as a needs assessment to accurately plan for and implement services that respond to the cultural and linguistic characteristics of the service area.
12. Health care organizations should develop participatory, collaborative partnerships with communities and utilize a variety of formal and informal mechanisms to facilitate community and patient/consumer involvement in designing and implementing CLAS-related activities.
13. Health care organizations should ensure that conflict and grievance resolution processes are culturally and linguistically sensitive and capable of identifying, preventing, and resolving cross-cultural conflicts or complaints by patients/consumers.
14. Health care organizations are encouraged to regularly make available to the public information about their progress and successful innovations in implementing the CLAS Standards and to provide public notice in their communities about the availability of this information.

Office of Minority Health, U.S. Department of Health and Human Services. (2000). *National Standards for Culturally and Linguistically Appropriate Services (CLAS) in Health Care.* **Federal Register, 65(247), 80865-80879.**
http://www.omhrc.gov/clas/finalcultural1a.htm

Fig. 2 National standards for culturally and linguistically appropriate services (CLAS) in healthcare

These guidelines not only address culturally competent care and language access, but also support protocol for organizations to develop.

Health Literacy

Currently, a person's literacy skills are the strongest predictor of their health status. According to the most recent national literacy study (Joint Commission 2008), a large portion of the American population have basic (29%) to below basic (14%) literacy skills. About 5% are illiterates. Half of all adults in the US have trouble reading to accomplish their daily tasks and their ability to use numbers is even lower. When low health literacy is coupled with being uninsured, health status is at risk.

Health literacy is the *ability* to read, understand and effectively use basic medical and act on health information (Institute of Medicine 2002). Upon review of literacy levels and the need for health literacy, the challenges to educate our patients, protect them in terms of their medical and health needs, and enhance their self-management skills are apparent. Lastly, adding the variable of being uninsured and most likely of low income, the picture darkens even more.

Several experts have estimated the cost of health illiteracy to be about $73 billion, annually. A study in Arizona of 400 Medicaid patients found that those with the lowest reading levels had medical costs almost 400% higher than those with higher reading levels. In addition, the low health literate individuals tended to have fewer primary care visits, more hospitalizations and less follow-through on recommended treatments and medications (NNLM 2009). The other costs of poorer health status and emotional stress are more difficult to document, but are present nonetheless. Some of the challenges for providers are that frequently patients will not ask their questions and hide their inability to read and understand from their providers. They also may not acknowledge various cultural beliefs and language differences. In addition, many of the educational materials provided for use in patient education, informed consent discussions, and self-management classes, are written at a level of literacy that is too *high* for many Americans, whether they are insured or uninsured.

Assessing Health Literacy Needs of Patients

The health literacy tool with which providers are familiar is the Test of Functional Healthcare Literacy in Adults (TOFHLA), considered the *gold standard* for health literacy testing. It measures both reading comprehension and numerical comprehension and is available in Spanish and other languages as well. However, since the TOFHLA can take up to 30 min to administer, some healthcare providers use a word recognition test instead. Some examples include the Rapid Estimate of Adult Literacy in Medicine (REALM), the Wide-Range Achievement Test (WRAT) and the Slossen Oral Reading Test (SORT) (*see* Fig. 3). Weiss et al. (2005) added a

Rapid Estimate of Adult Literacy in Medicine
REALM©

Terry Davis, PhD, Michael Crouch, MD, Sandy Long, PhD

Patient Name _____ Date of Birth _____ Grade Completed _____

Date _____ Examiner _____ Reading Level _____

List 1	List 2	List 3
fat _____	fatigue _____	allergic _____
flu _____	pelvic _____	menstrual _____
pill _____	jaundice _____	testicle _____
dose _____	infection _____	colitis _____
eye _____	exercise _____	emergency _____
stress _____	behavior _____	medication _____
smear _____	prescription _____	occupation _____
nerves _____	notify _____	sexually _____
germs _____	gallbladder _____	alcoholism _____
meals _____	calories _____	irritation _____
disease _____	depression _____	constipation _____
cancer _____	miscarriage _____	gonorrhea _____
caffeine _____	pregnancy _____	inflammatory _____
attack _____	arthritis _____	diabetes _____
kidney _____	nutrition _____	hepatitis _____
hormones _____	menopause _____	antibiotics _____
herpes _____	appendix _____	diagnosis _____
seizure _____	abnormal _____	potassium _____
bowel _____	syphilis _____	anemia _____
asthma _____	hemorrhoids _____	obesity _____
rectal _____	nausea _____	osteoporosis _____
# of (+) Responses in List 1: _____	# of (+) Responses in List 2: _____	# of (+) Responses in List 3: _____

Fig. 3 Rapid estimate of adult literacy in medicine

health literacy assessment to the standard healthcare vital signs by using a nutrition label with six questions to accompany it. This tool takes only 3 min to administer. Initial use of the nutrition label is reliable and correlates with the traditional TOFHLA (*see* Fig. 4). Results of health literacy measures serve as a guide for the creation of appropriate patient education and self-management tools.

In 2007, St. Elizabeth's Health Center in Tucson, Arizona, a faith-based community health center, administered 342 STOFHLAs with Spanish-speaking, uninsured patients at both their health center and in the community. Two hundred of these patients were diabetics. Inadequate functional health literacy has been determined by national standards to be a score of 0–16 on the STOFHLA. The percentage of uninsured patients with inadequate health literacy in the sample was found to be 32.2%, much higher than the national average of 14.0% (NAAL 2003) (*see* Fig. 5). As a result of this assessment, referrals are available for *all* patients at *no* cost, to meet with a community health worker for education and reinforcement of health education provided by the providers and/or diabetes educators. The community health workers also help develop other avenues for improved learning and understanding such as diagrams, audiotapes and revisions of written materials.

Nutrition Facts

Serving Size 1/2 cup

Servings per container 4

Amount per serving

Calories 250 Fat Cal 120

%DV

Total Fat 13g 20%

Sat Fat 9g 40%

Cholesterol 28mg 12%

Sodium 55mg 2%

Total Carbohydrate 30g 12%

Dietary Fiber 2g

Sugars 23g

Protein 4g 8%

* Percent Daily Values (DV) are based on a 2,000 calorie diet. Your daily values may be higher or lower depending on your calorie needs.

Ingredients: Cream, Skim Milk, Liquid Sugar, Water, Egg Yolks, Brown Sugar, Milkfat, Peanut Oil, Sugar, Butter, Salt, Carrageenan, Vanilla Extract.

Note; This single scenario is the fi nal English version of the newest vital sign. The type size should be 14-point (as shown above) or larger. Patients are presented with the above

scenario and asked the questions shown in Figure 1b.

Questions and answers score sheet for the newest vital sign — English.

ANSWER

CORRECT?

YES NO

READ TO SUBJECT: This information is on the back of a container of a pint of ice cream.

QUESTIONS

1. If you eat the entire container, how many calories will you eat?

Answer 1,000 is the only correct answer

2. If you are allowed to eat 60 g of carbohydrates as a snack, how much ice cream could you have?

Answer Any of the following is correct:

1 cup (or any amount up to 1 cup)

Half the container

Note: If patient answers "2 servings," ask "How much ice cream would that be if you were to measure it into a bowl?"

3. Your doctor advises you to reduce the amount of saturated fat in your diet. You usually have 42 g of saturated fat each day, which includes 1 serving of ice cream. If you stop eating ice cream, how many grams of saturated fat would you be consuming each day?

Answer 33 is the only correct answer

4. If you usually eat 2500 calories in a day, what percentage of your daily value of calories will you be eating if you eat one serving?

Answer 10% is the only correct answer

Pretend that you are allergic to the following substances: Penicillin, peanuts, latex gloves, and bee stings.

5. Is it safe for you to eat this ice cream?

Answer No

6. (Ask only if the patient responds "no" to question 5): Why not?

Answer Because it has peanut oil.

Total Correct

Fig. 4 Nutrition label health literacy assessment

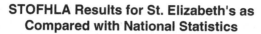

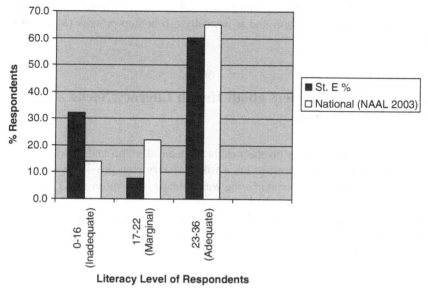

Fig. 5 Report of STOFHLA Examinations in St. Elizabeth Patients

Other recommended interventions in working with patients with literacy or language challenges, include using well-trained medical interpreters, use of plain language, use of drawings or models, teach back techniques, encouraging patients to ask questions, and regularly providing followup and outreach to assure understanding of health information and self-management skills. In addition, the National Patient Safety Foundation (2007) has promoted the use of "AskMe3." All patients should be reminded to ask their healthcare provider: (1) What is my main problem? (2) What do I need to do? and (3) Why is it important for me to do this? in order to ensure patient safety and improved health outcomes.

Patient Education Materials

Readability testing with patient education materials is another strategy to support patient safety and better patient understanding in order to improve health status. In working with uninsured populations, follow-up visits may not be affordable or available , therefore, the need for "take home" materials is essential. There are more than 40 different formulas for assessing readability and most of them use counts of language variables, such as work and sentence length. The Flesch-Kincaid formula is included in Microsoft Word and is a fast assessment of readability. In addition, the use of the SMOG (Simple Measure of Gobbledygook) grading formula is one of the simplest and fastest tests to administer without loss of accuracy. The SMOG takes about 15 min to perform and is basically a four-step process (McLaughlin 1969).

Learning from Providers about Health Literacy Needs of Uninsured Patients

Although many participants on the healthcare team develop and provide patient educational materials, the need to learn from primary care providers about their perceptions and needs in *communicating* with patients from various backgrounds is important to optimize literacy. A physician/provider survey was also developed at St. Elizabeth's Health Center to utilize in community health centers caring for the uninsured and underserved. The survey (Fig. 6) helps healthcare educators and other providers to identify the literacy needs of the patient population being served.

Summary

Traditionally, racial and ethnic disparities go hand-in-hand with the disparity of being uninsured. However, until medical coverage is provided for all, the disparity of being uninsured will impact timeliness of needed care, receiving quality care and needed treatments, and health outcomes. Healthcare providers can continue to develop skills providing culturally, linguistically and literacy appropriate care with assessment, planning and education.

Case Studies for Caring for the Uninsured to Reduce Disparities

The Concept of Refills

A young gentleman in his mid-thirties came to establish care with his sign language interpreter. He was deaf, could read lips, conveyed he understood English and was a recent immigrant from Odessa, Russia. He appeared to be in good health but had been referred to establish care from his counselor who had reported repeated high blood pressure readings over the past two months. As he was uninsured, he came to a local sliding fee scale community health center. He was found to be hypertensive and was started on medications with the instructions conveyed through the interpreter.

Health Literacy-Provider Survey

St. Elizabeth's Health Center

What are three things you find yourself explaining most often to patients?

1)_____

2)_____

3)_____

What are the three hardest things to explain to patients?

1)_____

2)_____

3)_____

Do you feel like you have an adequate understanding of what health literacy is?

_____yes   _____no

How it differs from general literacy?

_____yes   _____no

Are you able to readily identify patients of low health literacy? _____yes_____no

If so, how? _____

_____

Do you address health literacy with your patients? _____yes _____no

Fig. 6 Health literacy-provider survey

He nodded affirmatively about his new medications and indicated he would return for followup in 30 days. Two months passed and there was no sign of him. Upon contacting his interpreter, he indicated he had finished the pills prescribed and felt fine. The concept of refills and the chronic nature of hypertension had *not* been communicated in the initial visit. How might this have been avoided?

Parents of Bone Marrow Transplant Children

The home health nurse continued to bemoan the extra home visits made to families upon discharge of their child post-bone marrow transplant. Despite several educational sessions in the hospital, most parents required 2–3 home visits per week to assist with the care and medication administration with the parent or caregiver. The written materials were in English only and the multiple intravenous medications were confusing. Approximately 30% of the children were readmitted to the hospital. The nurse developed colored cards with matching colors on tubing and medications to assist the parent or caregiver and also created audiotapes that could be listened to for step-by-step instructions. The frequent calls for home visits thereby dropped by 50% in the initial year of the implementation. What might be the next steps for the nurse to continually improve in addressing the language and literacy disparities?

References

Agency for Healthcare Research and Quality (2007) Available at: www.hcup-os.ahrq.gov. Retrieved 1 May 2008

Ayanian JZ (2008) Health consequences for uninsured Americans and racial and ethnic disparities in healthcare. Testimony at Subcommittee on Health-US House of Representatives

U.S. Census Bureau (2008) Ethnic and racial disparities. Available at: www.uscensus.gov. Retrieved 23 Apr 2008

Centers for Disease Control and Prevention (2007) Racial and ethnic approaches to community health. Available at: www.cdc.gov/reach/about.htm. Retrieved 20 Apr 2009

Centers for Disease Control and Prevention (2009) The power to reduce health disparities: Voices from REACH communities. Available at: www.cdc.gov/reach/about.htm. Retrieved 20 Apr 2009

Cross M (2000) Cultural competency in the primary care setting. Arizona Association of Community Health Centers, Phoenix, AZ

Davis TC (1998) Louisiana State University Medical School. REALM health literacy Scale. Available at: tdavis1@lsumc.edu

DeLia D, Belloff D (2006) Disparity in health insurance coverage: Urban versus non-urban areas of New Jersey. Rutgers Center for State Health Policy, vii–ix

Institute of Medicine (2002) Unequal treatment: Confronting racial and ethnic disparities in healthcare. National Academy of Sciences, Washington, DC

Joint Commission (2008) Improving health literacy to protect patient safety. Available at: www. jointcommission.org Retrieved on 1 May 2008

Kaiser Foundation (2009) Race/Ethnicity and Healthcare Program. Available at: www.kff.org. Retrieved 23 Apr 2008

Kaiser Family Foundation (2003) Compendium of cultural competence: Initiatives in healthcare. Available at: www.kff.org. Retrieved on 1 Apr 2009, pp 2–17

McGuire TG, Alegria M, Cook BL, Wells KB, Zaslavshy AM (2006) Implementing the Institute of Medicine definition of disparities: An application to mental healthcare. Health Serv Res 41(5):1979–2005

McLaughlin GH (1969) Smog grading – A new readability formula. J Read 12(8):639–646

National Association of Adult Literacy (NAAL) (2003) Available at www.nces.ed.gov/. Retrieved 1 May 2008

National Committee on Preventive Priorities (2007) Preventive Care: A national profile on use, disparities and health benefits. Available at: www.prevent.org/content. Retrieved on 15 Apr 2009

National Healthcare Disparities Report (2007) Available at: www.hcup-os.ahrq.gov. Retrieved on 15 Apr 2009

National Network of Libraries of Medicine (2009) Health Literacy. Available at: http://nnlm.gov/outreach/consumer. Retrieved 15 Mar 2009

National Patient Safety Foundation (2007) Available at: www.npsf.org/askme3. Retrieved 1 May 2008

Office of Minority Health, US Department of Health and Human Services (2000) National standards for culturally and linguistically appropriate services in healthcare. Fed Regist 65(247):80865–80879

Shen JJ, Washington EL (2007) Disparities in outcomes among patients with Stroke associated with insurance status. Stroke 38:1010–1016

Shone LP, Dick AW, Klein JD, Zwanziger J, Szilagyi PG (2005) Reduction in racial and ethnic disparities after enrollment in the State Children's Health Insurance program. Pediatrics 115(6):697–705

Tervalon M, Murray-Garcia J (1998) Cultural humility versus cultural competence: A critical distinction in defining physician training outcomes in multicultural education. J Healthcare Poor Uninserved 9(2):117–125

Weiss B, Mays MZ, Martz W, Castro KM, DeWalt DA, Pignone MP, Mockbee J, Hale FA (2005) Quick assessment of literacy in primary Care: The newest vital sign. Ann Fam Med 3(6):514–522

Zuvekas SH, Taliaferro GS (2003) Pathways to access: Health insurance, the healthcare delivery system, and racial/ethnic disparities, 1996–1999. Health Aff 22(2):139–153

Providers of Care for the Uninsured

Nancy J. Johnson

Dr. Barbara James sat down at her desk at her private family medicine practice to finish documenting on her last patient for the afternoon. It was a warm fall day in her small town in North Dakota and the day was busy. Her last patient was a 48 year old man who had walked in unscheduled with a large laceration on his left arm from an accident at the farm where he was working. He was not a regular patient and had no regular physician or insurance. Dr. James spent the better part of an hour stitching the laceration, providing needed immunizations, and just checking on his overall health status. He had no insurance and little income, but it was an opportunity to help. Dr. James was used to receiving payment in many forms – insurance, produce from the farmers, and work provided at her home in exchange for care of a family's children – but also knew that she, along with the other primary care physicians in town, provided care for the uninsured in their community out of kindness.

Introduction

Despite the fact that the discussion in this chapter focuses on who the providers of care are for the uninsured in our country, it cannot ignore the many other contributing factors creating challenges in caring for the uninsured. More and more of our political, healthcare, and economic leaders are agreeing that the health care crisis for the uninsured and poor is beginning to impact many insured and middle class individuals and families too. In 2007, the United States spent $2.2 trillion on health care, which represents over 16% of the national economy (CMS 2008). In spite of this, nearly 46 million Americans are uninsured and another 16 million are underinsured (U.S. Census Bureau 2008). What we also recognize, as we identify care providers for the uninsured, is that many barriers to care exist for the insured population as well. Some of these include unaffordable deductibles on their health

N.J. Johnson
El Rio Community Health Center, Tucson, AZ, USA
e-mail: njohnson@ccs-soaz.org

N.J. Johnson and L.P. Johnson (eds.), *The Care of the Uninsured in America*,
DOI 10.1007/978-0-387-78309-3_5, © Springer Science+Business Media, LLC 2010

insurance plans, annual increases in premium costs, difficulty with access to care, shortages of primary care physicians in many parts of our country, and the usual challenges of life such as transportation, child care, caring for aging parents, and work schedules. Lastly, the economic difficulties in 2008 have resulted in a loss of 1.9 million jobs over the last year, causing many individuals and families to rely on the "safety net providers" in our communities (Department of Labor 2008). According to a recent Urban Institute study (Dorn et al. 2008), a one percentage point increase in the unemployment rate leads to a loss of employer-sponsored health insurance coverage for 2.5 million insured individuals. All safety net providers which primarily include hospitals, free clinics, and community health centers are especially stressed during economic hard times, as Medicaid is primarily funded through state tax revenues. As states struggle to balance their budgets in hard economic times, Medicaid funds and eligibility guidelines are frequently modified, resulting in less financial resources for the safety net providers. This is accentuated with the growth of those needing Medicaid enrollment. Correlations between Medicaid enrollment and unemployment is evident from the one percentage increase in unemployment leading to an increase of one million new Medicaid and State Children's Health Insurance members (Dorn et al. 2008).

Recently, a Robert Wood Johnson Foundation study (State Health Access Data Assistance Center 2008) illustrated that health care costs were rising faster than wages. The study released in April 2008, showed that health insurance premiums increased ten times faster than workers' wages between 2001 and 2005. Incomes in the United States increased by 3%, with health insurance premiums increasing by 30% over the same time frame. Average cost for an individual insurance policy had increased 61%, which was about $2,560 per year in 1996 and $4,118 in 2006 (State Health Access Data Assistance Center 2008). Therefore, as the assessment and discussion of the various providers, also known as the "safety net" providers, for the growing number of uninsured in our nation occur, it must be recognized that many Americans who are insured are not receiving the quality care they need for optimal health. The decrease in covered services, increases in premiums, economic hardships, and expensive medication costs, along with the shortage of healthcare professionals, are causing problems in access to care issues for the insured populations as well as the uninsured.

Who Cares for the Uninsured?

There are any number of providers of care for the uninsured including the hospital, the private practice physician, the community health center, the local free clinic, the emergency room, and many others. Most likely, nearly every provider in the current American healthcare system has provided care for someone who is uninsured at some point in time; however, the safety net providers absorb the majority of care for the uninsured. The safety net providers are a mix of hospitals, community health centers, and other healthcare providers who serve a disproportionate number of the uninsured in our communities. Some of these designated providers receive extra federal financial support to support the care of the uninsured. What is also apparent and important to note is that these providers are not linked in any formal sort of partnership or collaboration and all of them may not consistently provide care for the uninsured. This is one impeding factor to providing continuity of care as well as improving the health status of our uninsured population.

An additional challenge in providing care for the uninsured is their varying and sporadic use of the healthcare system. They may utilize a community free clinic, the hospital emergency room, clinics at the public health department, and various sources for prescriptions and other needed services. The choice of care may be based on the urgency of the need, geographic convenience, availability of funds, hours of operation, outstanding balances at a healthcare location, and past experiences with various healthcare organizations. All these factors also play a role in what the individual's health status is and will be in the future. Siegrist and Kane (2003) determined that although the uninsured were generally hospitalized for a similar level of severity of illness as the insured population, the uninsured were hospitalized more frequently and had a higher percentage of illnesses that were responsive to outpatient management and self management such as asthma and diabetes. This supports what we know about the lack of ongoing care management and preventive care strategies with the uninsured population, due to variable and sporadic use of the healthcare system. Improvement in these arenas could help minimize emergency room and hospital utilization.

Hospitals

Hospitals across the country are frequently the safety net providers as well as the providers when all else fails for the uninsured. Hospitals are currently providing about $34 billion in uncompensated care every year with most going to the uninsured (American Hospital Association 2009). Between 2001 and 2007, America's hospitals saw an increase in uncompensated care from $21.5 billion to today's $34 billion as reported by the American Hospital Association (2009). Although caring for people in need regardless of their ability to pay has always been a core element and value of our nation's not for profit hospitals, as the number of uninsured climbs, the strain upon hospitals attempting to provide an entire range of health and medical services continues to grow.

In 1986, Congress passed the Emergency Medical Treatment and Active Labor Act (EMTALA) as part of the Consolidated Omnibus Budget Reconciliation Act. It requires that hospitals and ambulance services must provide care to anyone needing emergency treatment regardless of citizenship, legal status, or ability to pay. There are no reimbursement provisions for the hospitals for this care. So, patients needing emergency treatment can only be discharged with their informed consent or when they need to be transferred to a hospital better equipped to deal with their needed type of care. Hospitals that must honor EMTALA include all those who receive payment from the Department of Health and Human Services, Medicare, and Medicaid. Therefore, the only hospitals who are exempt from EMTALA are Indian Health Services, military Veterans Administration hospitals, and the Shriners Hospitals for Children.

Because there are no direct funds for reimbursement, EMTALA is sometimes seen as an unfunded mandate as well as a reason for the over crowdedness in emergency rooms. For many uninsured individuals, the emergency room is the entry point for dental emergencies, psychiatric conditions, medical care, and substance use disorders. Since EMTALA was passed in 1986, the number of emergency rooms have decreased across the nation and more than half (55%) of the emergency care in the United States is uncompensated (Centers for Medicare and Medicaid 2008). Some consumer groups believe that the passing of this legislation has led hospitals to cost shifting; therefore, contributing to the higher cost of medical care. So, essentially, EMTALA requires hospitals to adhere to three obligations:

1. Patients requesting emergency care must receive a medical screening examination to determine whether an emergency exists. Examinations and treatments cannot be delayed while exploring whether a patient has a method of payment or insurance.
2. The emergency room must treat an individual with an emergency medical condition until the condition is resolved or stabilized. If the hospital does not have the appropriate standard of care available, they may transfer the patient to another hospital that can provide the needed care.
3. Hospitals with specialized capabilities must accept these transfers (EMTALA. COM 2008).

EMTALA has resulted in access to care for everyone with urgent health problems regardless of their insurance status, but has also resulted in less number of emergency rooms being available and over crowdedness in the existing emergency rooms. During the period from 1993 to 2003, the emergency room visits in the nation grew by 27%, but 425 emergency rooms closed in the same timeframe (Institute of Medicine 2006). In addition, the amount of uncompensated care grew from $6.1 billion in 1983 to $40.7 billion in 2004 (Kaiser Commission on Medicaid and the Uninsured 2004) with the percentage due to EMTALA legislation unknown. Various groups of people believe that illegal immigrants are causing the emergency room over crowdedness and uncompensated care. However, a report from the Kaiser Commission on Medicaid and the Uninsured (2009) reported that uninsured low-income non-citizens were the least likely to use emergency rooms, with only about 10% reporting a visit in the past year. However, many states such as Arizona, Florida, and other border states, report a much higher utilization of their emergency rooms and hospital stays by non-citizens (Florida Hospital Association 2003). The Florida Hospital Association is an example of a study group which collected data specifically related to uncompensated care in their state's emergency rooms, but also examined the amount of dollars spent on the subsequent follow up care. Their conclusions supported the emergency room as the access for urgent care for non-citizens, and the need for safety net providers to coordinate care management across the community, as well as country, at times, for uninsured patients as well. Lastly, the Medicare Prescription Drug, Improvement and Modernization Act of 2003 provides funding of $250 million per year through 2008 to reimburse providers for emergency health services provided to undocumented aliens (CMS 2008). Funds are still available for providers for reimbursement of emergency services in 2009 (www.trailblazerhealth.com, 2009). More about emergency care and refugees is discussed in Chapter 9 Uninsured Immigrants and Refugees.

On top of the challenging numbers of uninsured seeking care through community hospitals and emergency rooms, the physician shortage and physician availability compound the challenge. Recently, southern California reported more and more specialty physicians refusing to work in emergency rooms tdue to poor reimbursement along with the growing number of uninsured receiving care in the emergency rooms (Cover the Uninsured 2009). A survey completed by the American College of Emergency Room Physicians in 2006 reported that 73% of the nation's emergency rooms reported a shortage of specialty physicians to support the emergency rooms staffing needs (ACEP 2007). The problem of physician staffing worsens in smaller communities where the uninsured may comprise as much as 30% of the emergency room volume (Cover the Uninsured 2008).

On the basis of the EMTALA legislation as well as the community mission of many of our nation's hospitals, not only are the emergency rooms serving as a primary provider of care for the uninsured, the hospitals in their role as an outpatient and inpatient facility also provide hugely discounted care as well as a large amount of charity care for the uninsured. Hospitals, as providers of care for the uninsured, provide this community benefit through many classifications.

- Charity Care which is defined as care for which the hospital does not expect to receive payment from the patient or a third party payer such as an insurance company. An example is illustrated by Cook County hospitals which provided $152 million in charity care in 2004 (MCHC 2006).
- Bad Debt is for care provided with a bill generated and no payment received. Again, Cook County hospitals alone absorbed $640.9 million of bad debt in 2004 (MCHC 2006).
- Government sponsored indigent care which includes the un-reimbursed costs of federal, state, and local programs which assist individuals on the basis of their financial need. Some examples of these hospital subsidies are seen with Medicaid, Kids Care and other government funded programs.
- Government sponsored programs which have non-reimbursable components which are not indigent care such as Medicare.
- Subsidized health services which lose money for the hospital such as trauma centers, neonatal intensive care units, and burn care.

Hospitals as safety net care providers for the uninsured do carry a large portion of the care for the uninsured in communities due to their availability 24 hours per day, 7 days per week, and 365 days of the year. The Institute of Medicine (2006) concluded from its study that approximately 14% of emergency patients were uninsured, another 16% were covered by Medicaid, and an additional 21% covered by Medicare.

This results in over half of the emergency room volume leaving unpaid balances for emergency rooms and their hospitals to manage. However, a recent study completed by Arizona State University (2007) reported that 50% of the visits to hospital emergency rooms were for primary care needs such as upper respiratory infections, minor injuries, gastrointestinal problems, and minor illnesses.

On the basis of this information that many emergency room visits may be non-emergent, there is a need to expand community options for uninsured patients. Uninsured patients also need to be reached with the information about the appropriate source of care for non-emergencies in their communities. Uninsured patients need to be educated and assisted by establishing "medical homes" or "health homes" which frequently are the community health centers across the nation. The transition for the uninsured as it relates to the emergency room as the safety net needs to be a shift from acute, episodic care to community-based primary care.

As hospitals have attempted and continue to try to avoid growing financial losses from caring for the uninsured, they have developed services to help uninsured patients who come to the hospital via the emergency room as their initial contact with the health care system. Most hospitals have trained eligibility staff who help the uninsured apply for government assistance such as Medicare, Medicaid, State Children's Health Insurance Program, and any other program for which the individual or family may qualify. They help find birth certificates, pay stubs, process challenging eligibility forms, and frequently assist with electronic eligibility. In addition, most hospitals utilize counselors, social workers, and discharge planners to try to avoid future hospitalizations and emergency room visits by connecting the uninsured individual to community sliding scale or charity supported clinics. Most hospital systems provide these clinics as part of their community benefit initiatives. Hospitals generally try to help the uninsured through reduction of charges. For example, the Metropolitan Chicago Healthcare Council (2006) recommends that hospitals forgive charges for patients who earn up to 100% of the federal poverty guidelines and discount charges for patients earning up to 200% of the poverty level. Lastly, most hospitals work with uninsured patients to develop payment plans to pay the balance owed over time. These discounts and payment plans are beneficial, but many times, the uninsured patient does not qualify for assistance. This may be due to being over income and part of the "notch group" or "working poor." They may also fail to complete the needed application steps to qualify and remain qualified for assistance programs.

Critical Access Hospitals

The Medicare Rural Hospital Flexibility Program (Flex Program) was created by the Balanced Budget Act of 1997 (Rural Assistance Center 2009) and is in place to strengthen rural health care systems. In rural or near-rural communities, there is a greater likelihood that an individual will be uninsured. The Agency for Healthcare Research and Quality in 2002 compared the rural uninsured for a year (18.5%) to the urban uninsured (12.7%). Approximately a quarter of emergency room visits in the country are in rural communities and about 16% represent uninsured individuals (South Carolina Rural Research Center 2004). An estimated $8.8 billion was spent across the nation in rural communities for patients without insurance during a one year period of time in 2000 (South Carolina Rural Research Center 2004). In addition to the greater number of uninsured and low income people living in rural communities, the access and availability of services is also a challenge.

On the basis of these numbers, the Flex Program uses the Critical Access Hospital Program as an intervention to address the need of rural providers for the uninsured. A key component of the Flex Program is to create a statewide rural health plan. This plan should include the creation of a rural health network and a system for ongoing quality improvement. In many rural communities, hospitals have ceased to exist or have been scaled back to provide outpatient primary care services. Individuals living in rural communities may not have access to specialty services, inpatient services, or urgent and emergency services. The Critical Access Hospital Program is available to health care organizations that meet the following criteria:

- Located in a state that has established a Medicare Flex Program
- Has been designated a critical access hospital by the State
- Currently participating in Medicare as a rural public, non-profit, or for-profit hospital, or was a participating hospital that closed during the period of time from November 29, 1989 to November 29, 1999, or was downsized from a hospital to a health clinic or health center
- Located in a rural area or is treated as rural
- Located at more than a 35 mile drive from any other hospital – in areas with difficult travel such as secondary roads or mountains, the mile amount is 15 miles.
- Maintains no more than 25 inpatient beds with an average length of stay of 96 h for acute inpatient care.
- Complies with all critical access hospital conditions such as offering 24 hour per day, seven day a week emergency care services.
- May have "swing beds" which are used for post-hospital skilled care as well (Rural Assistance Center 2009).

The Critical Access Hospital Program is a benefit for the uninsured in rural communities. Individuals and families have access to emergency care as well as to other healthcare services and professionals in urban communities. They may still have the challenges of regular and continuous primary care services because of healthcare professional shortages. For hospitals in rural communities, the benefits of the critical access hospital program are many. Medicare provides cost-based reimbursement plus a percentage increase over cost, access to the Flex Program grants, and capital improvement costs are included in the allowable Medicare cost-based reimbursement. The program also provides more flexibility for rural hospitals in identifying and expanding services to address the community needs, such as services for the uninsured. Some states also provide a higher Medicaid reimbursement rate for critical access hospitals. Critical Access Hospitals is discussed in Chapter 13, The Rural Uninsured.

Government Programs

The Department of Health and Human Services is the federal government's key agency for protecting the health of our nation as well as providing human services. They provide over 230 programs and manage over 60,000 grants that fund public health, anti-terrorism, education, basic and applied science, special health programs, and child development. They also provide management for the Medicare and Medicaid programs.

As employer provided health insurance continues to decline as an offering by employers or as an affordable opportunity for many Americans, government resources become a source for seeking health care coverage. The Centers for Medicare and Medicaid (CMS) provide our current two national health care programs and have approximately 75 million Americans enrolled (Medicare.gor 2009). In addition, CMS provides the State Children's Health Insurance Program (SCHIP) that covers approximately 10 million children in our country (CMS 2009). As one looks at the government's support of Medicaid, they provide approximately 50–75% of the support in partnership with individual states. An additional Medicare Program added in 2006 was the Medicare Part D Prescription Program which assists with cost reduction on medication needs.

To begin with, Medicare Part A helps cover inpatient care in hospitals, skilled nursing care in nursing facilities, hospice care, and home health care. If the enrollees or their spouses paid Medicare taxes while working, there is usually no premium paid for Medicare Part A. However, for someone needing to pay a premium, the 2009 monthly premium cost was $443 monthly (Medicare.gov 2009). Medicare Part B helps cover medically-necessary services such as doctor's visits, outpatient care, and other medical services. Medicare Part B requires a monthly premium which is $96.40 in 2009. Medicare Part C represents Medicare Advantage Plans which provide managed care options provided by private insurance companies. These various plans have different rules and services covered and are not supplemental insurance for Medicare (Medicare.gov 2009). The last component of Medicare benefits is Medicare Part D which is the prescription benefit coverage. All individuals must enroll in Medicare Part D and can also apply for additional help from Medicare if qualifying by income and resources. However, for individuals with many regular medication needs, the annual funded discounted amount usually runs out prior to the end of the calendar year. This requires many low income Medicare recipients to seek help through prescription assistance programs and other discounted resources. Upon review of Medicare, the uninsured generally cannot afford the monthly premiums and fees associated with the program.

Fortunately, Medicaid is also provided as a match program between the federal government and the individual states for the low income uninsured population of all ages. Some Americans may also be "dual eligible" which means being able to receive Medicare Part A and B benefits, along with some services via Medicaid. The uninsured can apply for Medicaid services, for which there is no premium, but may have a co-payment due when services are accessed. Every state varies in how it manages the Medicaid program and eligibility is tied to the federal poverty guidelines annually. Again, the "working poor," also known as the "notch group" may not qualify for Medicaid, but do not have the funds or employment to access private health insurance. The Bureau of Primary Health Care provides services and funding for low-income uninsured individuals as well as for those with special health care needs. They are the source of funding for the federally qualified community health centers. The government also supports a Healthcare for the Homeless Program which encompasses an interdisciplinary team approach to delivering care inclusive of street outreach, case management, primary care, behavioral health, and patient advocacy. Human Resources and Services Administration (HRSA) also supports many grants and programs to help support health care for the uninsured and low income across the nation. Beyond these direct service funding programs or special projects funding, the government provides advocacy and resource direction for the uninsured. There are many hotlines and websites available at both the state and national level in which to gather information and are too numerous to list. However, they are simply informational services, without guidance for finding affordable and direct health care services.

Cover the Uninsured, a funded initiative of the Robert Wood Johnson Foundation, (Cover the Uninsured 2009) is a national project to highlight that too many Americans are living without health insurance. The second goal of the project is to present current data to leaders on a regular basis about the problem and the work being done to decrease the numbers of Americans who are uninsured. The target populations for the project include health care professionals, community and grass-roots groups, health policy-makers, business communities, and individual advocates. This website provides news, research updates, listings of activities and resources, and most importantly, a state by state resource for people seeking health insurance. Figures 1 and 2 illustrate the resources available for someone in the state of Idaho seeking health insurance as an example (Cover the Uninsured 2009).

Fig. 1 Idaho start-from covertheuninsured.org page 1 only (shrink)

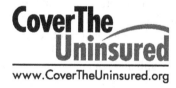

www.CoverTheUninsured.org

Fig. 2 Idaho steps to getting insured – from covertheuninsured.org (rest of pages-shrink)

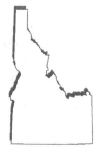

Another advocacy service related to access to healthcare for the uninsured includes the Department of Labor's explanation of COBRA coverage and policy, if one had insurance and is trying to avoid becoming uninsured. COBRA was passed in 1985 as the Consolidated Omnibus Budget Reconciliation Act and mandates an insurance program providing employees the ability to continue health care coverage after leaving employment. However, access to COBRA coverage is very expensive-and the episodic or chronically uninsured find the cost prohibitive. Most recently with the economic downturn of 2008, all Americans who were involuntarily terminated from employment between September 1, 2008 and December 31, 2009, and do not have an annual income greater than $125,000 for an individual or $250,000 for a family qualify for COBRA assistance. The federal government has authorized subsidies to cover 65% of the cost of health insurance premiums under COBRA for as long as nine months. This is an effort to maintain continuity of care for currently insured Americans and not add to the numbers of uninsured or the numbers seeking coverage through Medicaid (Cover the Uninsured 2009).

Two other resources offered by the government for the uninsured are access to the Insurance Commission in all states if you feel you are being denied coverage or payment for services as well as information about health savings accounts. Although these are worthy educational and resource efforts, they fail to address the basic needs for health care of the low income and uninsured persons in our country. (Ehealthinsurance Services 2008).

Health and Human Service Community Organizations

Most communities have local and regional health and human service organizations that are supported with various sources of funding to provide services for the uninsured and low income persons. Some of these target basic needs such as housing, food, transportation, job training, and other critical services. Generally, these organizations such as our homeless shelters and food banks serve as links to community clinics and other health-related services for the uninsured. A challenge in caring for the uninsured is the coordination of care and services among these many community health and human service organizations. In addition, the Department of Health and Human Services provides some targeted services as funding is allocated including vouchers for substance abuse treatment, immunization and vaccine availability, and low cost cancer screening for the uninsured (DHHS 2006).

Lastly, in many of our communities, there are Information and Referral Sources which are compiled and updated annually. These are excellent tools from which one may access many needed human services including low cost health care services. In 2004, the governor of Arizona created the Governor's Council on 2-1-1 to plan and build a statewide 2-1-1 system to facilitate the community's access to community health and human services as well as referrals and homeland security information. This is a web-based Information and Referral source which started as an online version of the traditional Information and Referral manuals from Arizona counties (Arizona 211 On-line, 2008). In addition, Fig. 3 provides an example of an Arizona webpage of resources for the community.

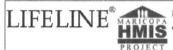 **LIFELINE®** required. Call 1-877-HIV-7020 or 1-800-448-7020.

Maricopa HMIS (Homeless Management Information System) Project
Assessing services provided to and unmet needs of homeless individuals in Maricopa County. This program is presented in cooperation with several agencies with support from the Department of Housing and Urban Development (HUD).

 Arizona Mortgage Foreclosure Helpline
With thousands of Arizonans facing foreclosure on their homes, Community Information & Referral has partnered with the Arizona Department of Housing to guide those people to agencies that can help them through the process and might be able to help them stay in their homes. Call 1-877-448-1211.

Valley Lifeline
In partnership with Lifeline Systems Inc., the nation's leading provider of personal emergency response services, we provide a way to help people remain independent in their own homes while maintaining a constant link to immediate emergency services should the need arise. This service is especially helpful to senior citizens and people with disabilities who might otherwise require constant supervision in an environment outside their homes. Call 602-263-8845.

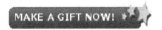 MAKE A GIFT NOW!

Get Help | Arizona Links | What We Do | Publications | About Us | Contact Us | Mailing List | Home

© Community Information & Referral

 For your clients, for your family, for yourself... You need these books!

click here to order yours today

Fig. 3 Arizona information and Referral Webpage

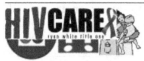 **Special Programs**
Updated June 18, 2008

Community Information & Referral offers several specialized programs for residents of Arizona. Please click on the name of the programs below to find out more about them including contact information.

24-Hour Helpline
Our English/Spanish bilingual Information & Referral Specialists are ready to help you 24 hours a day to assist you in finding the help you need. We are central and northern Arizona's *First Call for Help*. Call 602-263-8856 from anywhere or 1-800-352-3792 within area codes 520 & 928.

Childhood Immunization Hotline (Maricopa County only)
We refer callers living in Maricopa County to the closest clinic where they can get free immunizations for their children age 18 and under. Call 602-263-8856.

Community Voice Mail
Community Voice Mail assists homeless individuals in Maricopa County by giving them private telephone numbers to help them with job searches and keeping connected to family and friends. All clients must be referred by agencies that provide direct services to homeless individuals and/or families. Call 602-263-8845 x 108.

 CONTACS
The **CO**mmunity **NeT**work for **AC**cessing **S**helter helps domestic violence victims and homeless persons in Maricopa County find shelter in emergency situations 24 hours a day, 7 days a week. Call 602-263-8900 or 1-800-799-7739.

HIV CARE
HIV CARE is a **confidential** 24-hour information line for helping people with HIV/AIDS who need medical care. People can also get help with food, dental, counseling, social services and treatment. Services are available in English and Spanish. No insurance is

Fig. 3 (continued)

Faith-Based Organizations

The creation of the White House Office of Faith-Based and Community Initiatives in 2005 was positioned to expand the role of these organizations in addressing the nation's social programs as well as provide these organizations access to government-sponsored grants and programs. These faith-based organizations have become a frequent provider of medical and health care for the uninsured. The beginning of this White House Initiative focused on at-risk youth, ex-offenders, the homeless, the hungry, substance abusers, those with HIV/AIDS, and welfare to work families (DHHS 2005). They continue to focus on building local interventions and solutions to address community challenges.

Looking at the needs of the uninsured, faith-based organizations are key providers for medical, dental, and health care. They welcome all who need assistance or resources, and are well linked in their communities for collaboration, in addition to offering a spiritual perspective as a component of care. Many times, these organizations have access to community volunteers, contributions, and partnerships which optimize leveraging of their existing resources to expand service delivery. St. Elizabeth's Health Center in Tucson, Arizona is one such organization. Since its inception in 1961, the Health Center has cared exclusively for the uninsured with a small paid staff partnered with over 165 community volunteer physicians, dentists, and other healthcare professionals. In the most recent year, the volunteers provided nearly three-fourth of a million dollars in care for the sliding scale uninsured patient base of nearly 20,000 who see St. E's as their "medical home"(Catholic Community Services of Southern Arizona 2008). The faith-based mission of the Health Center presents a caring milieu in the community and an ongoing commitment for sustainability from its volunteers many of whom have volunteered for greater then ten years at St. Elizabeth's Health Center.

Faith-based organizations are also visible at the national level in advocating and providing care for the uninsured. Ascension Health is the nation's largest Catholic non-profit health system comprised of hospitals, medical practices, clinics, behavioral health, and residential care. Ascension Health is comprised of three faith based communities including the Sister of St. Joseph of Carondelet, the Daughters of Charity, and the Congregation of St. Joseph. Ascension Health's mission comprises four key strategic goals with one being "health care that leaves no one behind by 2020" (Ascension Health 2009). Ascension Health is active in driving health care policy with an outcome of 100% access and 100% coverage for all. Their website highlights their "Guiding Features" for a reform of health care policy (Ascension Health 2009).

One of the concerns about faith-based organizations is the potential to have a captive audience in need of service upon which to prostelytize. It appears that most faith-based organizations providing health care, at least, view their service to the uninsured and medically underserved as an extension of their mission, and not as a basis for pushing a religious point of view. Under the new federal administration, this expectation of not proselytizing is anticipated to harden to a policy (Patel 2009).

Federally Qualified Community Health Centers

Currently, Federally Qualified Community Health Centers are the largest primary care providers nationally caring for the uninsured, serving more than 18 million Americans (NACHC 2009). However, their history is important to reflect upon as one seeks creative models of care to address the needs of the uninsured in our communities. Community Health Centers were first initiated in 1965 under the leadership of President Johnson as part of the "war on poverty." The first community health centers were part of the Office of Economic Opportunity (OEO) and were to provide health and social services at convenient locations in poor and medically underserved communities. A secondary purpose was to inspire community empowerment around health care. The initial funds for the community health centers were awarded to local non-profit community organizations and avoided any sort of affiliation with state government. They were to be responsive to the needs of the community and the first two demonstration projects were located in Boston, Massachusetts in 1965 and Mound Bayou, Mississippi in 1967. President Johnson's administration also created the Medicare and Medicaid programs around this same time, but the two initiatives were not linked until nearly a decade later (Lefkowitz and Todd 1993).

In the early 1970s, the community health center program was moved to the Department of Health and Human Services and joined with the migrant health program. Finally, in 1996, the Health Centers Consolidation Act combined the community health centers, the migrant health programs, and the homeless and public housing programs all under 330 of the Public Health Service Act to create the consolidated health centers program. In order for a community health center to receive 330 status and be identified as a Federally Qualified Health Center (FQHC), it must be located in a medically underserved area (MUA) or serve a federally designated medically underserved population (MUP). Over the years, these designations are assessed at periods of time for population variances and the numbers of health professionals practicing in the areas. The data may result in revisions of the designations and geography.

In addition, community health centers must have nonprofit, public or tax exempt status, and provide comprehensive primary health care services, referrals, and any other services identified as necessary to provide access to care. They must have a governing board in which the majority are patients of the health center and provide services to all in the service area regardless of their ability to pay. All 330 community health centers must offer a sliding fee schedule that adjusts according to the family income (330 Public Health Service Act 2006). The community board membership is designed to help assure the community health center's responsiveness to their community rather than other potential influences.

Currently, about 80% of the government funding is awarded to community health centers with the remaining 20% divided between public housing, migrant, homeless, and school-based health centers. In addition, the government provides mandates on how much of the grant money can be allocated for capital and equipment, with the majority of the funds being reserved for direct patient care.

Today, FQHCs have grown and expanded dramatically with $2 billion funded annually through HRSA and over 16 million patients nationally (Hurley et al. 2007). Currently, there are approximately 1,200 federally qualified health centers nationally providing care through more than 7,000 geographical service locations (NACHC 2009).

Another safety net provider that is similar to the FQHC is the "Look Alike" model which is an outpatient clinic not receiving 330 funding, but operating and providing similar services to a FQHC. Some of the characteristics of a "Look Alike" include non-profit status, governed by users, no control or ownership by other entities, serving an entire or partially designated MUA or MUP, and meeting the statutory, regulatory, and program requirements for 330 grantees. "Look Alike" clinics must be open for a minimum of 32 hours per week, provide a sliding fee scale, have a Chief Executive Officer employed directly by the clinic, have management information systems available, and conduct an annual independent financial audit. The "Look-Alike" clinics must be or must apply to be a Medicare and Medicaid provider (HRSA 2009). Benefits to community health centers seeking "Look Alike" status include the following:

- Access to 340B drug pricing which allows them to purchase covered outpatient prescription medications for health center patients at reduced prices.
- Access to reimbursement under the Prospective Payment System (PPS) or other state-approved alternative payment methodologies, which are on the basis of cost-based reimbursement.
- Reimbursement by Medicare for "first dollar" of service rendered to Medicare beneficiaries if the deductible is waived.
- Safe harbor under the Federal anti-kickback statute for waiver of co-payments if the patient is below 200% of the federal poverty guidelines and therefore, eligible for a discount.
- Access to providers through the National Health Service Corps (NHSC) if located in a Health Professional Shortage Area (HPSA).
- Access to Federal Vaccine for Children program which provides vaccines at no charge for uninsured children (HRSA 2009).

The Tribal or Urban Indian FQHC which is operated by a tribe or Indian organization (Taylor 2004) is another provider of care for the uninsured and underserved which is managed under tribal governance. Figure 4 (www.raconline.org) provides a comparison of options for supporting primary care for the uninsured and underserved.

Rural Health Clinics

The Rural Health Clinic is another recognized model for provision of access to care for the uninsured and underserved. The purpose of the rural health clinic is to encourage the availability and accessibility of primary care in underserved rural areas which are defined as Health Professional Shortage Area, or areas designated

Governmental Options for Supporting Primary Care for the Uninsured

TYPE	BENEFITS
Federally Qualified Health Center	• 330 Grant • 340B Provider • FTCA Coverage • Eligible for additional Grants • Access to PPS reimbursement • Safe harbor for waiver of co-payments for those less than 200% of federal poverty level • Access to NHSC if a HPSA • Access to Vaccines for Children
Rural Health Clinic	• Use of midlevel providers in rural communities • Profit or not for profit • Provider based or independent • Access to PPS reimbursement
Critical Access Hospitals	• Access to PPS reimbursement • Able to address community urgent and emergent needs
Migrant Health Clinics	• 330 Grant • 340B Provider • FTCA Coverage • Eligible for additional grants • Access to PPS reimbursement
"Look Alike" Health Centerl	• 340B Provider • Access to PPS reimbursement • Safe harbor for waiver of co-payments for those less than 200% of federal poverty level • Access to NHSC if a HPSA • Access to Vaccines for Children

Fig. 4 Government option for support of primary care

by the U.S. Census Bureau as "non-urbanized" or as designated by a state's governor. Public Law 95-210, which is the Rural Health Clinic Services Act was passed in December 1977 and provided for cost-based Medicare and Medicaid reimbursement to qualified Rural Health Clinics for a set of regulated services delivered by a nurse practitioner or a physician assistant even in the absence of a physician (NARHC 2009). Rural Health Clinics may be for profit or not for profit may be part of an existing hospital system but not qualify for federal tort claim act coverage (FTCA) as an FQHC would (HRSA 2007). In 1992, Congress identified that community health centers had paid more than 40 million in malpractice insurance with less than 10 percent of that paid in claims on their behalf. At that point, FTCA was expanded to provide free malpractice coverage for health centers, thereby freeing more funds for primary care services.

In the past 6 years, FQHCs have received over $750 million in new funding which has decreased the population without access to care by more than 5 million (NACHC 2009). This new funding has helped to stabilize many community health centers as well as help provide medical homes for the growing number of uninsured with chronic diseases. Today, FQHCs provide care for over 18 million individuals in all fifty states. This includes 1 in every 7 uninsured, 1 in 8 of every Medicaid beneficiaries, 1 in 3 living below the poverty line, and 1 in 4 low income minority individuals. They work to not only improve outcomes for the uninsured, but also to provide cost effective care for patients, communities, and payers through a model of preventive primary health care (NACHC 2009). The research shows that a patient without insurance but having a regular "medical home" like a community health center actually receives better primary care than those who have insurance but no regular medical home (Phillips 2003).

However, there continues to be many challenges facing our nation's community health centers as the population of uninsured and low income people continues to grow. In addition, the healthcare professional workforce shortage creates recruitment and retention challenges for all community health centers. Another challenge on the horizon is seen with the report from the National Association of Community Health Centers and the Robert Graham Center (2007) that over 56 million Americans, many with insurance, do not have reliable access to primary care. Other facets of that study illustrate Americans are not getting the care they need, with numbers worsening as one factors in minorities and socioeconomic status (NACHC 2007). As these areas of concern are investigated, data exist on the proven effectiveness of community health centers. For example, medical expenses for community health center patients are 41% lower at $1,810 per person annually compared to patients seen in other locations, which is thought to be by avoiding the expensive use of emergency rooms. The utilization of this figure allows one to estimate a saving to the health care system between $9.9 and $17.6 billion nationally (NACHC 2007). As one looks at these savings, one can hypothesize that the improvement in cost effective care is a combination of many factors such as an integrated care delivery team, a sliding fee scale which may improve patient access for primary and secondary preventive visits, and community need focused care.

In addition to continuing to provide care for many Americans, community health centers are also working toward continually improving their service delivery and management. Focus today is on the implementation of electronic medical and health records, working to build integrated care models which improve clinical outcomes for patients, attempting to continually address regulation requirements and additional reporting requirements for the Bureau of Primary Health Care, Medicaid, and other third party payers, and identifying what are the most effective and appropriate quality improvement measures for community health centers. Some examples of clinical quality improvement include better management of diabetes, hypertension, chronic lung disease, and asthma.

The Health Care Safety Net Act of 2008 (Kaiser Commission On Medicaid and the Uninsured 2009a, b) was enacted in October of 2008 to reauthorize federally qualified health centers through 2012 in order to continue to grow their services to serve more than 25 million by the end of fiscal year 2012. This legislation also provides linkages with the NHSC and emphasizes major quality initiatives and growth of primary care in poorer communities.

The American Recovery and Reinvestment Act of 2009 has allocated over $2 billion for federally qualified health centers (NACHC 2009). This economic stimulus package provides $1.5 billion for community health center infrastructure needs such as health information technology, construction, renovation, and equipment, and an additional $500 million to fund community health center services. The approximately 1,200 federally qualified health centers in the nation are indeed the model of care for the uninsured and underserved in our communities, as shown by the ongoing federal commitment for expansion.

The review of the past 40 years of community health centers is interesting if one considers their origins to serve as a local health and human service resource for the poor, uninsured, and medically disenfranchised. Reviewing their amazing growth in funding, size, and evolution of their current appearance today as large primary care community based medical, dental, mental health, and health service facilities with many sites, one must reflect on the original mission and focus of the community health center. Although they continue to provide care for the uninsured, they also provide care for large populations of the insured. In addition, the community health center budget contains a payer mix of many insurance companies and community contributors. Community health centers are being viewed by many health planners as the best model for community based primary care, regardless of funding source.

Private Practice Providers and Volunteers

As noted in the opening chapter scenario, providers of the uninsured in our country also include private practice providers and many practitioners who volunteer outside their private practice or hospital setting. Although the numbers are not well documented, many practitioners provide assistance to the uninsured when presented with health needs or problems in the community. Some provide discounts via a sliding fee scale, while others provide services in kind. Volunteers in many free clinics and non-federally qualified health centers provide millions of dollars in medical and dental care for the uninsured across our nation annually, which is not well documented.

Health Care Professional Shortages

Another challenge in providing care for the uninsured is the national health care professional workforce shortage. Primary care practitioners such as family medicine physicians, pediatricians, internal medicine physicians, obstetricians/gynecologists, dentists, nurse practitioners, physician assistants, and dental hygienists are in demand in most community health centers and especially those in rural areas. The NHSC is committed to improving the health of the underserved and uninsured by addressing the primary care workforce shortage (HRSA 2009). The NHSC works to help communities recruit and retain primary care clinicians to serve across our nation. Since 1972, more than 27,000 health professionals have served with NHSC with approximately 4,000 clinicians practicing currently in underserved and uninsured communities. The federal government has currently funded $500 million for primary care workforce development with $300 million allocated to the NHSC.

The Area Health Education Center Program (AHEC) is another federally funded healthcare workforce development program. AHEC Programs are academic and community partnership programs funded between HRSA and various state and local funding sources. The mission of the AHEC program is to improve the supply, distribution, diversity, and quality of the healthcare workforce, ultimately increasing access to health care in medically underserved and uninsured areas (HRSA 2009). AHEC program links the resources of university health science centers with local planning, community, educational, and clinical resources. AHEC programs focus on recruitment and retention focusing on education for youth about health careers, placing health profession students for rotations in underserved areas, and providing retention resources for underserved and rural communities. AHEC programs were first funded in 1972 and reauthorized through the Health Professions Education Partnerships of 1998. There are approximately 53 AHEC programs across the country providing training for about 37,000 health professions students in a typical year and working about 1,500 community health centers nationally to place health care providers (HRSA 2009).

Many underserved and medically needy communities are also working to "grow their own" primary care providers by forging relationships with local schools, community organizations, and community health centers. Mt. Graham Regional Medical Center in Safford, Arizona is one such example of a small rural hospital connecting with the local high school to identify students entering the health sciences and staying in touch over the years through correspondence and community gatherings when students are home visiting family. In addition, Mt. Graham offers summer internships for high school students at the hospital to begin to build relationships for the future (Mt. Graham Regional Medical Center 2007).

Collaboration and Coordination

Upon review of the various providers caring for the estimated 46 million in our country without health insurance, it is apparent that all aspects of the healthcare system participate to some extent. Some are designated as providers for the uninsured,

Arranging Surgery for the Uninsured

Sponsor: Operation Access
Location: San Francisco, CA

Where would a non-English-speaking laborer with no health insurance go to have a hernia repaired? Too often, the answer is nowhere: the legions of working poor earn too much to qualify for Medicaid but can't afford a luxury like surgery. Those who don't speak English don't know where to go or how to seek help, so they soldier on, disabled and in pain. In the San Francisco Bay area, such an individual would have an option. Through Operation Access, his hernia could be repaired for free, he would be able to communicate with caregivers through an interpreter, and he could return to work quickly, his health restored.

The San Francisco-based not-for-profit is a matchmaker of sorts among 60 community clinics, 225 medical volunteers and 13 hospitals in seven Bay Area counties. It screens patients referred from the clinics for both medical and financial criteria, identifies surgical teams and hospitals that can perform outpatient procedures, then schedules operations and pre- and post-surgical appointments, and, if needed, arranges for interpreters.

Founded nine years ago, Operation Access is the brainchild of two Bay Area surgeons, who saw public hospitals stretched to their limits and steadily rising numbers of uninsured unable to pay for basic surgical procedures. Since then, it has arranged for about 900 surgeries and saved the public health system an estimated $3 million.

From the beginning, hospitals have been essential in supporting the program. Kaiser Permanente, San Francisco Medical Center was the pilot site, and five other Kaiser Foundation hospitals now participate. Along the way, "they've been instrumental in helping us recruit other hospitals. They make it easier for colleagues to see how the whole thing works," says Operation Access executive director Betty Hong. San Francisco General Hospital and St. Rose Hospital quickly followed suit; Santa Rosa Memorial Hospital joined in 2000.

Sutter Health came on board in 2000 and more than 100 Operation Access surgeries have since taken place at its four participating hospitals. "We see it as a unique example of how collaboration between the public and private sectors can work to the benefit of an entire community," says Cyndi Kettmann, senior vice president of public affairs for the Sacramento-based system.

Each hospital and volunteer interfaces differently with the program. Some commit to a certain number of surgeries each month, others do so quarterly; some offer operating room time on Saturdays, others, during the week. Operation Access collaborates closely with all parties to the benefit of needy and appreciative patients. "They're so grateful. Some have waited for such a long time," Hong says.

THE PROBLEM: Uninsured patients can't afford surgery.

THE PLAYERS: Operation Access, six Kaiser Foundation Hospitals, four Sutter Health hospitals, San Francisco General Hospital, St. Rose Hospital, Santa Rosa Memorial Hospital.

American Hospital
Association

Fig. 5 Collaborative Community Provider Model – San Francisco (arranging surgery)

THE PLAN: Coordinate efforts of hospitals, physicians and clinics to arrange free surgical procedures and related care.

THE RESULTS: Approximately 900 surgeries performed, saving the public health system an estimated $3 million; an average patient satisfaction score of 4.6 on a 5-point scale.

Caption
Operation Access executive director Betty Hong says some hospitals commit to a certain number of surgeries per month, others offer operating room time on Saturdays. Each hospital interfaces differently with the program.

Published by Hospitals & Health Networks Magazine
2002 NOVA Award Winners - July 2002

American Hospital
Association

Fig. 5 (continued)

as we see with the FQHCs and faith based organizations. Other providers address the needs of the uninsured as they present . In addition, the recognition that many other Americans who may be underinsured or medically disenfranchised are also not receiving needed care. Essential health care could empower them to optimize their health status and minimize the need for expensive urgent and emergent care. The notion of this challenge comes to the forefront. Community based safety net organizations continue to grow and creatively design care models to respond to the unique needs and concerns of communities and populations in all 50 states. Many are discovering unique strategies for care delivery and quality improvement utilizing a variety of healthcare professionals and community members. An example of a collaborative community model is described in Fig. 5. As these models and their healthcare providers are improved to offer quality medical, dental, and health care for the uninsured population, they may provide our best opportunities for a quality and cost effective healthcare delivery system for all Americans.

References

330 Public Health Service Act (2006) Available at www.dhhs.gov. Retrieved 10 April 2008

American College of Emergency Physicians (ACEP) (2007) ACEP reminds Americans during cover the uninsured week: Emergency care for the uninsured affects everyone's access to lifesaving emergency care. Available at: www.acep.org/pressroom.aspx?id=37912. Retrieved 10 April 2009

American Hospital Association (2009) Available at www.aha.org. Retrieved 15 March 2009

Arizona 211 On-line (2008) Available at www.az211.gov. Retrieved 10 April 2008

Arizona State University (2007) Emergency Department Visits. Available at: http://chir.asu.edu/ publications. Retrieved 10 April 2009

Ascension Health (2009) Available at: www.ascensionhealth.org. Retrieved 1 April 2009

Catholic Community Services of Southern Arizona (2008) Annual Report. Tucson, Arizona

U.S. Census Bureau (2008) Census bureau revises 2004 and 2005 health insurance coverage estimates. Available at www.uscensus.gov. Retrieved on 26 March 2008

Center for Medicare and Medicaid (CMS) (2008) Available at www.cms.gov. Retrieved 25 April 2009

Cover the Uninsured (2009) A Project of the Robert Wood Johnson Foundation. Available at: www.covertheuninsured.org. Retrieved 24 April 2009

Department of Labor (2008) Bureau of Labor Statistics. Current Population Survey. Available at www.bls.gov/cps. Retrieved 1 May 2009

Dorn S, Bowen G, Holahan J, Williams A (2008) Medicaid, SCHIP, and the economic downturn: Policy challenges and policy responses. Kaiser Commission on Medicaid and the Uninsured, Washington, Available at: www.kff..org/medicaid. Retrieved 1 April 2009

Ehealthinsurance Services (2008) Available at: www.ehealthinsurance.com Retrieved 12 May 2008

EMTALA.COM (2008) Available at www.emtala.com. Retrieved 26 March 2008

Florida Hospital Association (2003) Care of non-citizens in the emergency room. Florida Hospital Association Report, pp 1–8

Health Resources and Service Administration (HRSA) (2007) The Health Center Program. Available at www.bphc.hrsa.gov. Retrieved on 26 March 2009

Health Resources and Service Administration (HRSA) (2009) Available at www.bhpr.hrsa.gov/ ahec. Retrieved on 26 March 2009

Hurley R, Felland L, Lauer J (2007) Community health centers tackle rising Demands and expectations. Center for studying health system change, 116, Washington, DC

Institute of Medicine (2006) Quality through collaboration: The future of rural health care. National Academies Press, Washington, DC

Kaiser Commission on Medicaid and the Uninsured (2004) Retrieved on 24 March 2008, www.kff.org

Kaiser Commission on Medicaid and the Uninsured (2009a) Community Health Centers. Available at www.kff.org. Retrieved on 16 March 2009

Kaiser Commission on Medicaid and the Uninsured (KCMU) (2009b) Community health centers in an era of health system reform and economic downturn: Prospects and challenges. Available at www.kff.org. Retrieved on 31 March 2009

Lefkowitz B, Todd J (1993) An overview: Health centers at the crossroads. J Ambul Care Manage 22(4):1–4

Medicare.gov (2009) The Official US Government Site for People with Medicare. Available at: www.medicare.gov/. Retrieved 25 April 2009

Metropolitan Chicago Health Care Council (MCHC) (2006) Caring for their communities: A comprehensive report on the community benefits, 1–7

Mt. Graham Regional Medical Center (2007) Personal Interview with Linda Lopez, RN, 17 Jan 2008

National Association of Community Health Centers (NACHC) (2009) A sketch of community health centers: Chartbook 2009. Available at www.nachc.com. Retrieved 1 April 2009

National Association of Community Health Centers and the Robert Graham Center (2007) Access granted: The primary Care payoff. National Association of Community Health Centers. Washington, DC, Available at www.nachc.com. Retrieved on 26 March 2008

National Association of Rural Health Clinics (NARHC) Available at: http://www.narhc.org/. Retrieved 24 April 2009

Patel E (2009) Obama Should Be Bolder, The Washington Post On-Line. Available at: http://newsweek.washingtonpost.com/onfaith/eboo_patel/2008/07/obama_and_faith_the_speech_he.html. Retrieved 25 April 2009

Phillips B (2003) Why we need medical homes. Available at: http://www.aafp.org/afp/2003. Retrieved 30 March 2009

Rural Assistance Center (2009) Rural health. Available at: www.raconline.org. Retrieved 25 April 2009

Siegrist RB, Kane N (2003) Understanding the inpatient cost of caring for the uninsured. HealthShare Technology Available at: http://www.bcbs.com/issues/uninsured/research/Understanding-the-Inpatient-Cost-of-Caring-for-the-Uninsured.pdf. Accessed 28 Sept 2009

South Carolina Rural Research Center (2004) Available at: http://rhr.sph.cs.edu. Retrieved 1 April 2009

State Health Access Data Assistance Center (2008) At the brink: Trends in America's Uninsured 1994–2007. Minneapolis: University of Minnesota. Available at www.covertheuninsured.org. Retrieved on 30 March 2009

Taylor J (2004) The fundamentals of community health centers. George Washington University, Washington, DC, pp 2–28

Trailblazer Health Enterprises (2009) Available at: www.trailblazerhealth.com/Medicare.aspx. Retrieved 17 April 2009

U.S. Department of Health and Human Services (2005) Available at: www.hrsa.gov Retrieved 1 April 2009

U.S. Department of Health and Human Services (2006) Available at: www.hrsa.gov. Retrieved 1 April 2009

Chronic Disease and the Uninsured

Nancy J. Johnson

A community "Cover the Uninsured" health fair included many screening activities with individuals lined up early in the morning. An elderly gentleman sat down in front of the nurse with the concern of decreased vision of his right eye. Upon assessment, his blood pressure was 180/96, his left foot had two necrotic appearing toes, and his hemoglobin A1C was 10.2 upon fingerstick. He said he had no money for a doctor visit but was concerned when he started to have trouble with his vision and his toes. His last visit to a doctor had been about a year ago, when he was told he had diabetes and would need medication. The gentleman was assisted with a new eligibility application for sliding fee care at a nearby community health center and enrolled in its chronic disease program for patients with diabetes.

Chronic Disease Today

Chronic diseases are the leading cause of death in the United States representing 70% of all deaths. Seven of every 10 Americans or 1.7 million die of a chronic disease each year. Chronic diseases including heart disease, stroke, cancer, diabetes, and arthritis cause daily impairment to health, activity, and work for many Americans, in addition to pain, suffering, and financial hardship (CDC 2008). Some of the current information from the Center for Communicable Diseases (2008) supports the following points:

- Heart disease is the leading cause of premature, permanent disability in the US workforce and 66% of heart attack victims never fully recover.
- Sixty percent of leg and foot amputations unrelated to injury are among people with diabetes. Diabetes is the leading cause of new cases of blindness and kidney failure in adults.

N.J. Johnson
El Rio Community Health Center, Tucson, AZ, USA
e-mail: njohnson@ccs-soaz.org

N.J. Johnson and L.P. Johnson (eds.), *The Care of the Uninsured in America*,
DOI 10.1007/978-0-387-78309-3_6, © Springer Science+Business Media, LLC 2010

- Arthritis is the nation's most common cause of disability, resulting in activity limitations for nearly 19 million Americans.

Approximately 75% of the $1.4 trillion spent on annual medical care costs is for chronic diseases. We know that the rising costs of health care cannot be addressed without investigating the expenses incurred for chronic diseases. Again, the CDC (2008) reports as follows:

- In 2005, 133 million people lived with at least one chronic condition.
- Chronic diseases account for one-third of the years of potential life lost before 65.
- Direct and indirect care of diabetes is $174 billion a year.
- Arthritis results annually in medical care costs of nearly $81 billion and estimated total costs (medical care and lost productivity) of $128 billion.
- Estimated direct and indirect costs associated with smoking exceed $193 billion annually.
- In 2008, the estimated cost of heart disease and stroke in the US is projected to be $448 billion.
- Estimated total cost of obesity was nearly $117 billion in 2000.
- Cancer costs the nation an estimated $89 billion annually in direct medical costs.
- Nearly $98.6 billion is spent on dental services each year (CDC 2008).

More than one in five individuals with chronic disease or approximately 12.3 million lived in families that had challenges paying their medical bills (Center for Health System Change 2004). For the 6.6 million uninsured Americans identified in this HSC study, financial issues were very serious with nearly half of them reporting that they delayed or did not seek needed medical care because of the cost. More specifically, 42% went without needed care, 65% postponed needed care, and 71% did not fill a prescription in the past year because of the cost (Tu 2004). Other uninsured patients acknowledged that they cut pills in half to make them last longer and also determined which physician or service they needed the most – in essence, they self triaged on the basis of their perceived need for care (Johnson 2008a, b).

The cost of health care continues to rise and clearly creates problems for the entire population of the uninsured, but the uninsured with chronic illnesses are especially at risk because of the ongoing chronic disease expenses that are necessary on a monthly basis. The inability to fund these monthly out-of-pocket expenses results in expensive trips to the emergency room and hospital, which might be avoided with the ability to maintain monthly prescriptions and medical recommendations. The recognition that the chronically ill uninsured have difficulty paying their medical bills is apparent, but it is also apparent that the insured who are covered by private insurance are also struggling to pay the out-of-pocket costs in managing at least one if not more chronic illnesses (Tu 2004). Between 2001 and 2003, the low income chronically ill people with insurance who spent more than 5% of their income on out-of-pocket health care costs grew from 28 to 42%, which is nearly a 50% increase (Tu 2004). However, when we look at the uninsured with chronic conditions, 45%

reported spending more than 5% of their income consistently on medical care (Tu 2004). These findings are not a surprise, but for the uninsured chronically ill who are mostly low income, this is an expense that they cannot manage. A downward spiral occurs with chronic illness as those who are uninsured and become chronically ill continue to become more sick in terms of complications and life threatening scenarios because they are uninsured. Our community safety net providers see this on a regular basis with uninsured patients who are diagnosed with diabetes but have no funds for medication or treatment. These patients later appear with the need for lower limb amputations, or have lost their vision, or have symptoms of vascular disease. Other uninsured patients present with persistent warning signs of various cancers that they have not addressed either because of lack of funds or lack of knowledge regarding the significance of the symptoms. Consequently, these patients face the need for expensive treatment or even loss of life often, when an earlier diagnosis may have saved their lives. Some patients report finding death and disability preferable to leaving their family in a situation with large medical debts. The uninsured frequently put off or go without needed care.

Uninsured individuals with chronic conditions are left to attempt to pay high and rising costs on their own or rely on various community safety nets to simply avoid complications and hopefully, improve their health status. The increased governmental funding for community health centers has helped to some extent, but access to care is variable across the United States. However, even in communities where there are strong community health centers and other safety net providers, there is still difficulty with access to needed prescription medications and specialty services which are both critical and essential for those attempting to manage chronic conditions. The other point is that many of our uninsured Americans have undiagnosed chronic illnesses which are not treated and will eventually rob them of not only years of life but also quality of life as their condition remains untreated.

Our country has undergone many changes in lifestyle in the past few decades that are contributing to the increase in the number of Americans managing chronic illnesses. For example, some of these changes include less exercise in schools and homes, less access to fresh fruits and vegetables, sedentary employment, more fast food and "supersize" food consumption, urbanization, less walkable communities, and stress (CDC 2008). These various lifestyle and societal changes along with the increasing costs of medical care and prescription medications have helped to create an uninsured population with chronic illnesses that cannot begin to afford the optimal management of their diseases on their own.

Two Strategies – Prevention of Chronic Diseases and Self Management Programs

On the basis of the knowledge of the increasing number of uninsured Americans with chronic disease and the expensive nature of the management of chronic illness, there are two critical actions for adoption and study in working with communities.

The first is the cost-effectiveness and quality perspective of prevention of chronic disease. Not only does prevention improve the quality of life for individuals, but it also saves money for the individual and the health care system. For example, the CDC (2008) reports that for every dollar spent on water fluoridation, $38 is saved in dental restorative treatments. Implementing proven clinical smoking cessation interventions would cost an estimated $2,587 for each year of life saved, which is the most cost-effective of all clinical preventative services. The primary prevention interventions of healthy nutrition, regular exercise, and safe environments are known to save millions of dollars to the healthcare system in chronic disease prevention and direct medical care.

The second critical strategy for the uninsured population and the management of chronic disease is the development of self management programs targeted specifically for the uninsured population. Although disease management programs have been implemented by private insurance companies and large self-insured companies for their targeted populations, disease management and chronic disease management programs for the uninsured require some additional characteristics in terms of design, involvement of healthcare professionals, and strategies for health improvement.

Many community-based organizations and community health centers are collaborating to create effective programs and strategies that are accessible, culturally, linguistically, and literacy appropriate for various targeted populations, as well as being affordable and effective in improving health for the uninsured and underserved populations.

Conceptual Basis for Chronic Disease Management Programs

Common concepts in developing chronic disease management programs include the assessment and utilization of the chronic disease model, the development of a "medical" or "health" home, the definition of "access to care," self management skill development, and the facets of effective preventive screening tools. The review and integration of these components are illustrated in many developing, evolving, and effective chronic disease management programs for the uninsured in communities across the nation.

The Chronic Disease Model first appeared in an article by Wagner (1998) in the journal of *Effective Clinical Practice*. The model was further developed by the McColl Institute with the support of the Robert Wood Johnson Foundation and a panel of national experts (www.improvingchronicdiseaase.org, 2008). This model was designed by collecting and organizing all the literature about what might work in better management of chronic illness. Some of the challenges noted in managing chronic disease included the lack of care coordination, inconsistency in following evidenced based guidelines, lack of patient follow-up, and lack of patient skills to better manage their chronic disease. The Chronic Disease Model identifies the basic elements of a health care system that encourages high-quality chronic disease

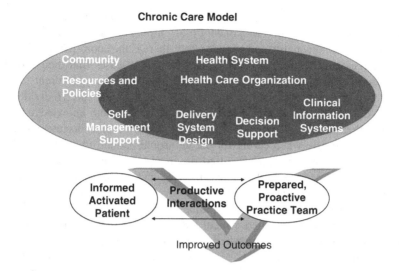

Fig. 1 Chronic Care Model

care through addressing these challenges. The components include the community, the health care system, self-management support, delivery system design, decision support, and clinical information systems (*see* Fig. 1).

Evidence-based change concepts help health care professionals work with their patients to take an active part in their care. The proposed bottom line is healthier patients, more satisfied providers, and cost savings. In 2003, the Improving Chronic Illness Care organization (ICIC) incorporated some new themes including patient safety, cultural competency, care coordination, community policies, and case management into the chronic disease model. As providers of care for the uninsured review the chronic care model, the issues of implementation and effectiveness in uninsured and underserved populations become a question for research and pilot models of care.

The first component of the Chronic Care Model is the community with its resources and policies. Historically, patients have received care within the health-care system without too much thought from the providers as to the patient's presence and status in the community. The care of the uninsured spotlights the importance of this component of the model in that many community resources are needed to ensure optimal management of chronic disease. For example, providers of care for the uninsured leverage and explore all potential partnerships with other organizations to address needed gaps in care and services as well as encourage patients to participate in community screenings, education, and support groups. Lastly, the role of advocacy in the community is not new to healthcare professionals working with the uninsured. For example, a community health center caring for the uninsured would have various resources in place for discounted supplies, food boxes, free health education presentations, advocacy, and low cost specialty care in collaboration with many in the community.

   The second component of the model is that of the Healthcare System and how care is organized. While this component of the chronic disease management model is heavily focused on quality and patient safety, there is the coordination of care and case management feature. All patients with chronic diseases find their use of the healthcare system to be laborious and complicated with many different locations and types of service providers. Imagine the process for an uninsured individual who may have language challenges, transportation issues, and knowledge deficits regarding their disease. This is a component of the chronic disease model that changes dramatically when caring for the uninsured patient. Physicians and other providers of care are challenged to find the most cost effective, yet high quality interventions and exponentially expand the role of the case manager. Most uninsured patients will need case management from a variety of disciplines in order to manage their chronic diseases at the optimal level.

   Another frequently identified critical feature in this second component of the model when caring for the uninsured is the creation of a "medical home" or a "health home." Part of the challenge in managing chronic conditions with the uninsured population is the infrequent or irregular use of the health care system depending on financial resources, acuity of the problem, and the current pending concerns for the individual and the family. Although family physicians have always known the value of the medical home, many today are using this term to describe the process of coordinating regular health care that is comprehensive and promotes improved health status with less expense for the individual and the health care system. The term "medical home" was first coined in 1967 by the American Academy of Pediatrics (AAP) as a way to improve care for children with special needs. In 2004, the American Academy of Family Physicians expanded this concept when they identified that every American should have a personal medical home (Backer 2007). The characteristics of a medical home include a personal provider, whole-person orientation, coordinated care, quality and safety, enhanced access, and adequate payment (www.aafp.org, 2007). As we look at the uninsured population, the characteristics of a medical home are not always in place or available in our current healthcare system depending on geography (rural vs. urban), workforce availability, financial resources, and community safety net. Community Health Centers most closely fit the model of "medical home" and have shown a 41% decrease in medical costs for patients having a community health center as their "medical home" (www.nachc.org, 2008). Interestingly enough, many "medical home" initiatives are being discussed and proposed through Medicare, private payers, and large self-insured employers. However, the population which may benefit the most health-wise as well as financially from the medical home concept is the uninsured, by identifying a location/provider that could monitor, coordinate, and address needed chronic condition and preventive health care needs on a regular basis. Beal et al. (2007) sponsored a health care quality survey that demonstrated that when uninsured and minority individuals had access to a "medical home," the rates of preventive screenings improved substantially and many disparities in access and quality were eliminated. Imagine, as an uninsured American, having a "health home" where you received your preventive care as well as chronic disease management with an integrated approach including medicine, nursing, dental, behavioral health, and pharmaceutical needs. The savings in avoiding duplication of services, unneeded emergency room visits, and hospitalizations along with a payment plan supportive of you or your family's income would characterize this "health" or "medical" home. A later chapter further develops and discusses the "medical" or "health" home.

Chronic disease management relies on available "access to care" for the uninsured population. With many community health centers and safety net providers having more patients than they can manage, access to needed care can be a challenge. Attention to regular care is a need in optimizing health for the uninsured with chronic illnesses. Access to health care has both a risk perspective as well as a quality perspective. The lack of access to care for the uninsured can result in a lack of continuity of care, late initiation of care, or a delay in diagnosis. The quality perspective is that access to care provides regular preventive care along with improved chronic disease management. Access to health care is basic to improve the care of the uninsured, and currently, has many regional variations as we look at the economy along with the workforce shortage in the health professions.

The third component of the chronic disease model is the development of Self-Management Support for patients and begins with the four aspects of care that are controlled at the practice level. This effort strives to educate and empower those with chronic conditions to improve their knowledge and become motivated to manage their disease as effectively as possible to avoid exacerbations and illness. Stanford University serves as the home for the Chronic Disease Self-Management Program (www.patienteducation.stanford.edu, 2008) which is a 6-week workshop provided in community settings such as senior centers, churches, libraries, and hospitals. The workshops are attended by people with different chronic diseases and facilitated by healthcare professionals and non-healthcare professionals who may or may not have chronic diseases themselves. The self-management content and skills developed include the ability to deal with frustration, fatigue, pain, and isolation, appropriate exercise to improve energy and quality of life, appropriate use of medications, communicating effectively with family, friends, and healthcare professionals, nutrition, and evaluation of new treatments. The program participants receive a book, "Living a Healthy Life with Chronic Conditions" and an audio relaxation tape called "Time for Healing." Although the content developed by Stanford supports the chronic disease model, the methods in which the group is taught and conducted are most noteworthy. Group members all participate and support one another in managing their chronic illnesses, thereby improving their self-management and self-efficacy skills. The results of the initial study of the Program showed that the participants when compared to the non-participants demonstrated improvement in exercise, cognitive symptoms management, communication with physicians and other healthcare professionals, self-reported health status, fatigue, disability, and less number of outpatient visits and hospitalizations. The cost to savings ratio was approximately 1:10 with these results persisting for up to 3 years (Lorig et al. (1999). The use of this model of education and self-development with some adaptation for the uninsured population is developing in community settings across the country. Historically, an enabling model of working with the uninsured is evolving to models of self-management which are moving toward empowerment, no matter whether insured or uninsured. The self-management support points to the patients as being central in managing their health, helps to develop support and resources, and enhances problem solving skills for individuals living with chronic illnesses.

The chronic disease model advocates for Designing Care Systems which are effective and efficient for clinical care and self management. For the uninsured population, this mandates case management, engaging others to be part of the health care team, and overcoming geographic barriers by making access to care reachable. For example, many clinics and communities caring for the uninsured have added community health workers to the clinical team to assure that outreach and follow up are in place with a communication loop of important data back to the healthcare team. Other health centers have added clinical pharmacists to the care system to assure access to needed medications, as well as an understanding of the potential side effects and interactions. The diversity of the uninsured population mandates that the design of the care system is culturally, linguistically, and literacy appropriate for the population with instructions, methods of communication, and care delivery.

Decision support through evidence based guidelines for clinical practice is a crucial component of the chronic disease model to ensure that providers have the latest and most effective interventions to optimize the health of patients with chronic diseases. In caring for the uninsured, these guidelines are sometimes challenging to operationalize with the mobility of the uninsured population and the lack of continuous care at times.

Clinical information systems are the last component of the disease management model and are essential to manage chronic diseases. Particularly, in caring for the uninsured, who may access care at various locations in the community, a clinical information system can improve continuity and standardization of care, and avoid duplication of testing and diagnostics. Today, most clinic and practice locations are on the road to electronic health records and the HIPAA compliant sharing of patient information. This path may help to optimize chronic disease management.

The outcome of the chronic care model hopefully leads to an informed, activated patient able to interact productively and proactively with a prepared team of healthcare professionals. This model is our best hope for learning to provide better chronic disease management with patients and is indeed challenging to implement with insured patients. Working with uninsured populations necessitates the tailoring of the model to address special needs, access to resources, and other conflicting priorities of patients.

Essential Tools in Managing Uninsured Patients with Chronic Diseases

A consideration in the management of chronic conditions with the uninsured population is the selection of screening tests which are most effective in terms of disease prevention and healthcare expenditures. An effective screening test available (Brill

2007) should be one that reflects a disease that is a substantial health care burden, that has a recognizable non-symptomatic, non-metastatic phase, and results in a much better outcome when diagnosed early in the disease process; in other words a screening test that is directly related to improved mortality statistics.

One such example is colorectal screening with a colonoscopy, wherein even insured Americans do not adhere to the recommendations for colorectal screening. However, a screening colonoscopy is effective with much improved mortality outcomes and reasonable cost, and provides relief to the healthcare burden of treating advanced colon cancer. Colorectal screening qualifies as a good initiative in working with uninsured populations. Mountain Park Community Health Center (2008) in Phoenix, Arizona found that the use of a patient navigator added to the health care team doubled the number of patients returning stool card kits for colorectal screening. The modification to the care delivery system, based upon a large uninsured, mostly Hispanic target population, improved their ability to prevent chronic disease in this group (Mountain Park Health Center 2008).

Another effective screening tool for identifying the uninsured with or at risk for chronic diseases in the community or at a first encounter can be easily completed with seven questions (*see* Fig. 2). These are completed verbally and allow a quick assessment of who may be most needy for assistance with chronic disease management. Figure 3 presents a Carle Clinic (Shelton et al. 2000) similar risk assessment screening tool.

Assessing and teaching self-management skills with the uninsured to support chronic disease management can be challenging with other barriers such as transportation, financial resources, and conflicting priorities for patients and their families. Developing a variety of tools and intervention can best help optimize patients' success and efficacy in managing chronic diseases. There are three components for development of self-management protocols for use with uninsured patients, which

At Risk Assessment

- Do you have a doctor?

- Have you seen the doctor in the last year?

- Do you have a chronic or long term illness?

- Do you take more than 3 medications daily?

- Are you over 60? Have you fallen in the past three months?

- Have you been in the hospital or emergency room in the last 3-6 months?

- What do you believe your health to be?(poor,fair,good,excellent)

Fig. 2 Brief Risk Assessment Tool

The Community Assessment Risk Screen (CARS)

1. Do you have any of the following health conditions?

                                                                                    Yes   No

    a. Heart disease?   ____   ____

    b. Diabetes?   ____   ____

    c. Heart attack or myocardial infarction?   ____   ____

    d. Stroke?   ____   ____

    e. Chronic obstructive pulmonary disease?   ____   ____

    f. Cancer?   ____   ____

    (Score: If two or more conditions are "YES" score = 2)   SCORE ___

2. How many prescriptions medications do you take?   ___

    (Score: If "5 or more" medications score = 3)   SCORE ___

3. Have you been hospitalized or had to go to an emergency room or

    urgent care center in the past six months?

                                                                                    Yes ___   No ___

    (Score: If the answer is "YES" score = 4)   SCORE ___

                                                                                    TOTAL ___

Carle Clinic, Urbana, Illinois

Fig. 3 The community assessment risk screen (CARS)

include training providers and other key staff on how to help patients with self-management goals, use group visits to support self-management, and use self-management tools that are evidence based.

Initially, training providers and other key staff to support self-management requires team building for role identification, standardization of educational content and tools, and assurance of consistent follow-up and documentation. Group care visits are a common strategy with chronic disease management. Group visits are comprised of the individual patient visit as well as group education, support, and interaction.

Group Chronic Care Visit Tips

- Start small —train all care team members on self - management strategies.

- Keep group visits informal and as interactive as possible.

- Identify quality as well as culturally, linguistically and literacy appropriate patient education tools.

- Test assessment and educational tools with a small group of patients to pilot usefulness.

- Best tools are those that assist patients with the disease as they live with it, rather than educational curriculum.

- Patient priorities start the group visit conversation.

- Avoid lecturing at group visits --- place open questions with participants and facilitate discussion.

- Reinforce positive behavior changes and decisions.

Fig. 4 Group chronic care visit tips

Two different types of group visits are used in working with chronic disease patients. The first type is a group visit model that generally last about 2 to 3 hours and includes up to about 15 patients with a common chronic disease at a time. A variety of practitioners are involved and clinical care, as well as education, is provided along with creating behavior change action plans (*see* Fig. 4). The second sort of group visit is the drop-in group medical appointment which lasts about 90 min and engages any chronic disease patient who has an immediate need for care, support, or help with behavior changes (Jaber et al. 2006).

Self management assessment tools are plentiful in the literature and need to be tailored to address the cultural and literacy needs of the uninsured population (*see* Fig. 5).

These various characteristics and attributes of the chronic disease model can be interwoven into innovative models of care delivery for our uninsured patients with chronic conditions, which may not only improve quality of life and health status but also assist in minimizing expenses and use of the tertiary healthcare system.

Evolving Models of Chronic Care Management with the Uninsured

St Elizabeth's Health Center – Diabetes Group Day, Tucson, Arizona

As noted earlier, one of the areas in which we stand the most to gain is improvement of quality of life, decreasing complications, and savings in healthcare expenditures with the diabetic uninsured population. The development of chronic care models around uninsured patients at risk or those having diabetes is one of the first targets for many community safety net providers as well as private practice medical groups. Many community health centers and community hospitals have targeted their efforts around this population in the past decade. In addition, the incidence of diabetes type II is nearly at epidemic proportions in many populations and also geographically situated across our nation. In 2000, St. Elizabeth's Health Center in Tucson, Arizona who cares exclusively for the uninsured with a rather unique model of care pairing a small paid staff with community volunteer physicians, dentists, and other healthcare professionals elected to begin to focus on the diabetic population. The chronic disease model was reviewed with initial attention focusing on the delivery system design. Within the health center, all new patients registering for care also completed a pre-diabetes risk assessment (Figs. 5 and 6) and all existing diabetic patients were reviewed for compliance with self management guidelines along with improvement in clinical outcomes.

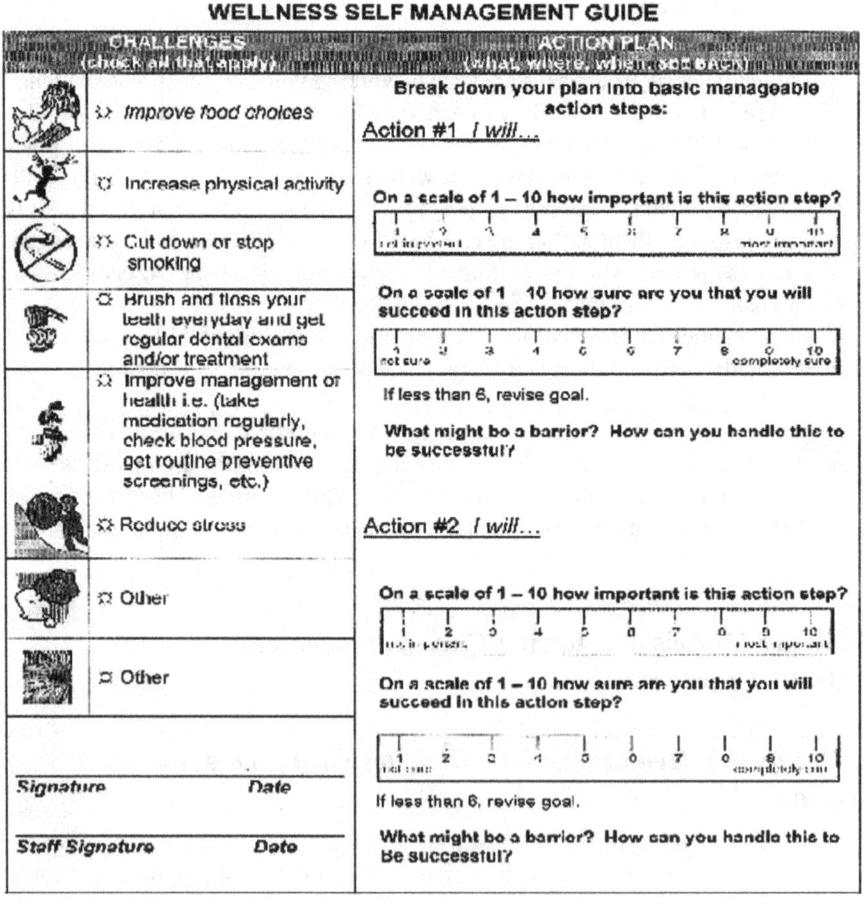

WELLNESS SELF MANAGEMENT GUIDE

CHALLENGES (check all that apply)	ACTION PLAN (what, where, when ...)
☐ Improve food choices ☐ Increase physical activity ☐ Cut down or stop smoking ☐ Brush and floss your teeth everyday and get regular dental exams and/or treatment ☐ Improve management of health i.e. (take medication regularly, check blood pressure, get routine preventive screenings, etc.) ☐ Reduce stress ☐ Other ☐ Other Signature Date Staff Signature Date	Break down your plan into basic manageable action steps: Action #1 *I will...* On a scale of 1 – 10 how important is this action step? 1 2 3 4 5 6 7 8 9 10 (not important … most important) On a scale of 1 – 10 how sure are you that you will succeed in this action step? 1 2 3 4 5 6 7 8 9 10 (not sure … completely sure) If less than 6, revise goal. What might be a barrier? How can you handle this to be successful? Action #2 *I will...* On a scale of 1 – 10 how important is this action step? 1 2 3 4 5 6 7 8 9 10 (not important … most important) On a scale of 1 – 10 how sure are you that you will succeed in this action step? 1 2 3 4 5 6 7 8 9 10 (not sure … completely sure) If less than 6, revise goal. What might be a barrier? How can you handle this to be successful?

Fig. 5 Wellness self management guide

a

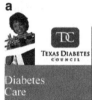

TEXAS DIABETES
COUNCIL

Diabetes
Care

Diabetes Risk Assessment Tool

Are you at risk for diabetes? Take a test to find out.

Millions of people have diabetes and don't even know it. If you have it and you don't know it, you could become very sick. Diabetes can damage the heart, arteries, eyes, nerves, and kidneys and lead to serious health problems. But if you know you have it, you can get the treatment you need to stay healthy.

Take this test to determine your risk for diabetes, and see your doctor to find out for sure.

Risk for diabetes	Yes	No
I am African American, Hispanic, Native American, or Asian American.		
I have a sister, brother, parent, grandparent, aunt, or uncle with diabetes.		
I have high or low blood sugar.		
I am overweight (20% or more over ideal weight).		
I usually have no daily exercise.		
I am 45 or older.		
I previously had diabetes during pregnancy or had a baby weighing more than 9 pounds at birth.		
I have high blood pressure (greater than 140/90) .		
I have high cholesterol.		

b

I have the following symptoms of diabetes:		
Blurred vision		
Fatigue, lack of energy		
Extreme thirst, hunger		
Frequent trips to the bathroom (urination)		
Unexplained weight gain or loss		
Slow-healing sore or cut		
Numbness, pain, or tingling in hands or feet		
Frequent infections		
Depression		

The more boxes you checked "Yes," the more likely you are to have diabetes.

Only your doctor will know for sure.

This test can only tell you if you **might** have diabetes. The only way to know for sure is to see your doctor. If you do not have a doctor, a public health clinic can also help you. Early detection and proper treatment of diabetes can lead to a longer and healthier life!

Fig. 6 Diabetes risk assessment tool

The initial findings illustrated that continuity of care was a problem and many patients had not completed an annual eye examination, foot exam and were not in compliance with needed laboratory monitoring. The existing health care team designed a monthly diabetes group care day for the patients to attend. For a small co-payment based on a sliding fee schedule, patients could arrive in the morning, have their laboratory work drawn, share a mid-morning healthy snack, have short appointments with the registered dietitian, podiatrist, ophthalmology, clinical diabetic educator, community health worker, and counselor, and receive a summary treatment plan from the physician. Patients were encouraged to come to the group day visit at a minimum of once a year, but were welcome to attend as frequently as they felt they needed to in order to manage their diabetes. Also, monthly, the group self-management topic would vary. Some months it might present the dietitian discussing healthy adaptations for their usual recipes and other months, it might feature the counselor discussing depression and coping strategies, or the physician reviewing self management strategies. This group model was specifically designed to build strong relationships between the providers and the patients. The initial project was grant supported, but it has continued as the "best practice" standard of care as both provider and patient satisfaction results are high. The initial data review from this sample in 2003 illustrated that from a sample size of 272 diabetes, over 50% had improved their HgbA(1)c readings a minimum of one point (Fig. 7).

Medications and access to affordable medications, glucometers, and test strips which are essential to optimal management are addressed in a variety of ways. A volunteer registered nurse assists patients with Prescription Assistance Programs by completing the online applications. Other medication access grants are written and funded through the health center as additional resources for the diabetic patients.

Functional and Clinical Outcomes

• Diabetes Group Day Visits

	Baseline 1/03	Actual 12/03	Target
HbA1c < 7.0	18%	38%	70%
LDL < 100	40%	74%	70%
B/P < 130/80	55%	55%	75%
Flu Vaccine	46%	57%	90%
Self Man Goals	78%	98%	90%

*Analysis of data by HSAG for Continuing Care Clinic Project Demonstration

Fig. 7 Functional and clinical outcomes

In addition, St Elizabeth's Health Center partners with the local community hospital in a large purchasing group to access the test strips at the lowest cost for uninsured patients. Other facets of the program that developed to address the health promotion and preventive aspects of chronic disease management were the development of a walking group for diabetes with patients as group leaders and the creation of a "novella" style educational video to teach the management of blood sugar and exercise. Overall, the model has the lowest unit cost for care in the state of Arizona for the care of uninsured diabetic patients. Two components of this program that support cost effectiveness are the use of the community health workers (promotoras) who serve to provide patient follow up, group day and/or appointment reminders and educational reinforcement, and the use of the specialty physician volunteers (podiatry, ophthalmology, dentists, endocrinologists) from the community. The Community Health Workers are instrumental in building self management skills with the diabetic patients to reinforce their knowledge, help them with lifestyle modification, and develop assertiveness in communicating with the healthcare system. Currently, in addressing the clinical information system component of the chronic disease model, the health center is converting to electronic medical records for not only the medical care, but also the interdisciplinary team's documentation of education program attendance, visits with the dietitian, walking group attendance, etc to begin to note differences in participation and differences in clinical outcomes and healthcare utilization.

Clinica Amistad and the Role of Outreach in Chronic Disease Management-Tucson, Arizona

The uninsured populations seek health and medical care wherever they can find it and afford it. Many communities feature free clinics that operate once a week in a church or office building when not being used for its primary purpose. For an acute illness or minor injury, these free clinics provide episodic care and may address the need appropriately. However, for the chronic illness patient who frequents the free clinic when not feeling well or having an acute illness or exacerbation, the lack of continuity of care is a problem. Community health workers attend the weekly clinical session of Clinica Amistad and provide health education in the waiting area. These informal sessions are "platicas" or small groups which reach those who may learn better in small group settings. Their messages are short, informative, and offered in both English and Spanish. Literacy appropriate materials are left with the invitation for patients with diabetes, hypertension, asthma, or other chronic illnesses to call to arrange a tour of the local community health center and establish care. The community health workers speak of the fact that many times, they will talk with an individual over a few months before they are comfortable to come and establish care. Some express concern over the system of health care and the medical bills they believe they will receive, while others simply lack the knowledge of community safety net services.

This outreach is very valuable in reaching the chronically ill uninsured as it achieves the following:

- Increases health education in the community.
- Decreases the number of unnecessary emergency room visits.
- Maximizes the availability of effective health services for the uninsured.
- Makes personal connections and helps to build relationships which then can influence patient health behaviors.
- Empowers individuals to recognize, treat, and manage their illnesses on a daily basis.
- Provides culturally competent advocacy to improve access to care.

The Community Health Workers also serve to create the milieu at the community health center which is welcoming and includes "infomercials," cooking demonstrations, children's indoor and outdoor playroom with adult supervision, and screening opportunities while patients are waiting for services.

Komen Foundation for the Cure – Leveraging Resources to Provide Chronic Care Treatment for the Uninsured, Tucson, Arizona

Over the past two decades, the Komen Foundation for the Cure in Southern Arizona has raised dollars exclusively for breast cancer treatment for the uninsured and underserved in five southern Arizona counties. During the past year, Komen collaborated to partner with local community health centers, the state health department and community oncologists, surgeons, and community hospitals to leverage funding anticipated to provide treatment for four uninsured women with breast cancer ($40,000 per woman) increased to providing care for thirteen women. This was done by creating a prepared, proactive practice team and a focus on the community and the health care system. The community provided discounts, volunteer providers, and easy access to treatment with advocacy and support. The health system worked to make connections across the five counties, provide needed decision support for the patients and their families, and help with follow up support groups for self-management. Most currently, a photo journaling self management group is in place for the uninsured women receiving breast cancer treatment as well as for the uninsured survivors. This example of operationalizing the chronic disease model illustrates modifying the health care delivery system, building advocacy in the community, and developing self-management and self-efficacy skills for the patients.

Project Access: Caring for the Uninsured, Dallas County, Texas

This program was initiated in 1998 to provide care for the uninsured working poor in Dallas County, Texas. Project Access worked to create and coordinate a group of community-based health clinics, volunteer primary and specialty care physicians, local hospitals, and pharmacies, and faith based organizations to care for the uninsured. Currently, they are monitoring the care coordination to see if there is a decrease in emergency room utilization along with increases in preventive screenings for chronic illnesses. The focus is on integrating primary, secondary, and tertiary preventive services with community-based health care to manage chronic conditions.

Creating Interdisciplinary Teams for the Care of the Uninsured with Chronic Obstructive Lung Disease (COPD), Tucson, Arizona

Another aspect of the chronic care model is the focus on clinical decision making (evidenced based practice guidelines) as well as developing resources for the uninsured patient. Uninsured patients with chronic lung disease generally have challenges in terms of resources for medication and oxygen, along with access to other members of the health care team to improve stress management, energy and nutrition. In 2007, the Arizona Department of Health Services funded community grants to develop a clinical delivery system to improve the health of patients with chronic obstructive lung disease which is the fourth leading cause of death in Arizona (www.azdhs.gov/phs/cdpc/pdf/chronic_disease_plan.pdf 2006). In addition, there was a need to document clinical care guidelines for the care of uninsured patients with COPD. Baseline tools were selected, including the PHQ to assess depression (Fig. 8). As seen in the COPD clinical flow sheet, (Fig. 9) protocol has been established and measurement initiated to determine if the use of the interdisciplinary chronic disease model can improve the health status of the uninsured with COPD. The integration of this protocol into the electronic medical record will also provide trending and clinical outcome data for this patient population.

Alive and Lively: Coastal Medical Access Project, Brunswick, Georgia

The CMAP Program in Georgia initiated a chronic disease management program for their clinic population of uninsured and underserved in 2002. The model of care is patient driven (Fig. 10) and focuses on clinical, fiscal, psychological, and social care. Registered nurses case manage the patients enrolled who receive clinical care, education, and support. The goals of the program are to have participants who are physically healthier and have improved quality of life. Participants will have reduced medical costs, as well as tracking and monitoring of their improvements with their providers online through the use of a personal electronic health record. This program utilizes clinical information systems for patients with diabetes, asthma, and cardiovascular disease and is staffed by a combination of employed and volunteer healthcare professionals.

PHQ (English)

Name _____

Physician _____ Date _____ Chart #

_____

1. Over the _last two weeks_, how often have you been bothered by any of the following problems?	Not At All (0)	Several Days (1)	More Than Half the Days (2)	Nearly Every Day (3)
a. Little interest or pleasure in doing things?	☐	☐	☐	☐
b. Feeling down, depressed, or hopeless?	☐	☐	☐	☐
c. Trouble falling or staying asleep, or sleeping too much?	☐	☐	☐	☐
d. Feeling tired or having little energy?	☐	☐	☐	☐
e. Poor appetite or overeating?	☐	☐	☐	☐
f. Feeling bad about yourself--or that you are a failure or have let yourself or your family down?	☐	☐	☐	☐
g. Trouble concentrating on things, such as reading the newspaper or watching television?	☐	☐	☐	☐
h. Moving or speaking so slowly that other people could have noticed? Or the opposite--being so fidgety or restless that you have been moving around a lot more than usual?	☐	☐	☐	☐
i. Thoughts that you would be better off dead or of hurting yourself in some way?**	☐	☐	☐	☐
2. If you are experiencing any of the problems on this form, how **difficult** have these problems made it for you to do your work, take care of things at home or get along with other people?				
☐ Not difficult at all ☐ Somewhat difficult ☐ Very difficult ☐ Extremely difficult				

> _**If you have thought that you would be better off dead or of hurting yourself in some_
> _way, please discuss this with your doctor, go to a hospital emergency room or call 911._

Fig. 8 PHQ (English)

Building Self-Management Skills in the Uninsured

As seen in the studies from Stanford University, self-management skills can lead to increased confidence and self-efficacy in patients with chronic disease. It may, indeed, be the most powerful of the components of the chronic disease model. But how do we build self management in the uninsured population to manage chronic

Chronic Obstructive Pulmonary Disease (COPD) Quality Indicators, Clinical

Patient _____ DOB_____

MR #_____ PCP _____

Date/Initials	Frequency	Baseline	3 months	6 months	9 months	12 months
Spirometry: FEV1/FVC % Predicted	Q 6 months					
Height Weight BMI If < 18%, nutritional counseling	Q 6 months					
GOLD Class See Back of Sheet	Q 6 months					
QOL Scale	Q 6 months					
Dyspnea Scale	Q 6 months					
*Smoker/ Pack yrs; Referral recommended	Once Q visit					
Pneumovax	Once					
Influenza	Q 12 months					
SABD **						
LABD **						
Anticholinergics						
Theophyllines						
Inhaled Steroids						
Systemic Steroids						
O2 assessment	prn					
Resp Therapy	Series					
Nutrition Therapy	Series					
Exercise Therapy	Series					
Behavioral -Depression -Anxiety	Q 3 months					
COPD Self Care	Q 6 months					
Group Session	Q 3 months					
Emergency Rm Visit	Q visit					
Hospitalization	Q visit					

*Smoking: assess and suggest cessation program each visit.

** Drugs per stepped GOLD Protocol; document if considered

Signature	Initials	Signature	Initials

Fig. 9 Chronic obstructive pulmonary disease (COPD) quality indicators, clinical

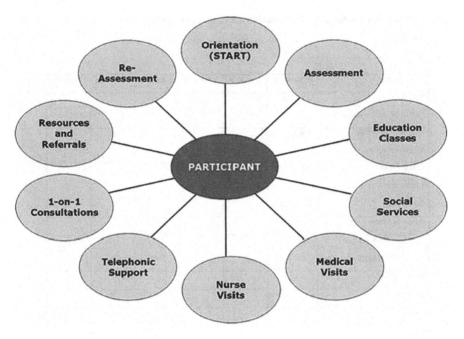

Fig. 10 CMAP

conditions? Although all members of the health care team can encourage self management, the relationships between patients and community health workers or patient navigators can strengthen and reinforce knowledge, behaviors, and attitudes. Community health workers or patient navigators can spend the time to assess cultural, linguistic, and literacy skills of the patient to improve the acquisition of needed knowledge to manage chronic disease.

Benefits of Chronic Disease Programs for the Uninsured and Next Steps

The use of the chronic disease model in managing the care of the uninsured is a very effective intervention to weave through out clinical care. Initial outreach in the community can help with identifying the chronically ill uninsured and work toward the establishment of a "medical" or "health" home as the point of coordination. The interdisciplinary team supports the co-management of chronic illness and assures coordination of care. In addition, we know that when uninsured individuals have a medical home they have improved medical compliance leading to improved outcomes. When patients gain control of their chronic illnesses, they become empowered to recognize, treat ,and manage their illness on a daily basis. In addition, the personal follow up allowed by some of these evolving models of care also leads to improved outcomes (www.improvingchroniccare.org, 2008).

Some recent articles supported by the CDC (Slonim et al. 2008), identify a call to integrate the various disease specific chronic care models being developed across the nation to care for the insured, the low income, and the uninsured groups. This is a very reasonable path to take to optimize resources, build consensus and validity for various evolving models of chronic care management, and improve clinical outcomes across populations. Some of the areas of chronic disease management that are all traveling the same paths include the preventive health behaviors such as sound nutrition, regular physical activity, and minimization of stress. Whether we are addressing asthma, diabetes, cancer, or heart disease, these primary prevention strategies make sense along with the use of a core set of self management skills as identified in the Stanford self-management workshops. However, the needs of differing populations are addressed, as in this case for the uninsured, and specific interventions and use of resources as described in pilot programs must be tailored to suit their needs.

Finally, our measurements for chronic disease improvement with the uninsured populations must include and focus on utilization of urgent and emergency room visits, specialists' visits and hospital days, clinical quality as measured by disease specific indicators, improved access to the "medical" or "health" home, patient satisfaction, and provider satisfaction. Improvement in the management of the uninsured with chronic diseases is a crucial strategy to improve quality of life and reduce health care expenditures.

References

Backer LA (2007) The medical home: An idea whose time has come … again. Fam Pract Manag. Available at: http://www.aafp.org/fpm/20070900/38them.html. Accessed 11 April 2009

Beal AC, Dory MM et al (2007) Closing the divide: How medical homes promote Equity in health care. Commonw Fund. Available at: www.commonwealthfund.org

Brill J (2007) What makes an effective screening test? Arizona Cancer Coalition, Phoenix, AZ

Center for Communicable Disease (2008) Chronic disease costs. Available at: www.cdc.org. Accessed 1 May 2008

Center for Studying Health System Change (2004) Rising health care costs, medical debt and chronic conditions. #88

Jaber R, Braksmajer A, Trilling J (2006) Group visits for chronic illness care: Models, benefits and challenges. Fam Pract Manag 13:37–40

Johnson LP (2008a) Personal Interview regarding uninsured patients. Tucson, Arizona

Johnson NJ (2008b) Personal interview regarding chronic disease management. Tucson, Arizona

Lorig KR, Sobel DS, Stewart AL, Brown BW, Ritter PL, Gonzalez VM (1999) Evidence suggesting that a chronic disease self-management program can improve health status while reducing utilization and costs: A randomized trial. Med Care 37(1):5–14

Mountain Park Community Health Center (2008) Colorectal screening programs: Patient navigators. Presentation, December 2008

Shelton P, Sager MA, Schraeder C et al (2000) The Community Assessment Risk Screen (CARS): Identifying Elderly Persons at Risk for Hospitalization or Emergency Department Visit. Amer Jour of Mang Care 6(8): 925–933

Slonim AB, Callaghan C, Daily L et al (2008) Recommendations for integration of chronic disease programs: Are your programs linked? Available at www.cdc.org. Accessed 11 April 2009

Tu HR (2004) Rising health costs, medical debt and chronic conditions. Center for studying health system change. Available at: www.hschange.org. Accessed 28 March 2008

Wagner EH (1998) Chronic disease management: What will it take to improve care for Chronic illness? Eff Clin Pract 1:2–4

www.aafp.org (2007) Accessed 1 April 2008

www.azdhs.gov/phs/cdpc/pdf/chronic_disease_plan.pdf (2006). Accessed 28 Sept 2009

www.improvingchroniccare.org (2008) The chronic care model. Accessed 1 April 2008

www.nachc.org (2008) Accessed 30 April 2008

www.patienteducation.stanford.edu (2008) Chronic Disease Workshops, Accessed 1 April 2008

Medical Homes *(preferably "Health Home")* and the Uninsured

Nancy J. Johnson

Michelle entered the evening Free Clinic in the church basement to see someone about her earache. For the past 3 days, the pain in her ear had gotten worse, especially after working all day. Without any health insurance, the emergency room was too expensive and getting an appointment at a doctor's office in the evening was impossible. The volunteer nurse practitioner checked her ears, listened to her chest, and gave her an antibiotic with enough pills for the needed ten day course. Michelle left her donation of $5 for the help. Fortunately, her ear pain resolved over the next week, but she continued to have a cough and felt like she was running a fever. She called a community health center but was unable to get an appointment that day as a new patient. At work, the next day, she felt exhausted and fainted while putting away supplies. Her boss took her to the emergency room, where she was examined, had a chest x-ray which diagnosed pneumonia, and was sent home with antibiotics and an order for at least a week in bed. Unfortunately, she was also sent home with a bill of over $800 and discharge instructions to follow up with her regular doctor. Michelle did not have a "regular doctor" – or a "medical home" for help with preventive health behaviors or acute health problems.

About Medical Homes

The concept of a "Medical Home" is not a new idea, despite the many recent articles and publications supporting its adoption and potential benefits in terms of quality improvement and cost savings. Initially, the American Academy of Pediatrics (AAP) first presented the concept of medical home in 1967 with the target population being children with special medical needs (Backer, 2007). Today, the National Center of Medical Home Initiatives for Children with Special Needs (2009) provides support to physicians, families, and other healthcare professionals who care for children and youth with special needs. Each state has its own webpage which identifies resources, partnerships, and work in progress to help assure that all children with special needs have a medical home. The scenarios and realities for children with special needs clearly identify why this group of children catalyzed the

N.J. Johnson
El Rio Community Health Center, Tucson, AZ, USA

N.J. Johnson and L.P. Johnson (eds.), *The Care of the Uninsured in America*,
DOI 10.1007/978-0-387-78309-3_7, © Springer Science+Business Media, LLC 2010

need for the original medical home concept. For example, children with special needs comprise 80% of the healthcare dollars spent on children (AAP 2009) and the realities for families are daunting. Approximately 13% of families with special need children identify spending more than eleven hours weekly, coordinating care and services for their children and nearly 25% report having to cut back on their work hours because of their child's condition. An additional 28% actually quit work due to their child's condition. Many of these families struggle with managing their finances and staying employed and insured (AAP 2009).

Healthy People 2010 (2009) references access to a medical home as a specific objective for all special needs children. In addition, the recognition that our health care system is fragmented, more families lack health insurance, and more children are living with chronic health conditions, supports AAP's continued expansion of their medical home concept. The goal is that all children, uninsured or insured, have a medical home. AAP (2009) defines a medical home as a system in which high quality, comprehensive, and cost effective health care services can be provided by a primary care physician with collaborative partnerships from other health care professionals and the family. This is the standard of care and addresses well child care, acute care, and chronic care for children from birth until adulthood. As the concept has been further discussed, presented, and published, the addition of the community concept has occurred along with a focus on optimizing the health of the child (AAP 2009). A recent review of past studies investigating the effectiveness of medical homes for children with special health care needs (Homer et al. 2008) provided support that the existence of a medical home related positively to better health status, timeliness of care, a focus on the family, and improved family functioning.

In March 2007, AAP collaborated with the American Academy of Family Physicians (AAFP), the American College of Physicians (ACP), and the American Osteopathic Association (AOA) to produce a consensus statement on medical home characteristics and positioning in the healthcare system. These professional groups encompass the primary care physicians within our healthcare system across the country. They produced the "Joint Principles on the Patient-Centered Medical Home" which addresses the medical home for children, youth, and adults. The joint position statement identifies a medical home as having primary care that is accessible, family-centered, continuous, comprehensive, coordinated, compassionate, and culturally effective (Guidelines for a Medical Home 2009). Figure 1 describes each of these defining characteristics for a medical home. These characteristics cluster around three different pillars including community-based systems, transitions, and value. Community-based systems support the medical home including the family and community networks of health and support services for healthy development and well being. Transitions speak of the ability of the medical home to change and shift as individuals grow, change, or age and have differing health needs. The last pillar of value recognizes the outcomes of the medical home resulting in high quality, cost effective care which is highly satisfying to the patient, family, and health care provider.

Medical Home Characteristics

ACCESSIBLE

- Care provided in the community
- All insurance, including Medicaid and uninsured, is accepted and changes are accommodated.
- Families/youth are able to speak directly to their medical home provider when needed.

FAMILY-CENTERED

- Mutual responsibility and trust exists between patient and family and the medical home
- Family is recognized as the principal caregiver and center of strength and support for the child
- Clear, unbiased, and complete information and options are shared on an ongoing basis with the family

CONTINUOUS

- Same primary care providers are available from infancy to young adulthood
- Assistance with transitions is provided
- Medical home provider participates to the fullest extent allowed in care and discharge planning when the child is hospitalized

COMPREHENSIVE

- Available 24hrs a day, 7 days a week
- Preventive, primary, secondary and tertiary care needs are addressed
- Medical home provider advocates for the child and family in obtaining needed comprehensive care

COORDINATED

- Plan of care developed with physician, child, family and shared with other providers
- Central record or database of all pertinent information is maintained at the medical home.

COMPASSIONATE

- Concern for well-being of the child and family is expressed and demonstrated in verbal and nonverbal interactions.
- Efforts are made to understand and empathize with the feelings and perspectives

CULTURALLY EFFECTIVE

- Culturally, linguistically and literacy appropriate interactions/interventions

The Medical Home. (2002). *Pediatrics.* 110: 184-186.

Fig. 1 Medical home characteristics

The "Joint Principles on the Patient-Centered Medical Home" (2007) identifies the following general guidelines for a medical home across the lifespan:

- Patients have a continuous relationship with a personal physician in a physician-directed practice. This personal physician provides continuous and comprehensive care and leads the team who collectively take responsibility for the care of the patient.
- Practice has a whole person orientation which means across the life span and includes health maintenance, and acute and chronic care management.
- Care is integrated and coordinated, which occurs across facilities such as hospitals, home health agencies, pharmacies, community agencies such as churches, health clubs, etc as well as across health care specialties.
- Quality and safety are hallmarks which mean evidence-based protocols, involving the patient and his/her family and measuring health outcomes.
- Enhanced access to care is available through systems and new communication options such as open scheduling, expanded hours, and electronic communication.

(http://www.aap.org, 2009)

Upon review of these general characteristics, the health care system, particularly primary care, has the framework in which to specify and develop protocols and best practices.

Part of the movement behind this consensus statement endorsement for medical homes in 2007 was the growing shortage of primary care physicians due to adverse practice conditions. Currently, physicians are pressured to see more patients in less time and are swallowed in administrative and clinical documentation. These challenges of and struggles with financial management conflict with the development of trusting, compassionate relationships with patients. In addition, the increasing prevalence of chronic diseases in the United States and poor health outcomes as compared to that in other industrialized countries have stirred the passion to redesign our American healthcare systems. Currently, more than half of Americans report one or more chronic diseases and 75% of healthcare spending is for chronic disease. Only 56% of those with chronic diseases receive clinically indicated care and only about 27% of adults reported having full access to a well-organized source of health care (Commonwealth Fund 2006). Bodenheimer (2008) reported that these patients with multiple chronic conditions may visit a physician up to 16 times per year, in addition to having duplicative screenings and diagnostic tests due to lack of coordination of care. These less than optimal health outcomes documented in the American healthcare system are at least somewhat related to the poor coordination of care among providers in a community. The health care system has an opportunity to reorganize and prepare for the shift from acute care to chronic care management as our population ages. The Institute of Medicine's (IOM) report, "Crossing the quality chasm: A new health system for the twenty-first century", (Berwick, 2002) recognized the fragmentation of the health care system and the challenges presented for patients in order to get the needed care to maintain or improve their health. The IOM report ascertained that future health care needed to focus on safety, effectiveness, patient-centeredness, timeliness, efficiency, and equity. The need for coordination of care was a primary concern in the IOM report.

Futhermore, the identification that the existing health care system would not work to meet these areas for improvement fueled the medical home movement.

The Future of Family Medicine Project (2004) presented the idea that every American regardless of age, sex, socioeconomic status, or health status receives care through a medical home. This comprehensive report defined characteristics of the medical home, recommendations for family medicine residency training and the various services inherent in a medical home model (http://www.annfammed.org, 2009). The concept of medical home continued to expand as a comprehensive model of care for all Americans of all ages. The timeliness of the medical home concept is apparent as a valuable tool today as we look to appropriately utilize limited resources, continually improve the quality of care, be as cost effective and efficient as possible, and cover the uninsured. Other names for the "medical home" concept which show up in the literature include "patient-centered medical home" and "health home". The "health home" targets that health is much more than what happens in the exam room or clinic setting. The need to engage a team that is representative of health care professionals and community resources unique to the needs of the patient is indicated in the "health home" model.

The research, policy papers and draft recommendations also discuss the need to address physician compensation in developing the attributes and systems to provide an effective and measurable medical home. The Joint Principles of the Patient-Centered Medical Home (2007) also provides a framework for payment for care in a medical home setting. The payment structure should assess and take into account the following:

- Value of the physician and non-physician staff care management that is not face-to-face care with the patient and/or family
- Need to pay for services associated with coordination of care with various providers and entities
- Need to support adoption and use of health information technology for communication and quality improvement
- Need to support secure email communication and telephone consultations
- Need to reimburse separately for face-to-face care as well as payment for care management services
- Differences in patient populations for which medical home care is provided such as the uninsured, chronically ill, elderly, special needs children, etc

As the concept of medical home is piloted with governmental, private, and public organizations, tools for outcome measurements and payment methodologies will also develop.

Evolving Models and Demonstration Projects for the Medical Home

Section 204 of the Tax Relief and Health Care Act of 2006 (http://www.medicare.gov, 2009) requires the development of demonstration projects that redesign the health care delivery system to provide targeted, accessible, continuous, coordinated, and family-centered care to high need populations. "High need" populations are defined as those with prolonged or chronic illnesses that require regular care, medical monitoring, treatment, or education and advice. One of the demonstration projects to redesign health care delivery currently under development is that of the Medical Home Demonstration Project which was presented in a Special Open Door Forum on October 28, 2008. As noted, the defining characteristics of the Medical Home closely match with the original work of the American Academy of Pediatricians. The current motivation is on the basis of the growing Medicare population, the growing incidence of chronic diseases, and the need to cost effectively manage quality chronic care management. Between 2009 and 2012, over 400 medical practices (representative of over 2,000 individual physicians) will participate in the Medicare Medical Home demonstration project. The evaluations will be completed with the National Committee for Quality Assurance (NCQA) Physicians Practice Connections, a set of tools designed explicitly to monitor these medical home demonstration projects. The NCQA tools include ten measurement standards for the demonstration projects which are as follows:

- Written standards for patient access and patient communication
- Use of data to show standards for patient access and communication
- Use of paper or electronic charting tools to organize clinical information
- Use of data to identify important diagnoses and conditions in practice
- Adoption and implementation of evidence-based guidelines for three chronic conditions
- Active patient self-management support
- Systematic tracking of test results and identification of abnormal results
- Referral tracking, using a paper or electronic system
- Clinical and/or service performance measurement, by physician or across the practice
- Performance reporting, by physician or across the practice (http://www.ncqa. org, 2009)

Additional components of NCQA's revised measurement sets include language preferences, planning for patient transitions to other care providers, and electronic family/patient communication standards. The demonstration projects will utilize a new payment code from Medicare which is the monthly "care management fee" which will be based upon the attributes of the medical practice in providing medical home services and skills. Medicare has created two tiers of medical home criteria tied to the amount of the monthly care management fee received by the physician. Examples of items included in the tiers are systematically tracking tests and follow ups, use of e-prescribing, interactive websites for patients and families, and coordination of referrals. Currently, a total of 28 items are represented in the two tier system. This demonstration project creates a financial incentive for medical practices to develop the needed resources and standards to qualify as a medical home and provide coordination of care and care management services. Unfortunately,

Medicaid recipients and uninsured individuals are ineligible for these medical home demonstration projects.

Other private insurance companies are also beginning medical home pilot programs offering participating physicians a per-member-per-month care management fee. One such insurer is Blue Cross Blue Shield of Michigan which has implemented a "Patient-Centered Medical Home Initiative Plan for Coordination of Care". (http://www.bcbsm.com, 2009). This initiative is optional for contracted providers and includes incentive payments for performance and participation in the initiative. The overall goal is to have all providers receive full competency in implementing core competencies of the medical home. Figure 2 lists the beginning draft of the Coordination of Care Initiative tasks for primary care providers. As noted, the initial strategies are focused on selecting one chronic condition and developing protocols for care coordination. Blue Cross Blue Shield is structuring a 6 month planning phase, an initial performance phase, and an ongoing performance phase for measurement.

United Health and IBM announced a collaborative pilot project in February 2009 (Abelson, 2009) to implement the medical home concept with the IBM workforce. Physicians will receive additional compensation to closely monitor patients who are IBM employees and a consultant has been added to help physicians change their practice patterns to support the medical home concept. This pilot will also assess if single practitioners can serve as medical homes as effectively as group practices. Interestingly, the pilot was initiated by IBM, who is anxious to improve health care for its employees.

Another organization, The Patient-Centered Primary Care Collaborative (PCPCC) (http://www.pcpcc.net, 2009), has adopted the term "patient-centered care". This collaborative is comprised of major employers (representing over 50 million workers), consumer groups, patient quality organizations, health plans, labor unions, healthcare professionals (over 300,000 physicians), hospitals, and clinics, which are also focusing on building the patient-centered medical home. Their design of the medical home concept does not differ from the models earlier described, but they are primarily focusing on exploring alternative methods to compensate physicians and help control the costs of health care. The PCPCC recognizes the crucial role of primary care providers in helping people optimize their health and live longer. The PCPCC hopes to encourage large self-insured employer groups to pilot the medical home with their employee groups. They also propose that medical homes improve patient and provider satisfaction as well as cost effectiveness of primary care. They support primary care providers as advisors, partners in care, and overall coordinators of the health care team (www.pcpcc.net, 2009).

TransforMED (2009) is a national demonstration project that is developing a new model of care that contains the medical home concept as the centerpiece. This project is a private partnership of various corporations supporting the Joint Principles of the Patient-Centered Medical Home through the development of this new not-for-profit initiative (2007). TransforMED's mission is to transform health care delivery

---

Coordination of Care Initiative Tasks – DRAFT 2009

13.1 For every patient with chronic condition selected for initial focus, mechanism is established for being notified of each patient admit and discharge or other type of encounter, at facilities with which the physician has admitting privileges or other ongoing relationship.

- Standards for information exchange have been established to enable timely follow up with patients

13.2 Process is in place for sending necessary medical records and discussing continued care arrangements with other facilities for all patients with chronic condition selected for initial focus

- Patients are encouraged to request that PCMH Practice Unit be notified of any patient encounter with health care facilities.

13.3 Systematic approach is in place to use patient registry to systematically track care coordination activities for each patient with chronic condition selected for initial focus. Fields are structured to allow care coordination across other settings of care as well.

- Facility name
- Admit date
- Origin of admit(ED, referring physician, etc.)
- Attending physician
- Discharge Date
- Diagnostic findings
- Pending tests
- Treatment plans
- Complications at discharge

13.4 Systematic approach is in place to flag for immediate attention any patient registry data that indicates a potentially time-sensitive health issue for all patients with chronic condition selected for focus.

13.5 For patients leaving the practice (e.g., moving, changing providers, going into a nursing home, etc.) written transition plans are developed in collaboration with the patient and their caregivers for patients with chronic conditions selected for initial focus.

- Patients are assisted with finding a new primary care provider and/or specialists.

13.6 Capability is in place to coordinate care with health plan case manager(s) regarding extra-contractual benefits and services for all patients with chronic condition selected for initial focus.

13.7 All members of care team are adequately trained on care coordination processes as determined by each Practice Unit, and have clearly defined roles within that process.

- Practice Unit will develop written policies on how to communicate with patients/caregivers and how all coordination tasks will be delineated (e.g., using a flow sheet).

13.8 Care coordination capabilities are extended to all patients with chronic conditions that need care coordination assistance.

13.9 Care coordination capabilities are extended to all patients that need care coordination assistance.

www.bcbsm.com (2009). PatientCentered Medical Home Initiative Plan for Coordination of Care.

Fig. 2 Coordination of care initiative tasks – DRAFT 2009

to achieve optimal patient care, professional satisfaction, and success of primary care practices (www.transforMED.com, 2009). They are focused on translating the model of care into operational processes with measurable outcomes using research and science. Figure 3 identifies the various components of their task forces including

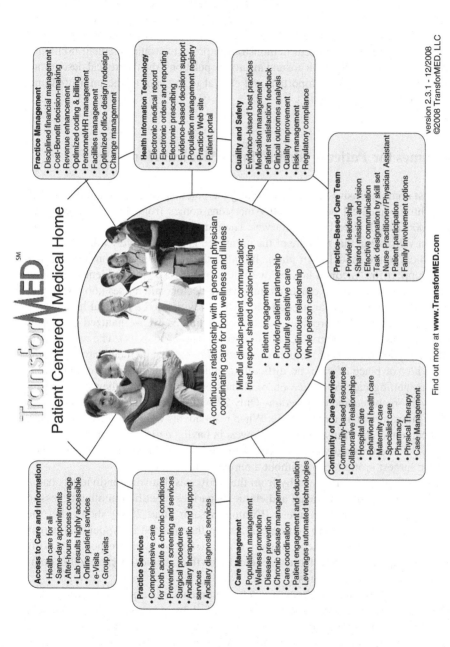

Fig. 3 TransforMed Model

TransforMed℠
Patient Centered Medical Home

A continuous relationship with a personal physician coordinating care for both wellness and illness

- Mindful clinician-patient communication: trust, respect, shared decision-making
  - Patient engagement
  - Provider/patient partnership
  - Culturally sensitive care
  - Continuous relationship
  - Whole person care

Practice Management
- Disciplined financial management
- Cost-Benefit decision-making
- Revenue enhancement
- Optimized coding & billing
- Personnel/HR management
- Facilities management
- Optimized office design/redesign
- Change management

Health Information Technology
- Electronic medical record
- Electronic orders and reporting
- Electronic prescribing
- Evidence-based decision support
- Population management registry
- Practice Web site
- Patient portal

Quality and Safety
- Evidence-based best practices
- Medication management
- Patient satisfaction feedback
- Clinical outcomes analysis
- Quality improvement
- Risk management
- Regulatory compliance

Practice-Based Care Team
- Provider leadership
- Shared mission and vision
- Effective communication
- Task designation by skill set
- Nurse Practitioner/Physician Assistant
- Patient participation
- Family involvement options

Access to Care and Information
- Health care for all
- Same-day appointments
- After-hours access coverage
- Lab results highly accessible
- Online patient services
- e-Visits
- Group visits

Practice Services
- Comprehensive care for both acute & chronic conditions
- Prevention screening and services
- Surgical procedures
- Ancillary therapeutic and support services
- Ancillary diagnostic services

Care Management
- Population management
- Wellness promotion
- Disease prevention
- Chronic disease management
- Care coordination
- Patient engagement and education
- Leverages automated technologies

Continuity of Care Services
- Community-based resources
- Collaborative relationships
  - Hospital care
  - Behavioral health care
  - Maternity care
  - Specialist care
  - Pharmacy
  - Physical Therapy
  - Case Management

version 2.3.1 - 12/2008
©2008 TransforMED, LLC

Find out more at **www.TransforMED.com**

access to care and information, information systems, redesigned offices, quality and safety, management, point of care services, and a team approach.

The concept of the medical home is tied closely to two facts: first, that many Americans live with chronic illnesses and second, the desire to compensate primary care providers differently to attempt to improve health status and manage costs. Despite the fact that the current demonstration projects around medical home are focused on caring for the Medicare and insured populations, the theoretical descriptors of medical home are most important and crucial to the care of the uninsured and underserved in our country.

Outcomes for Patients Identifying a Medical Home

The most comprehensive research regarding the potential outcomes and benefits of establishing a medical home for all Americans comes from the Commonwealth Fund 2006 Health Care Quality Survey. The comprehensive nature of this survey has been valuable in that the care of the uninsured is also positively impacted when the medical home model is in place. Initially, the study demonstrated the strong public support for "medical homes" with 80% of the respondents identifying it as very important to have one practice/clinic where doctors and nurses know you, and provide and coordinate your needed care. The study defined a medical home as "a health care setting that provides patients with timely, well-organized care, and enhanced access to providers" (Commonwealth Fund 2006, p. ix). The respondents to the survey identified four features of a medical home that included having a regular provider or place of care, no difficulty contacting their provider by phone, no difficulty getting care or advice on weekends or evenings, and their office visits being well organized and on schedule. Only 27% of the respondents identified have all four indicators of a medical home. When respondents were queried about having a medical home, the uninsured ranked lowest in having a medical home as depicted in Fig. 4. The uninsured were least likely to have a medical home (16%) and they were the largest group (45%) without a regular source of care.

What was also very noteworthy from the study was that when individuals had a regular medical home, the racial and ethnic disparities identified in other access to care studies disappeared. Figure 5 (Commonwealth Fund 2006) shows that the percentages of those always getting care, when they needed it, is identical across race and ethnicity when a medical home is reported upon by the respondents. This is a strong support for the establishment and growth of medical homes within community health center structures.

A feature of the medical home model recommended is a patient recall system and reminders regarding preventive screenings, follow up appointments, and health advice. The Commonwealth Fund Survey (Fig. 6, 2006) also demonstrated that patients with reported medical homes also reported reminders for preventive screenings provided for insured and uninsured patients. The feature of a "reminder" provided by a medical home resulted in increased rates of preventive screenings

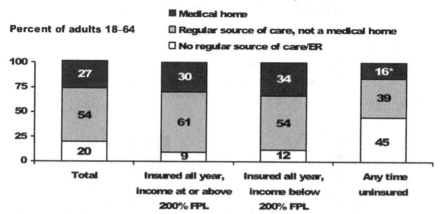

Fig. 4 Uninsured are least likely to have a medical home and many do not have a regular source of care

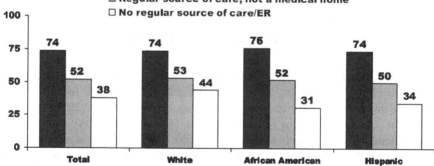

Fig. 5 Racial and ethnic differences in getting needed medical care are eliminated when adults have medical homes

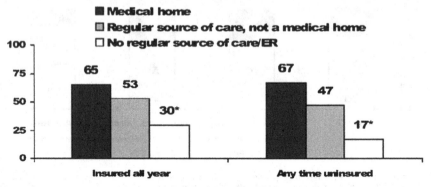

ES-6. Patients with Medical Homes—
Whether Insured or Uninsured—Are Most Likely
to Receive Preventive Care Reminders

Percent of adults 18–64 receiving a reminder
to schedule a preventive visit by doctor's office

■ Medical home
☐ Regular source of care, not a medical home
☐ No regular source of care/ER

Note: Medical home includes having a regular provider or place of care, reporting no
difficulty contacting provider by phone or getting advice and medical care on weekends
or evenings, and always or often finding office visits well organized and running on time.
* Compared with medical home, differences are statistically significant.
Source: Commonwealth Fund 2006 Health Care Quality Survey.

Fig. 6 Patients with medical homes – whether insured or uninsured – are most likely to receive preventive care reminders

completed for both insured and uninsured patients. Two thirds of both insured and uninsured adults with medical homes received preventive care reminders, compared with half of insured and uninsured adults without medical homes (Commonwealth Fund 2006).

Community Health Centers and Medical Homes

The Commonwealth Fund study (2006) identified that community health centers and public clinics were serving about 20% of the uninsured and 20% of low income adults in this sample. They also were providing care for about 13% of African Americans and more than one of five Hispanics. However, the survey showed that these patients receiving care in a community health center or public clinic were less likely to have the features of a medical home available. In fact, only 21% reported that they had a regular doctor, no difficulty accessing their doctor by phone, no problems getting care or medical advice on weekends or evenings, and that their doctor was on time and organized (Commonwealth Fund 2006). Safety net providers, such as community health centers, or other providers caring for vulnerable populations, have the most to gain by adoption of the medical home model. As a general rule, safety net providers see all who seek care, provide comprehensive primary care services, and have a majority patient population comprised of the uninsured, low income, and Medicaid populations. The medical home model is very important for those who have no insurance, struggle with multiple chronic diseases, have low literacy, are challenged with language barriers, and have other issues which make receiving care and coordination of care a challenge. Based upon this recognized need, the Commonwealth Fund (2008) initiated technical assistance to safety net providers in developing more characteristics of the medical home. Four regional coordinating councils will be selected to collaborate with 12–15 safety net providers on building medical homes for vulnerable and uninsured populations in 2009. This funding initiative should lead to more expertise and provision of medical home features within primary care safety net providers. The National Association of Community Health Centers (NACHC 2008) partnered with various organizations in March 2009 to offer a National Medical Home Summit featuring a medical home training program. This program included the basics of a medical home combining perspectives and thoughts of various groups. In addition, processes for accreditation, legal considerations, and involving patients in the development of their medical home were offered. (http://www.medicalhomesummit.com 2009).

Describing the Medical Home

Upon review of the characteristics of the medical home documented by various organizations, a key shift is the partnership formed between primary care physicians and their patients. The medical home emphasizes the ongoing relationship between the patient and the physician to build health, discuss options, learn self-management skills, and utilize community resources. It is not just an interaction when an illness or acute need requires a physician intervention. A medical home is not simply a disease management system. Disease management has been a health care system initiative driven by insurance companies and actual disease management organizations. The medical home is distinctly different from disease management programs in that disease management programs assign a case manager who interacts with the patient about the other members of the health care team. The growing concept of medical home places the physician as the leader for optimizing health for all individuals in our health care system, rather than assigning a case manager. The medical home focuses on the whole person, across the life span as various health opportunities and challenges occur.

Some of the needed components for a medical home include an organized interdisciplinary health care delivery system, evidence-based support for clinical decisions, information systems, relationships with community resources, and enhanced involvement and self-management of patients in regard to their health. For medically focused clinics and practices, the lack of seamless interdisciplinary teams and the relationships with existing community resources present the greatest challenge. As more health information technology is adopted, the partnerships between physicians, patients, and other needed resources will and can change more readily to build an ongoing medical home care delivery system.

So, practically, what does a medical home look like in terms of behaviors and best practices? What processes would need to be in place to address different medical home criteria or standards? How do we turn the research and standards into procedural guidelines, systems, and daily activities? And more so, how do we monitor these activities and ascertain areas for improvement, desired outcomes reached and, dollars saved?

Initially, the development of a medical home practice would begin with the clarity around mission, vision, and values. The physician as well as staff members, all need to practice and work from the same value base which assures the focus on the patient's needs and optimal health. The process would include a practice assessment to identify strengths of the organization possibly in terms of infrastructure, patient-friendly environment, service delivery, and many other potential attributes. Areas for improvement as mentioned earlier for many primary care practices would be the need for resource network development in the community to assure smooth transitions for other services for the patient and family. This is just an example of the preliminary planning process for establishing a beginning level medical home for patients. Leadership commitment, as with any change, is crucial. Service to the patient may be a key factor as the medical home develops and resources for communication evolves. For example, the new patient who is establishing care would receive a guide of information including the physicians and healthcare providers available, the location and hours of service, the philosophy of the practice, how appointments are made, the fees and financial policies, and a tour with personal introductions to key staff members. Medical homes may have an advocate assigned for every patient to address challenges in navigating the system or reaching their provider. So, in addition to this new patient orientation, a detailed patient history, background, and current health care needs would be established in the electronic health record of the practice. Medical homes would have established networks of various specialty providers who would assist with medical and surgical needs. Patients would be assured that referrals were completed and the specialty provider would be informed of all needed data required to coordinate care. Medical homes would present with an integrated seamless model as seen in community health centers providing primary medical and dental care, behavioral health providers, as well as laboratory, radiology, and nutritional services.

Medical homes would ensure that patients are aware of and receive reminders for preventive screenings, keep logs of their care management, follow up visits, and have access to ongoing health education and health improvement opportunities. Group visits for patients with chronic conditions would be provided as a method of improving self-management skills as well as for building self-efficacy. Same day appointment systems or patient driven scheduling methodologies would be available to further empower the patient in their medical home. Increasing access to data and communication via email and the internet would further develop the patient and physician relationship. The overarching concept of the medical home is the development of the relationship with the patient which mandates excellence in patient service and communication to yield the most effective care management. Currently, evidence around best practices is beginning to be collected. Variability around best practice criteria for medical homes will vary based on the population demographics, the health status, and the percent of underserved and uninsured in the community.

In the medical home model, the care and care management resides with the physician and his/her heath care team. As a medical home is established and the key attributes are in place and measured, evaluating effectiveness is essential. Monitoring the effectiveness of the medical home is part of the needed development. Some of the measurements would include patient satisfaction, provider and staff satisfaction, as well as clinical process and outcomes measures,

Moving Organizations toward the Medical Home Model

The medical home concept seems like a natural fit in caring for the uninsured and underserved in our communities. The uninsured are likely to benefit the most in terms of access to preventive care, acute care, and chronic care management. The first step in assuring a medical home for all uninsured individuals is the engagement and commitment of healthcare professionals and leadership to design current health care delivery systems. Education based upon the earlier noted consensus statements, demonstration projects, and current research on reducing and eliminating disparities regarding access to care are powerful catalysts for change for providers and organizations caring for the uninsured and underserved. Baseline assessments of already existing practice components that support the medical home must be completed with a priority list of next steps to add. Figure 7 presents an initial list of "must-haves" in creating a medical home for uninsured individuals in our community. Lastly, financial structures and payment must acknowledge the needed changes in reimbursement and funding, recognizing the long term savings for our health care system, as well as the improved health status and outcomes for both the insured and uninsured populations.

Medical Home Programs for the Uninsured

Healthy San Francisco was initiated in July of 2007 to provide an inclusive safety net for all uninsured residents. The program provides affordable access to basic and ongoing health care services for uninsured residents regardless of their immigration status, employment status, or pre-existing conditions. The Healthy San Francisco program covers all residents who have been uninsured for at least 90 days and do not qualify for other public programs. The use of medical homes is a key component of the Healthy San Francisco program. However, the San Francisco Community Clinic Consortium has been providing culturally, linguistically, and literacy appropriate medical homes for individuals for over 30 years. Healthy San Francisco is expanding this work to hopefully provide care for the entire uninsured city population estimated at 72,000 (http://www.sfccc.org, 2009). An individual enrolls and

"Must Haves" for developing a Medical Home for the Uninsured

1. Patient guide with contact information that includes the phone number, fax number, office hours, web address, email policies and hours of operation using linguistically and literacy appropriate methods.
2. Share special needs information such as physical navigation, visual or hearing impairments, etc.
3. Description of how tests are ordered and results communicated within what timeframe. Communicate the system for screening and follow up reminders of the health center.
4. Communicate the guidelines for emergency and after hours care.
5. Identify methods and process for medication refills and reporting side effects, medication contracts, etc.
6. Location including address, public transportation and parking information
7. Appointment information including patient driven scheduling(open scheduling) directions, no-show and cancellation guidelines, and estimates of reasonable waiting times.
8. Expanded hours for appointments
9. Protocol or welcome to bring a family member or caregiver as needed to the medical visit.
10. Registration and eligibility information via brochures, phone messages and websites. Include "live" people to help with the process of eligibility to establish care and expanded hours of assistance at various locations within the targeted geography service areas.
11. Create personal health cards with identified primary care provider, key phone numbers, regular medications, chronic health problems and individual payment protocol.
12. Assist with process to retrieve past medical records, history, etc.
13. Utilize an electronic health record to establish connectivity with other members of the care delivery team
14. Personal primary care physician assigned with a designated health care team
15. Integrated health care delivery team comprised of primary care, dental care, behavioral health, wellness and health improvement services, registered dietitians, advocates, laboratory, radiology, and other specialists that communicates electronically and is available to meet for care management as needed.
16. Health coaches, community health advisors and community support groups available to support chronic disease management and health promotion behaviors.
17. Electronic systems to manage patient recall, follow up and tracking for both preventive and chronic care management
18. Creation of a comfortable physical environment, rich in service and respect which provides access to health information and resources
19. Systems to provide prompt response to patients by a team member or primary care physician.
20. Attention to patient names, preferences and relationship building as part of the care delivery system
21. Use of e-prescribing
22. Creation of electronic disease registries
23. Opportunities for group visits
24. Opportunities for home visits and outreach to address barriers to care such as transportation, child care, etc.
25. Education Classes which help build empowerment and self-management skills
26. Monitoring of health indicators and health improvement based upon characteristics of the population served

Fig. 7 "Must-Haves" for a Medical Home

chooses a medical home from the 29 participating clinics. The clinic then takes the leadership in assigning a specific physician or clinical provider for the enrollee. Each patient is also assigned a care coordinator who helps monitor preventive screenings, treatment management, and self-management goals. While other cities in the country have established health care access programs, San Francisco is the first to provide services for all uninsured using a medical home model. Most of the medical homes are community health centers that have successful track records with quality and cost. The program provides universal access and cost sharing based upon income. As the program approaches its second anniversary, further outcomes will be reviewed in terms of health, reduced disparities, and reduced expenditures for tertiary care (http://www.kff.org, 2009).

Community Care of North Carolina (CCNC) is a coordinated medical system that provides care for the Medicaid and uninsured population throughout the state of North Carolina through a medical home approach. For the past ten years, CCNC has worked to replace the traditional episodic health care visit with the medical home model. Primary care physicians and case managers, who review claims data from Medicaid and complete chart audits, work together to manage care across over 1,200 medical practices that are providing care for over 884,000 Medicaid recipients. For the past two years alone, the medical home model has saved the state of North Carolina over $150 million each year through better management of asthma and diabetes treatment. CCNC started with a small pilot study in 1988 in rural Wilson County. Medicaid agreed initially to pay participating physicians in two medical groups a small additional fee to manage the care for their patients and the program has grown and developed from there. In 2005, the program went statewide but the government made a decision to have the program managed with local networks. This has allowed local teams to evolve, set their own health improvement and medical home goals, and have access to an electronic database to identify patient histories, utilization, and risk factors. Much of the success has occurred due to the local community team working to supply patients with the resources they need to optimize their health. On the basis of the cost savings to date, the state of North Carolina has asked CCNC to focus more of their efforts on managing Medicaid recipients with multiple chronic conditions. The use of the medical home is notable in North Carolina, not only from a cost savings perspective and improved health indicators for individuals with diabetes and asthma but also for the work of the team. The team of the medical home model works collaboratively to address root causes of patient problems, rather than simply increase the quantity of health care. CCNC illustrates that we need better quality of care which is personalized and relationship oriented, rather than providing more care.

Unity Health Care in the District of Columbia is another implementation of the medical home model. Two federally qualified health centers collaborate with the local correctional institutions to assure the assignment of a medical home for inmates after release from the correctional unit. Unity has found that the use of discharge planners, nurse case managers, and medical providers who work both in the jail as well as in the community led to the sharing of the treatment plan and less disruptions in chronic care medication and treatment management. Unity Health

Care has utilized the coordination of care component to manage a high risk population and shares connectivity and electronic health records with the local correctional institutions (NACHC Policy Institute 2009).

Access Across Vermont Plan: Advancing a Medical Home Model began with a grassroots group of community members who were working to add more satellite federally qualified health centers in rural areas of Vermont. These communities are serving as "blueprint pilot communities" to test the medical home model. They have various pilot components of the medical home model underway such as a pediatric mobile clinic, electronic health records, behavioral health integration with primary care, telemedicine child psychiatry, and various outreach and eligibility work to enroll individuals in the medical home model (www.bistatepca.org, 2009).

References

Abelson R (2009) United Health and IBM test health care plan. The New York Times. February 7, 2009

Access across Vermont plan (2009) Available at http://www.bistatepca.org. Accessed 1 Apr 2009

American Academy of Family Physicians (2009) Available at http://www.aafp.org.Accessed 20 March 2009

American Academy of Pediatrics (2009) Available at http://www.aap.org. Accessed 1 Mar 2009

American College of Physicians (2009) Available at www.acp.org. Accessed: March 1, 2009

Backer LA (2007) The medical home: An idea whose time has come….again. Fam Pract Manag 14:38–42

Berwick D (2002) Crossing the quality chasm: a new health care system for the 21st century. Available at http://www.healthaffairs.org. Accessed 1 Mar 2009

Blue Cross Blue Shield of Michigan (2009) Patient-centered medical home initiative plan for coordination of care. Available at http://www.bcbsm.com. Accessed 1 Apr 2009

Bodenheimer T (2008) Coordinating care-A perilous journey through the health care system. N Engl J Med 358(10):1064–1071

Commonwealth Fund (2007) Closing the divide: How medical homes promote equity in health care: Results from the Commonwealth Fund 2006 Health Care Quality Survey. http://www.commonwealthfund.org. Accessed 1 Apr 2009

Community Care of North Carolina (2009) Available at http://www.ccnc.org. Retrieved 1 Apr 2009

Grumbach K, Bodenheimer T (2002) A primary care home for Americans: Putting the house in order. J Am Med Assoc 288:889–893

Guidelines for a Medical Home (2009) Available at http://www.medicalhomeinfo.org. Accessed 3 Apr 2009

Healthy People 2010 (2009) http://www.healthypeople.gov. Accessed 24 Feb 2009

Homer CJ, Klatka K, Romm D, Kuhlthau K, Bloom S, Newacheck P, Van Cleave J, Perrin JM (2008) A review of the evidence for the medical home for children with special health care needs. Pediatrics 1222(4):922–937

Kaiser Commission on Medicaid and the Uninsured: Healthy San Francisco (2009) Available at http://www.kff.org. Accessed 31 Mar 2009

McAllister J, Presler E, Cooley WC (2007) Medical home practice-based care: A workbook. Center for Medical Home Improvement, Greenfield, NH

Medical Home Demonstration Project (2009) Available at http://www.medicare.gov Accessed 1 Mar 2009

Moore G, Showstack J (2003) Primary care medicine in crisis: Toward reconstruction and renewal. Ann Intern Med 138:244–247

Murphy J, Chang H, Montgomery JE, Roger WH, Safran DG (2001) The quality of the physician–patient relationships: Patients' experiences: 1996–1999. J Fam Pract 2001(50):123–129

National Association of Community Health Centers (2009) A nationally recognized discharge planning program: Linking inmates with a medical home. Presented by Diana Lapp, Policy Institute, Washington, DC

National Medical Home Summit (2009) Available at http://www.medicalhomesummit.com. Accessed 3 Apr 2009

Patient-Centered Primary Care Collaborative (2009) Available at http://www.pcpcc.net. Accessed 31 Mar 2009

Physicians Practice Connections (2009) Available at http://www.ncqa.org. Accessed 3 Apr 2009

San Francisco Community Clinic Consortium (2009) Available at http://www.sfccc.org. Accessed 3 Apr 2009

The Future of Family Medicine Project (2004) Available at http://www.annfammed.org. Accessed 3 Apr 2009

TransforMED (2009) Available at http://www.TransforMED.com. Accessed 1 Mar 2009

Medication Assistance for the Uninsured

Nancy J. Johnson and Janet S. Smith

Case Study on Best Practices and Future Opportunities

St. Elizabeth's Health Center, in Tucson, Arizona is the largest faith based community health center in Southern Arizona. For the past 47 years, St. Elizabeth's has provided medical, dental, and health care exclusively for the uninsured, using a unique model of care partnering, a small paid staff with over 165 volunteer physicians, dentists, nurses, and other healthcare professionals. Prescription assistance is a daily challenge for the majority of the patients, ranging from children through the elderly, who make St. E's their "medical home." In addition, emergency room patients are referred regularly to St. Elizabeth's for needed prescriptions. Various community collaborations and strategies keep the resources in place for the patients. Initially, St. Elizabeth's has established two grants for medication assistance. One is with the City of Tucson for $50,000 annually, and one is with the County for $40,000 annually. Each of these grants has eligibility restrictions along with a capped amount per individual. In addition, the local electric company provides an unrestricted small grant for medications. The many volunteer physicians provide needed samples for patients as well. Over 40 physicians have their office staff "on call" when sample medication is needed, and is not in St. Elizabeth's sample closet. Lastly, but most noteworthy to the community collaboration, is the service of a volunteer retired registered nurse, who spends 16–20 hours weekly, preparing and managing the Prescription Assistance Program. In 2007, her efforts provided over $1 million in prescriptions for St. Elizabeth's uninsured patients. The continual assessment and gathering of resources, assures that uninsured patients will have access to needed medications. On the education side of the equation, the physician and nurse practitioner soon become proficient in knowing the medications that are less expensive, as well as which will be most likely adhered to and managed effectively by the patient population.

Introduction

Medication prescription costs are escalating each year in the United States due to the growth of the older population, as well as the many various and new treatment options available which necessitate ongoing prescription medications. Equally, the

N.J. Johnson (✉)
El Rio Community Health Center, Tucson, AZ, USA
e-mail: nancyj@elrio.org

N.J. Johnson and L.P. Johnson (eds.), *The Care of the Uninsured in America*,
DOI 10.1007/978-0-387-78309-3_8, © Springer Science+Business Media, LLC 2010

number of uninsured and under-served individuals is also growing. This population lacks the resources to pay for their short term and long term prescription medications. Many entities including the government, pharmaceutical manufacturers, nonprofit organizations, and communities are identifying strategies to address the medication needs of the uninsured. These diverse groups are attempting to decrease the number of acute and chronic medical conditions going without treatment. In addition, these groups are also working to decrease emergency room visits and hospitalizations for chronic conditions, for which the continuity of medication could have possibly avoided expensive tertiary care utilization.

Status of the Need

As we consider the 47 million Americans who lack healthcare insurance, we frequently discuss the need for access to care along with the dramatic costs of emergency rooms and hospitalizations. However, the challenge of funding medications for the uninsured population as well as the low income and under-served individuals and families is continuing to escalate. The Agency for Healthcare Research and Quality (AHRQ 2008) reports that consumer spending for prescribed medicines rose from $103 billion in 2000 to $177.7 billion in 2003. There are various facets to this continually growing expense as we analyze the components of the population. The Medicare population continues to grow and represents 75.3 billion of the total expenditures in 2003. Over 50% of the individual total expenditure was being paid out of pocket, if no Medicare supplementary policy was owned. For the non-Medicare insured population, approximately 40% is paid out of pocket. However, when we review the uninsured population, we recognize they spend the least amount annually ($488/year), but also pay the greatest percentage out of pocket (88% or $428) when compared to those with public insurance only ($768 and $226, respectively), or those with any private insurance ($697 and $271, respectively) (AHRQ 2008).

Nearly one-fourth (24%) of adults aged 19–64 lacked prescription drug insurance coverage at some point in 2001 (Schur et al. 2004). Nearly two-thirds of this group lacked health coverage of any kind. Although, most had prescription coverage if insurance was purchased through their employer, many had no prescription coverage when insurance was purchased in the marketplace. The most recent study available, completed in 1996, illustrated that individuals with incomes between 100 and 300% of the federal poverty level were most likely to lack coverage for medications (Schur et al. 2004).

The absence of prescription coverage has significant consequences. Based on Schur et al. (2001), non-elderly adults without drug coverage were almost twice as likely to report not filling a prescription due to cost. They were also less likely to see a doctor when sick, or to skip recommended preventive tests or follow up care. Some of this behavior may be due to knowing that a prescription will be difficult or impossible to fill. Other studies also support the behavior of less adherence to much needed medications, for the treatment of chronic conditions in the uninsured and low income populations. In addition, research also looks at the effect of capped medication benefits which are offered in some Medicare and Medicaid plans. Two studies of monthly limits showed that the lower numbers of prescriptions filled resulted in more emergency room visits, more nursing home admissions, and more visits to community mental health centers (Johnson et al. 1997). In addition, about one-third of Medicare beneficiaries report not filling a prescription or altering the dosage due to out of pocket costs. The results included under-use of needed medications especially for those with lower incomes or poorer health (Johnson 1997).

An additional illustration of what happens when people do not have access to drug coverage can be seen from the state of Oregon. Some of Oregon's residents, who were enrolled in the state Medicaid program, lost drug coverage due to short-falls in the state budget in 2003. An assessment of these patients showed that about one-half reported not taking prescriptions due to out of pocket costs, one-third surveyed reported that they switched to a different less expensive drug, and about one-fourth reported getting assistance from pharmaceutical assistance programs. Lastly 7% reported getting free samples from their physician. Respondents also reported cutting back on their food budget, delaying payment of bills, and borrowing money for prescribed medications. In summary, the implications for the uninsured who do not have prescription insurance coverage can be medically and financially damaging (Zerzan 2004).

Governmental Response to Medication Assistance for the Uninsured

Historically, Medicaid has offered various levels of benefits as they relate to medication coverage from state to state. These can be included as a paid benefit, or require a co-pay of various amounts depending on the administering state. The formularies of medications are predetermined, and pre-authorization must be granted to prescribe outside the formularies. However, as we look at Medicare, prescription coverage had never been an included benefit prior to the implementation of Medicare Part D:so many seniors were part of the uncovered or uninsured population as it related to prescription coverage. Medicare identified that approximately one-quarter of seniors and people with disabilities in Medicare had no drug coverage.

The Center for Medicare and Medicaid estimated that nearly 11 million beneficiaries with limited income would receive help from a Medicare Prescription benefit. In addition to the 75% subsidy that would be provided for medication costs, the low income beneficiaries would receive an additional benefit of nearly $2,300 in the first year of 2006. The concerns over the many new medications available for treatment, their prices, and the limits with pharmaceutical assistance programs led to the enactment of this Medicare prescription coverage for Medicare beneficiaries. In 2004, Medicare released the final rules for the prescription drug benefit.

The benefit began in 2006 and allowed all Medicare beneficiaries to sign up for drug coverage through a prescription drug plan or Medicare health plan. This was a step toward decreasing the number of uninsured as defined by prescription coverage (CMS 2004).

Each Medicare drug coverage plan can vary in the cost and what medications are covered. When you join you pay a monthly premium. However, if an individual chooses not to join when they are first eligible, the individual may have to pay a penalty for joining at a later date. Enrolled individuals can make changes to their Medicare drug plan each year, during the period from November 15 through December 31. This governmental response has assisted the Medicare population, after they have met the $250 deductible, by providing a safety net. They are then eligible for up to an initial $2,250 of medications per year. For many low income Medicare beneficiaries, the $250 deductible is a barrier to prescription medication coverage. As is apparent, this medication benefit is of value to the Medicare beneficiaries, but still does not address the needs of the uninsured and their prescription needs.

Current efforts by legislators are underway to pass legislation that allows the government to negotiate with drug manufacturers to obtain lower drug prices for Medicare beneficiaries. For Medicare beneficiaries who have limited incomes and resources, they may qualify for extra help with their prescription costs. The National Council on Aging (2009) provides an application for possible assistance if your income is less than $16,245 if single, and $21,855 if married, and your resources are less that $12,510 if single, and $25,855 if married. These Medicare beneficiaries may qualify for lower or no deductibles and no coverage gaps ("donut holes").

Although, we frequently first think of older adults needing access to affordable medications, uninsured children are also at risk. They may require short term treatment for acute illnesses or have a chronic disease requiring medications, such as diabetes or asthma. However, the Vaccines for Children Program (VFC) was passed in 1994 as legislation in response to a national measles outbreak from 1989 to 1991. This epidemic resulted in tens of thousands of cases of measles and hundreds of deaths. When the Centers for Disease Control (http://www.cdc.gov, 2009) investigated, more than half of the children with measles were not immunized. VFC is a federally funded program that provides free immunizations for uninsured or under-insured children up to and including age eighteen. Eligible children must meet one of four criteria, which includes: being Medicaid eligible, being uninsured, being under-insured, or being either American Indian or Alaska Native. These vaccines are funded with federal funds, therefore, they are always free of charge. Providers and health centers can charge an administrative fee which may not exceed $15.00 for each vaccine. However, providers and health centers can also lower or waive the administrative fee as well (http://www.needymeds.com, 2009).

The federal government has also provided access to prescription drugs for uninsured individuals, through the 340B program which was established in the Veterans Health Care Act of 1992. The 340B program requires drug manufacturers to provide outpatient drugs at a reduced price for certain covered entities, as defined in the Veterans Health Care Act statutes. The 340B program allows physicians and providers employed in federally qualified health centers (FQHCs), and FQHC look-alikes, HIV/ Ryan White Programs, state operated sexually transmitted disease programs, hemophilia treatment centers, tuberculosis clinics, Title X family planning clinics, urban/638 tribal programs and certain disproportionate share hospitals, to operate pharmacies. These are sometimes known as the "safety net providers" who provide care for the uninsured. A couple of these qualified programs warrant additional comments. For example, the FQHC's provide health care for one of every eight uninsured in our country, and one in every five low income Americans. The disproportionate share hospitals are either government owned or non-profits who have a government commitment to care for the uninsured. They must have a share adjustment percentage of over 11.75% over other hospitals to qualify. The 340B price is defined in the legislation and is considered the ceiling price. All covered providers and clinics can negotiate below the ceiling with the manufacturers (http://www.aphanet.org, 2009). These providers can purchase medications at a lower price and then fill prescriptions for the uninsured, either free of charge or at a reduced cost. The 340B program is administered by the Health Resources and Services Administration (HRSA) and all agencies desiring to participate in the program must register with HRSA. Drug manufacturers must make the 340B prices, which are estimated to be about half of the "list price" paid by retail customers, available to all registered entities. The estimated volume for the 340B plan in 2006 was about $4 billion (HRSA 2006).

Another governmental intervention to address medication assistance for the uninsured comes in the form of the Prime Vendor Program which contracts with the federal government to administer a component of the 340B Program. The current contract for the Prime Vendor Program is held by HealthCare Purchasing Partners International (HPPI), which is a group purchasing organization in Texas. They work to negotiate prices below the usual retail prices, as well as work to provide improved distribution methods and costs to those who participate. In addition to the lower cost medications, HPPI offers diabetic test strips, meters, and vaccinations. The HPPI currently purchases about $2.2 billion in medications each year.

There are two restrictions to the 340B Program which are, that the drugs cannot be used for resale to anyone other than a patient of the participating entity and that a Medicaid rebate cannot be used in addition to the already discounted drug price. The other barrier identified by possible participants is the complexity of the 340B plan in terms of administration as well as the need to have a pharmacy in order to participate. In the past few years, HRSA has begun to encourage and look at innovative ways in which to expand the 340B Program to reach more uninsured and under-served individuals.

There are currently demonstration projects underway to link small clinics together to share a pharmacy. One demonstration project to improve the management of diabetes was conducted at El Rio Community Health Center in Tucson, Arizona. The project goal was to show positive results in clinical outcomes in diabetes by providing access to pharmacists. Arizona law was modified to allow pharmacists to initiate and modify medications consistent with approved written physician protocols.

This allowed the pharmacist to not only provide 340B Program medications and diabetic supplies to patients, but to also monitor their diabetes and provide diabetic education. The outcomes lowered blood pressure, cholesterol, and improved their blood glucose (El Rio Community Health Center 2007). These various demonstration programs as well as the continual group pricing discounts have the potential to enroll more patients into 340B medication programs. The larger challenge is the need to identify more participating organizations who provide care for the uninsured and under-served.

Community Interventions for Medication Assistance for the Uninsured

When an uninsured person needs health care, they may go to the hospital emergency room, the health department, or a community health center for assistance. However, many times, a prescription is written without consideration to the cost involved or the uninsured individual's ability to pay for the prescription. Communities frequently find that many programs, interventions, and resources must be in place to assure that health care problems can be treated promptly before they worsen in complexity or care needs.

In addition to the government's programs, including Medicare Part D and the Federal 340B Medication Program, communities across the country have developed many programs with various characteristics to address medication assistance for the uninsured. The most common are the pharmaceutical companies', Prescription Assistance Programs (PAPs). Many pharmaceutical companies have established PAPs to provide low income and/or uninsured people the ability to obtain medications they cannot afford to purchase. There are approximately 219 manufacturer-sponsored programs. Historically, many of these programs have been around for over 50 years, but have often been difficult to access for the low income and uninsured due to literacy and language issues. Today, many of the applications are becoming easier to complete and are available in Spanish. In 2005, the Pharmaceutical Research and Manufacturers of America reported donated drugs totaling an estimated wholesale value of approximately $5 billion (PhRMA 2007). Most prescribed medications are offered by the manufacturers and PAPRx, an example of a software package for prescription assistance use (2007) reports that over 1,500 medications are available for patients. Unfortunately, these prescription assistance programs are designed to be a "last resort" effort for patients, but many use them as their "only resort" to maintain treatment regimes for chronic illnesses.

The eligibility and guidelines for these many programs vary, but the majority requires US citizenship and incomes below 200% of the federal poverty guidelines. In addition, most require that the patient have no prescription drug coverage, except for the Medicare patients when they hit the "doughnut hole" of their Part D coverage. The "doughnut hole" refers to the gap in coverage once the Medicare beneficiary has reached their maximum of $2,330 and before they exceed the $3,600 out of pocket cap. Most of the programs ship the medications directly to the clinic, health center, or physician office. Generally, the patient is not charged, but some programs do charge the patient a co-pay, dispensing fees or postage/shipping fees. Some programs send vouchers which patients can redeem at the local pharmacies. This can be preferable in that the clinic or medical practice avoids the need to store the medication for the patient after its arrival and prior to the patient's arrival to pick it up. There continues to be a wide variability in the response times from the various pharmaceutical manufacturers. Some are able to respond within a week's time to a patient's application, where others take nearly 6 weeks to respond with the needed medication. A sample patient application for AstraZeneca is included in Table 2.

The numbers of participants in the PAPs are mere estimates, in that, individuals are counted even when they simply seek information about the prescription assistance program. However, over 36 million prescriptions were filled in 2005 (PhRMA 2007). Some PAPs require a physician or patient advocate to complete the application and some large medical groups often use a staff member to facilitate the process for the patient. This is especially true when medications are quite expensive, as in oncology treatment, or when there are literacy and language issues. However, many medical groups are not supportive of staff completing the application due to the lengthy nature of the process.

One study cited in Hoadley's report (2007) indicated that clinic staff spent an average of 111 hours per month in processing applications. Imagine the hours spent in our safety net organizations who care for the majority of the uninsured and under-served in our communities. Lastly, two-third of the clinics and practices that reported not using PAPs, cited that they were too time-consuming and complex. How could we expect our uninsured patients to wrestle with such a process on their own in order to access needed medications? Electronic submissions are mostly used by safety net providers which help to simplify the application, but also manage the processes of working with multiple pharmaceutical companies and one patient's prescriptions, tracking renewal/reapplication dates, and other aspects of program management.

Despite the abundance of these manufacturers' prescription assistance programs, the uninsured patient faces barriers in attempting to utilize them. Initially, the uninsured patient may not know they exist, may not have a regular primary care provider, and may not know what medications they need. In addition, they may need multiple applications for differing manufacturers, making the process difficult. Most recently, pharmaceutical manufacturers have worked to promote their PAPs via television, radio, celebrity spokespeople and even, traveling buses called the "Help is Here Express." Upon reviewing Needy Meds, which was established in 1997 and serves as an informational resource for saving money on prescriptions, there were 219 different prescription assistance programs available via the online application as well as many other assistance programs, including free and low cost clinics and disease-based assistance. The manufacturers included both brand name and generic medications and also discount coupons for medications. This Web site also offers assistance with the applications and the PAPRx Tracker, which allows the applicant to monitor the progress of their applications. Lastly, advocacy services are offered and donations encouraged for medication assistance for the uninsured and under-served (http://www.needymeds.org, 2009).

Table 1 Medication assistance for the uninsured – St. Elizabeth's Health Center

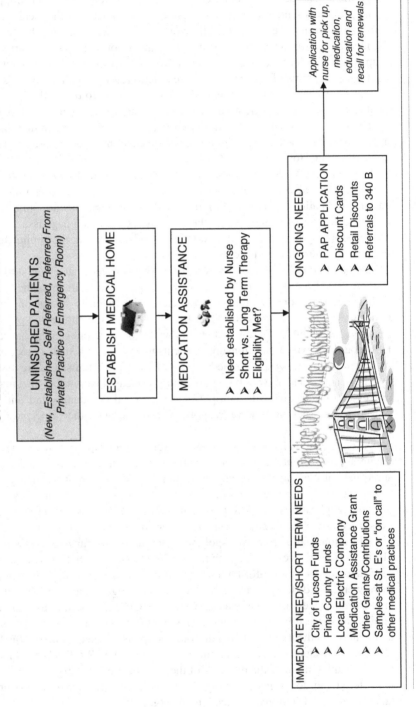

MEDICATION ASSISTANCE FOR THE UNINSURED
ST. ELIZABETH'S HEALTH CENTER

UNINSURED PATIENTS
(New, Established, Self Referred, Referred From Private Practice or Emergency Room)

ESTABLISH MEDICAL HOME

MEDICATION ASSISTANCE
➤ Need established by Nurse
➤ Short vs. Long Term Therapy
➤ Eligibility Met?

ONGOING NEED
➤ PAP APPLICATION
➤ Discount Cards
➤ Retail Discounts
➤ Referrals to 340 B

Application with nurse for pick up, medication, education and recall for renewals

Bridge to Ongoing Assistance

IMMEDIATE NEED/SHORT TERM NEEDS
➤ City of Tucson Funds
➤ Pima County Funds
➤ Local Electric Company
➤ Medication Assistance Grant
➤ Other Grants/Contributions
➤ Samples-at St. E's or "on call" to other medical practices

Currently, there are prescription assistance programs to access generic medications. Generic medications are generally less expensive than the pharmaceutical companies' name brands. In the past 2 years, large retailers such as Walmart, K-Mart, Target and Sam's Club have offered formularies of prescribed generic medications for a flat $4 per prescription. However, some generic medications still have higher costs, especially for specialty care. Rx Outreach was founded in 2004 by Express Scripts which is one of the largest pharmacy benefit managers in the country. Their web site offers about 120 generic medications to individuals with household incomes below 250% of the federal poverty level. There are no other restrictions and patients pay either $20 or $30 for a 3-month prescription with the medication sent to the patient's home, clinic or physician's office. Another similar program is offered by Xubex Pharmaceutical Services and provides about 250 generic drugs. The patient, again, pays a $20 or $30 co-pay for a 90-day supply and is also charged a $3.95 shipping and handling fee. The family must also be at below 250% of the federal poverty level, but cannot be enrolled in Medicare Part D. In addition, Xubex requires a pay stub as proof of income. Based upon the fact that these two generic programs do have fees associated with their access to medications, it is unclear how beneficial they are to the truly uninsured and poor. The local retail programs for $4–$8 per prescription may be more affordable for the individual.

A variation on the Prescription Assistance Program is the Manufacturer-Sponsored Discount Cards which patients can receive from the state government, retail pharmacies and other organizations. Many of these cards were originally marketed to the senior population, but the focus has expanded to the uninsured population. The only qualification is being uninsured for prescription coverage and having income at somewhere between 200 and 400% of the federal poverty level. Discounts vary from as little as a 15% discount, to as much as 60% discount off of the retail price. Discount cards can be free or can have a fee attached to them. For example, AARP offers a free or low-cost discount drug card to its members, which tends to provide an average of a 20% discount on pharmaceuticals for a fee of $19.95 (http://www.aarp.org, 2009). In addition, some of the discounts have conditions attached to them, such as only available through mail order services, must have 3 months prescriptions at a time, as well as other annual renewal fees, which may outweigh the cost savings. (http://www.needymeds.com, 2009).

Other community interventions to provide medication assistance for the uninsured come in the forms of grants and contributions. Not only do grant opportunities arise that will fund prescription assistance, relationships with community private physicians and organizations can provide help. Many Community Health Centers have "sample partnerships" with private practice physicians, who regularly provide extra manufacturers' samples for patients without insurance. At times, samples can provide the entire course of treatment or at least, serve as a bridge until a prescription assistance program application can be completed and approved. Other private practices of various specialties may be, resources to contact when a certain medication is needed, that a particular medical practice may have. For example, for cardiac and blood pressure medications, the local groups of cardiologists may be willing partners for needed samples.

Innovative Programs and Initiatives

With the extensive process required to apply and qualify individual uninsured patients for the various prescription assistance programs, large community health centers as well as many community hospitals and governmental organizations are looking for opportunities to simplify the process, as well as expand the medication safety net for uninsured and low income individuals. Some examples include:

- *Communicare* – Located in South Carolina, it involves a network of physicians who see uninsured patients at no charge. In order to assure that prescriptions needed are filled, they have negotiated agreements with some drug manufacturers to donate free medications. The network of physicians is approximately 2,300 and they see approximately 15,000 patients annually across the state. They have been operating a central pharmacy that dispenses the donated medications by mail to patients' homes, physician offices, or clinics. The patients must be uninsured and have incomes below 200% of the federal poverty guidelines.
- *Kaiser Medicare Drug Benefit Calculator* – Kaiser Network provides a Medicare drug benefit calculator online, which was designed in 2006 to help determine out of pocket costs for a variety of Medicare drug plans. Low income beneficiaries can also assess their additional benefits. Although this has not been updated to reflect accurate out of pocket costs, Medicare now provides a "Medicare Prescription Drug Plan Finder" at http://www.medicare.gov (2008) to compare plans (http://www.kaisernetwork.org, 2008).
- *RxPartnership* – Initiated in 2003, with funding from the Virginia Health Care Foundation to make free prescriptions available for participating free health centers and clinics in Virginia. GlaxoSmithKline was the first company to join the partnership and has provided over $3.8 million in free prescriptions to uninsured Virginians.
- *Central Louisiana Medication Access Program (CMAP)* – Opened in 2001, to provide medication assistance and education for uninsured rural poor. All prescriptions are somewhere between $3 and $15 per prescription and includes the pharmacist visit. The medications are funded through pharmaceutical companies. The initial 2 years enrolled 5,307 patients and they received over 140,000 prescriptions at a cost savings of greater than $2.5 million.
- *MEDBANK* – Since 2001, has connected patients to a variety of PAPs and in the first 5 years helped nearly 35,000 patients with over 400,000 prescriptions and medications worth over $100 million. Eligibility for one person is a minimum of $926.01 with those having lower incomes referred to state Medicaid. They cannot have a source of medication coverage. This program has been replicated in New Mexico.
- *PatientAssistance.com* – This new Web site can find over 1,000 different PAPs for patients to choose from, with the medications listed and eligibility requirements. The Web site is totally free of charge and patients can build their own medication profiles with reminders for reordering dates.

Another concern with medication assistance and management of the uninsured and under-served as mentioned earlier, are the challenges around language, education, and health literacy. Although medications may be made available through various low cost resources, healthcare professionals need to ascertain that the individual or caregiver understands the dosage of the medication, the rationale for the prescription, the possible side effects, and the length of duration for the prescription medication. The diverse cultures and backgrounds of the United States can lead to stopping medications prior to completion, not understanding the concept of "refills" and dosing the medications incorrectly. Many health centers are developing simple medication educational handouts in various languages with pictures, as well as making follow up telephone calls or home visits to check on medication adherence to the prescriptions provided. Currently, a nurse with a pediatric home care agency serving the uninsured and low income, observed the lack of adherence as well as the various errors made by parents in caring for chronically ill children at home. This led to the development of medication education tools that include pictures, audiotapes, and color coding of various medication bottles, syringes, and tubes, prepared for the parents. Consequently, the nurses experienced less follow up visits to the home for medication errors and questions (Jones 2009). The provision of necessary prescription medications may sometimes just be the beginning of improving health for the uninsured in our communities.

Best Practices Guidelines for Medication Assistance for the Uninsured

There are currently many resources available to assist the uninsured in accessing needed prescriptions, whether for a short course of therapy or on an ongoing basis for chronic conditions. The best practices for communities in addressing the needs of the uninsured, suggest having a multitude of strategies and resources in place to assure ongoing treatment. These multiple strategies and resources can assist with making sure diabetic patients are well-managed, children with asthma have consistent use of needed inhalers, patients with infections are treated early and complete a full course of medication, along with many other care scenarios. These multiple strategies and resources should include:

- Access to PAPs electronically, and the human resources to assist patients with applications and re-enrollment as needed, being cognizant of the complexity as well as literacy and language challenges for some patients.
- Awareness of various community programs, Web sites, PAPs for generic medications and retail discount programs to ensure patient access to the most cost effective prescriptions.
- Knowledge of local and regional 340B Programs and methods of patient referrals and/or innovative program collaborations.
- Relationships with local private physicians with access to samples for uninsured patient scenarios that may arise, along with regular donations of samples.
- Ongoing grant and contribution development to establish unrestricted funds for patients with emergency prescriptions and other medication needs.

- Ongoing program management to identify and monitor the numbers and demographics of patients in need of prescription assistance, as well as the various strategies employed, most needed classes of medications and the success of the strategies (Table 2).

Table 2 Application for prescription assistance

Application *for* Free
AstraZeneca Medicines
PO Box 66551, St. Louis, MO, 63166-6551

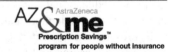

Prescription Savings™
program for people without insurance

What is the AZ&Me Prescription Savings™ program for people without insurance?

- The AZ&Me Prescription Savings program for people without insurance (the Program) is a program offered by AstraZeneca that allows you to get free medicines if you qualify. It is not a government program or an insurance plan.

- If you qualify, you will get free medicine for up to one year. At the end of that year, AstraZeneca will send you an application for renewal.

- Most medicines will be sent to your home. Some medicines will be sent to your doctor's office.

- Most medicines are sent in a 90-day supply.

The Program can be changed or stopped by AstraZeneca at any time or for any reason.

Who is AstraZeneca?

- AstraZeneca is a company that makes prescription medicines.

- AstraZeneca has offered prescription savings programs to people who qualify since 1978.

Do you qualify for the Program?

You probably qualify for the Program if:

- You don't have other insurance that helps pay for your medicines.

- You meet the income limits in the table below.

How do you get started?

- Fill out this application.

- If you have trouble filling out this application, call 1-800-424-3727

- Mail the completed application to:
  PO Box 66551
  St. Louis, MO, 63166-6551

Income limits in order to qualify

Current income limits are based on 2007 program guidelines and might change; income limits may be higher in Alaska and Hawaii.

No. of people in your household	Total monthly income	Total yearly income
1 person	less than $2,500 a month	less than $30,000 a year
2 people	less than $3,333 a month	less than $40,000 a year
3 people	less than $4,166 a month	less than $50,000 a year
4 people	less than $5,000 a month	less than $60,000 a year
5 people	less than $5,833 a month	less than $70,000 a year

eset Fields

From Your Doctor *Please print clearly in black or blue ink.*

Doctor's Name:_____ Phone ( )_____

DEA or State License # (ask your doctor) _____ Fax ( )_____

Address _____

City_____ State _____ Zip _____

[ ] *Include prescription with this application*

Questions? Call 1-800-424-3727 or visit www.azandme.com

Personal Information

Name _____ Date of Birth ___/___/_____ (mm/dd/yyyy)

Address_____ City_____ State_____ Zip_____

Phone ( ) _____ ☐ Male ☐ Female

Marital status:
☐ Married
☐ Single
☐ Divorced
☐ Widow/Widower

U.S. Veteran:
☐ Yes   ☐ No

Disabled:
☐ Yes   ☐ No

Primary language spoken (optional):
☐ English
☐ Spanish
☐ Other_____

Ethnic origin (optional):
☐ Asian
☐ Black
☐ Hispanic
☐ White
☐ Other_____

Please provide your **Social Security Number** if you have one.
This information will only be used to determine if you are eligible and once qualified as described below.

☐ ☐ ☐ — ☐ ☐ — ☐ ☐ ☐ ☐

If you don't have a Social Security Number you must provide
one of the following:

☐ Green Card Number _____

☐ A copy of the confirmation letter from the government stating that
you have applied for a US Green Card

☐ Work Visa Number _____

Medicines

List any medicines you are **taking**:

_____

_____

_____

_____

List any medicines you are
allergic to:

_____

_____

_____

_____

Attach a separate piece of paper if you need more space.

Questions? Call 1-800-424-3727 or visit www.azandme.com

Insurance

Do you have any form of prescription drug coverage?

☐ Employer furnished or private drug coverage

☐ VA or Military Benefits

☐ Medicaid

☐ Medicare Part B (covers some medicines)

☐ Medicare Part D

☐ State assistance program for medicines_____

☐ Other _____

☐ None

Have you applied for Medicaid in the past and been denied?

☐ Yes   ☐ No   *If yes, please attach a copy of the Medicaid denial letter.*

Income

Number of people in your household
*(yourself, your spouse, and dependents):*_____

Total combined income for yourself, your spouse, and dependents:

$_____ Monthly   **or** $_____ Yearly

Proof of Income

Do you have a copy of your federal income tax return from last year?

YES

Please send us a copy of last year's **Federal Income Tax Returns** for yourself, your spouse, and dependents

NO

If you didn't file a federal income tax return last year, you **must** send a copy of:

☐ All income statements from jobs (W2 or 1099)

or

☐ Social Security Income Yearly Benefits Statement

If you don't have any of these documents, please call 1-800-424-3727

Questions? Call 1-800-424-3727 or visit www.azandme.com

Consent Information

I **give** AstraZeneca, the Program, the Program administrators, and my doctor permission to:

- Check my information to make sure it is true and complete
- Share my information with the pharmacists that may supply my medicine
- Share my information with the people helping with the Program
- Contact me by mail or phone about the Program and about other products, programs, or services that might interest me
- Contact me in order to make sure that I have received the medicines sent by the Program

I **promise** that:

- All the information in this application, including all copies of documents proving my income, is true and complete
- I am authorized to sign this application
- I do not have any assistance or insurance that would help pay for my medicines
- I will contact the Program if any of my information about my prescription drug coverage or insurance changes

I **understand** that the Program will only use my information to:

- Decide if I qualify to participate in the Program
- Administer or improve the Program
- Communicate with insurance plans, including Medicare Part D plans
- Share my information with the Centers for Medicare and Medicaid Services

I **understand** that I can call 1-800-424-3727 at any time to:

- Withdraw from the Program
- Cancel my permission to use my information and withdraw from the Program
- Get a copy of the AstraZeneca Privacy Statement

I **understand** that:

- The Program can ask for more information from me at any time
- AstraZeneca can change or stop the Program at any time or for any reason

I **give** the Program, and the Program administrators permission to contact the person named below with follow-up questions about my application (this only applies if someone completed this application for you).

Signature of Applicant or Legal Guardian

X_____ Date_____

If someone helped you with this application, and you want them to answer questions for you, please give us their name and phone number.
Helper's Name:_____ Helper's Phone: (____)_____

Before you mail this application

You must:

- ☐ Attach your prescription
- ☐ Attach a copy of last year's federal income tax returns for yourself, spouse, and dependents (or other proof of income)
- ☐ Include your doctor's license number (ask your doctor)

Mail completed application to:

AZ&Me Prescription Savings Program
PO Box 66551
St. Louis, MO 63166-6551

Questions? Call 1-800-424-3727 or visit www.azandme.com

AZ&Me Prescription Savings is a trademark of the AstraZeneca group of Companies.
©2007 AstraZeneca LP. All rights reserved. 255057 9/07

References

Agency for Health Research and Quality (2008) Available at http://www.ahrq.gov

Center for Medicare and Medicaid (2008) Available at http://www.medicare.gov

Chrisholm MA, Reinhardt BO, Vollenweider LJ, Kendrick BD, Dipiro JT (2000) Medication assistance reports: medication assistance programs for uninsured and Indigent patients. Am J Health Syst Pharm 57(12):1131–1136

El Rio Community Health Center (2007) Interview with Arthur Martinez, MD, Medical Director

Harmon GN, Lefante J, Roy W, Ashby K, Jackson D, Barnard D, Smart A, Webber L (2004) Outpatient medication assistance program in a rural setting. Am J Health Syst Pharm 61(6):603–607

HRSA Pharmacy Services Support Center (2009) http://www.aphanet.org

Johnson R (1997) The effect of increased prescription drug cost sharing on medical care utilization and expenses of elderly health maintenance organization members. Med Care 35(11):1119–1131

Jones L (2009) Unpublished paper: improving parental education with medications in the home through health literacy assessments, pp 1–21

Kaiser Network (2008) Available at http://www.kaisernetwork.org

National Council on Aging (2009) Available at http://www.ncoa.org

Patient Assistance (2008) Available at http://www.patientassistance.org

PhRMA, Pharmaceutical Industry Profile (2007) Available at http://www.phrma.rog/files/profile/2007

Resources for Prescription Medications (2009) http://www.needymeds.com

Schur CL, Doty MM, Berk ML (2004) Lack of prescription drug coverage among the under 65: A symptom of underinsurance. Issue brief, Task force on the future of health insurance, The commonwealth fund

St. Elizabeth's Health Center (2008) Interview with Estela Garcia, RN, Director of Nursing

Vaccines for Children (2009) http://www.cdc.gov

Zerzan J (2004) Oregon's medically needy program survey. Summary report, Available at http://www.oregon.gov/DAS/OHPPR/RSCH/docs/medicallyneedy.pdf. Accessed April 1, 2009

Medically Uninsured Refugees and Immigrants

Lane P. Johnson

Lola and Raul Rodriquez, and their 16 year old daughter Lolita, immigrated legally to the US from Peru in the mid 1990s, following their son, Raul, who had come alone earlier and who had permanent residency status. Raul, Sr., 50, a professor at a dental school in Peru, spoke very little English. He helped Lola in caring for children at their home. When Raul had a heart attack 3 years later, they had no insurance. The cardiologist waived his fee and continued to follow Raul for free, but they continued paying $50 a month to the hospital for many years, and struggled to buy his five daily medications.

Eventually, Lola found work supervising at a commercial cleaning business, but still did not have insurance. Raul began work as a caretaker for the elderly, with an agency. They have both become American citizens; now make too much money to be eligible for Medicaid, and still do not have insurance through their work. They are hoping to have enough eligible quarters of work to be eligible for Medicare when Raul retires.

Background

Despite the fact that in the United States, 99% of the population are either immigrants or their descendents, immigration remains one of the most divisive and difficult political issues in contemporary American society. During the 1990s, over one million immigrants entered the United States each year from other countries. Immigration reforms enacted in 1996, and further restrictions following the terrorist attacks of 9/11/2001 have made it more difficult for people from other countries to immigrate to the United States. Nonetheless large numbers of immigrants continue to enter the US each year, and diverse immigrant populations represent an increasingly greater percentage of people in the US (Table 1).

L.P. Johnson
Arizona Health Sciences Center, Tucson, AZ, USA
e-mail: lpj@email.arizona.edu

N.J. Johnson and L.P. Johnson (eds.), *The Care of the Uninsured in America*,
DOI 10.1007/978-0-387-78309-3_9, © Springer Science+Business Media, LLC 2010

Table 1 Percent of foreign-born in the US by region of their birth (2003)

Central America (includes Mexico)	36.9%
Europe	37%
Asia	25%
Caribbean	10.1%
South America	6.3%
Other Regions	8%

Larson (2004)

Statistics suggest that legal and illegal immigrants provide a far more positive economic effect, and a far less negative health impact than immigration critics would admit. Nonetheless, immigrant populations make up about 25% of the medically uninsured in the United States; and 70% of immigrants lack health insurance. This represents a significant impact on the US health system. While current federal policies are mostly directed at restricting health services to immigrants, there are a number of state and local efforts to increase health services to these populations. *Legal Immigrants* are people who have attained citizenship, have permanent resident (green card) status, have a temporary residency status (amnesty), or temporary protected status due to civil conflict or natural disaster in their home county, or are refugees or asylees.

Refugees apply to come to the United States from another country, to which they have fled from their home country. After being in the United States for a year, they are eligible for permanent resident status, and may seek citizenship after 5 years. Asylees have been granted political asylum once they have entered the United States, having left their home country due to fear of persecution. They are usually eligible for citizenship within 1 year.

Non-immigrant foreign nationals are granted visa for study or work. They must claim they do not intend to stay in the United States permanently, and can demonstrate an ability to support themselves (Morales 2007).

Demographics

Over the history of the United States, waves of immigrants have come to the US for educational and economic opportunities; fleeing religious persecution, political and social unrest, or personal danger. Immigrants represent a diverse mix of social, cultural, political, economic, geographic, religious, and health backgrounds. Over the years, many immigrants and immigrant populations have acculturated in the melting pot, while many others have not.

In 2005 new immigrants (not native born) represented approximately 36 million people, or 12% of the US population. This percentage has doubled since 2000, and shows no sign of decreasing (Derose et al. 2007). During the 1990s almost one million persons immigrated legally each year, and another 200,000–300,000 illegally (including those who overstayed legal visas). The number of refugees allowed in the United States, however, has decreased. Despite expanding numbers of refugees globally, only 30,000 were allowed to enter the US in 2007 (Morales 2007)

About 1/3 of immigrants are in each of the three principal legal status groups (naturalized citizens, legal permanent residents and undocumented immigrants). Current immigration policy that places more restrictions and delays than in the past, means that the number of undocumented immigrants is likely to continue to increase (Derose et al. 2007).

The distribution of the foreign-born population (especially from Latin America and Asia) are predominantly in the Western United States (37.3% of foreign-born vs. 21% of the native population). Almost 45% of the foreign-born population live in a central city in a metropolitan area, compared with about 27% of the native population. The percentage of foreign-born living in non-metropolitan areas is significantly less than the percentage of natives (5.3% vs. 20.2%)(Larson 2004).

The age distribution of the foreign-born population in the US in 2003, between the ages of 18–64, was 80% compared to 60% of the native born population in this age group. The percentage of foreign-born, over the age of 65 is about the same as native born (11.1 vs. 12.1). The percentage of foreign-born, less than 18 years of age, is 8.9% compared to 27.8% of native born. This may be due to the children of foreign-born adults being born in the US (Larson 2004).

Over 16% of the foreign-born population in 2002 were living in poverty compared to 11.5% of the native born population. The poverty rate is highest for foreign-born populations from Central America (23.6%), Latin America (21.6%), and the Caribbean (18.9%); intermediate for foreign born populations from South America (14.5%) and Other Regions (14.1%); and lowest for foreign-born populations from Asia (11.1%) and Europe (8.7%) (Larson 2004).

About 5 million immigrants are in the labor force working predominately in construction, the restaurant industry, and agriculture. About 50% of new labor force growth in the US in the last two decades, is new immigrants (Morales 2007). It is estimated that immigrants add about $10 billion to the US economy each year. Social Security reports that workers without a valid Social Security number contribute $8.5 billion to Social Security and Medicare annually. A 1998 study by the National Academy of Science, concludes that the average immigrant pays $80,000 more in taxes than they consume in government services over a lifetime (Bahadur 2000).

The Personal Responsibility and Work Opportunity Reconciliation Act (PRWORA), the 1996 welfare reform bill, have made most legal immigrants ineligible for public funded services such as Medicaid for the first 5 years of residency, although states can provide eligibility by fully funding services. Undocumented immigrants are ineligible for publicly funded services (Derose et al. 2007). This act also required medical examination and immunization for immigrants, and those seeking asylum. These exams must be performed by designated Civil Surgeons certified by the Bureau of Citizenship and Immigration Services (BCIS) (Morales 2007). This exam is usually not covered by medical insurance (if the immigrant has it) and can cost upward of $500.

Immigrant's access to health care resources is directly or indirectly related to educational attainment, type of occupation and earnings, and proficiency in speaking English. Immigrants are less likely to have graduated from secondary school, more likely to work in service occupations, and more likely to live in poverty, though this is less true for immigrants from Asia and Africa, in contrast to immigrants from Mexico or Central America (Derose et al. 2007). Legal status, health beliefs, trust of the system and providers, and financial issues all effect immigrant access to health care in the United States.

New immigrants and their children make up about ¼ of the nations uninsured. Most are legal immigrants (Appleby 2000).

Health Status

In addition to the issues that can affect immigrant access to health care, there are a number of factors that can affect immigrant's health status directly.

Diseases that are prevalent in their home country must be a primary consideration. These include infectious diseases such as tuberculosis, HIV, hepatitis, parasitic diseases, malaria, and rheumatic heart disease. There may (or may not) be a greater likelihood of lack of immunization. Environmental conditions such as elevated lead level, respiratory disease, and malnutrition are also common. Immigrants and their families may travel back and forth to their country of origin and contribute to the spread of these conditions in that way.

Health beliefs and culture can also affect health. Immigrants may use traditional healing methodologies in lieu of, or in addition to standard health measures. The use of medications available without a prescription in the immigrant's home country (such as antibiotics), medications banned or considered dangerous in the US (Refecoxib, a painkiller), and adulterated or contaminated traditional remedies (Chinese traditional remedies have been found to contain heavy metals, steroids, or actual pharmaceutical products) have all been found.

Diet, exercise, sexual practices, and other cultural beliefs may have either good or bad effects on health, based on US standards. Immigrant families and communities may be closely tied, providing a source of support and caring, but also increasing stress by the added responsibility of caring for ones' relatives or others in the community (Morales 2007).

Of particular concern in immigrant populations are issues of mental health. By definition, immigrants are leaving home and relatives to come to a new country where they have to learn to deal with a new language, culture, social isolation, poverty, and are often at the bottom of the social strata, no matter how successful they may have been in their home country.

For refugees and asylees this situation may be exacerbated by conditions of violence, intimidation, rape, torture, or other horrors they escaped in their home country. They may have relatives and friends left behind, whom they cannot help or even find out how they are faring.

Coupled with this is a lack of cultural competency in the mainstream of community mental health services, along with a paucity of publicly funded services, that add to immigrant fear, and lack of trust of government health services in general (Mutaner 2006).

Anne Fadiman's book *The Spirit Catches You and You Fall Down*, is a poignant picture of the clash of the medical culture in the United States with an Immigrant population (Fadiman 1998)

Despite all the negative factors associated with immigrant health and lack of access to health services, some studies suggest that many immigrants, because they are often younger and coming to the United States to work, are relatively healthy and experience better health outcomes (less morbidity and mortality; both adult and infant) than similar populations in the United States (Derose et al. 2007; Morales 2007).

The perception that the US health care system is over-utilized by immigrant populations is also questionable. Immigration critics claim widespread hospital closings are the result of hoards of immigrants crowding in to emergency rooms, that so called "anchor babies" are the foundation of generations of immigrants taking advantage of the health and welfare system, and that the United States will soon be overwhelmed by fatal diseases (such as polio, cholera, or Typhoid fever), thought long gone in the US, but teeming within immigrant populations (Cosman 2005). Far right political invective continues to fuel the anti-immigrant fire, and make real reform even more unlikely (Schepers 2007).

Studies have suggested that immigrant per capita health care expenditures are 55% lower than US born citizens, uninsured and publicly insured immigrants have half the health related expenditures, and immigrant children have 74% per capita health expenditures than US born children. Emergency department expenditures, however, are 3 times higher for immigrant children (Mohanty et al. 2005). Specific reasons for this are debatable; it is likely both a combination of avoidance of the health care system due to issues outlined above, as well as financial, cultural, and other issues. Increased emergent expenditures suggest delay of care as well as a lack of insurance.

The concerns regarding immigrant use of hospitals have led to ethically questionable practices on the part of some hospitals. At least one Southwest hospital has a policy of busing or sending by air, Hispanic immigrants to the Mexican border once they have been stabilized in the Emergency room per EMTALA regulations. What is not clear is whether these patients have clearly been determined to be illegal immigrants, or if they are only from Mexico. It also appears claims of uncompensated care may be wildly inflated by utilizing full billing costs of services, and not including cash payments made by, or on the behalf of, immigrant patients (Lee 2009).

This same hospital has also been accused of telling illegal immigrants if they do not pay their hospital bills, the hospital will provide their demographic information to the immigration authorities (Lopes 2008).

A recent series of articles in the New York Times further documents repatriation practices by hospitals across the country These programs remain furtive, with some high profile cases of neglect shining a light on the practice. There are varying degrees of coordination between the treating hospital and the immigrant's home facilities prior to repatriation (Sontag 2008).

In contrast, some hospitals continue to make an effort to acknowledge both the need and a responsibility, to provide appropriate accessible continuous care for patients without consideration of their national origin. Lee Memorial Hospital System in Florida emphasizes a community-based approach, with a community coordinator to work with community providers to obtain subsidized prescriptions, social work services, rehabilitation, outpatient services, and beds at local shelters (Lee 2009).

Programs

Since the 1996 welfare reform law denied Medicaid eligibility to most new immigrants, a number of states and communities have developed programs to try to assist immigrant access health care locally (Sherman 1999). Nearly 22 states and the District of Columbia used state or other funds to provide at least some services to legal immigrants. Some states have also provided services to illegal immigrants; primarily women and children. These efforts have been effective in lowering the uninsured rate among immigrants in these states (Kaiser Commission on Medicaid and the Uninsured 2004).

One of the local alliances, in Alameda County, California attempted to provide affordable medical, dental, vision, pharmacy, and alternative health services through premium payments by enrollees. The "No Wrong Door" project used health promoters providing community outreach to help immigrants travel the bureaucratic jungle of enrollment through a variety of programs that could provide coverage (Morales 2007). What this, and other programs, have discovered, is that these local or regional programs are financially unfeasible without federal support (Hirota et al. 2006).

A federal, comprehensive bipartisan immigration reform proposal in 2007, that proposed a guest worker program and a path for citizenship, along with tougher border and workplace security, went absolutely nowhere, felled by backroom agreements prior to debate, and an inability to overcome far right efforts to defeat it (Schepers 2007; Associated Press 2007).

While the new Administration has provided at least some rhetoric on immigration reform, and with it, immigrant health reform, immigration will likely take a back seat to the economic crisis (Boston.com 2009). The current divisive political climate makes it less likely that the federal government will be able to broker improving the situation for supporting immigrant health care, any time in the near future.

Nor is it likely that overall, the influx of immigrants and refugees to the US will decrease, although the current economic crisis and anti-immigration legislation is causing some changes. Recent anti-immigrant legislation enacted in Arizona has resulted both in a manpower shortage in the agriculture, restaurant, landscape, and construction industries, as well as a significant negative impact on local businesses, and apartments and rental properties, as even long time immigrants have returned home (Howley 2008).The ferocity of this continued struggle in a land of immigrants is ironic, to say the least.

References

Appleby J (2000) Studies look at issues immigrants, insurance. USA Today, July 18, 2000

Associated Press (2007) Immigration bill suffers major defeat in Senate. Available at http://www.msnbc.msn.com/id/19475868/. Accessed 29 Mar, 2009

Bahadur G (2000) Immigrant medical coverage is lacking, Austin American-Statesman July 19, 2000

Boston.com (2009) Obama puts immigration reform on docket. Available at http://www.boston.com/news/nation/articles/2009/03/19/obama_puts_immigration_reform_on_docket/. Accessed 29 Mar 2009

Cosman MP (2005) Illegal aliens and American medicine. J Am Phys Surg 10:1, Spring:6–10

Derose KP, Escarce JJ, Lurie N (2007) Immigrants and health care: sources of vulnerability, Health Affairs 26:5 Sept/Oct 2007 1258–1268

Fadiman A (1998) The spirit catches you and you fall down. Farrrar Straus and Giroux, New York

Hirota S, Garcia J et al (2006) Inclusion of immigrant families in US health coverage expansions. J Health Care Poor Uninsured 17(1 Supplement):81–94

Howley K (2008) The one-man wall. Reason on-line. Available at http://www.reason.com/news/show/128890.html. Accessed 29 Mar 2009

Kaiser Commission on Medicaid and the Uninsured (2004) Covering new Americans: a review of federal and state policies related to immigrant's eligibility and access to publicly funded health insurance. Available at http://www.kff.org/medicaid/upload/Covering-New-Americans-A-Review-of-Federal-and-State-Policies-Related-to-Immigrants-Eligibility-and-Access-to-Publicly-Funded-Health-Insurance-Report.pdf. Accessed 28 Mar 2009

Larson LJ (2004) The foreign-born population in the United States, 2003. Current Population Reports U.S. Census Bureau, Washington, DC. Available at http://www.census.gov/prod/2004pubs/p20-551.pdf. Accessed 28 Mar 2009

Lee M (2009) Local, State, National and International Immigrant Health Care Policy. Unpublished Master's in Public Health Internship Report, University of Arizona College of Medicine, March, 2009

Lopes P (2008) Arizona State Representative District XX, Personal Communication, February, 2008

Mohanty SA, Woolhandler S, Himmelstein DH, Pati S, Carrasquillo OH, Bor D (2005) Health care expenditures of immigrants in the United States: a nationally representative analysis. Am J Public Health 95(8):1431–1438

Morales S (2007) Immigrant health issues. In: Medical management of vulnerable and underserved patients, McGraw Hill, New York, pp 255–264, Chapter 25

Mutaner C, Geiger-Brown J (2006) Mental Health. In: Levy BS, Sidel VW (eds) Social injustice and public health. Oxford University Press, pp 277–293, Chapter 16

Schepers E (2007) What happened to immigration reform? politicalaffairs.net. Available at: http://www.politicalaffairs.net/article/view/5578/1/272/. Accessed 28 Mar 2009

Sherman R (1999) Unfinished business: the restoration of immigrant health access after welfare reform. States Health 9:1–8

Sontag D (2008) Immigrants facing deportation by US hospital. New York Times. Available at http://www.nytimes.com/2008/08/03/us/03deport.html?scp=1&sq=Immigrants%20deportation%20sontag&st=cse. Accessed 28 Mar 2009

Medically Uninsured and the Homeless

Jennifer Vanderleest

Alice Crowley is a 34 year old who lives out of her car. She lost her house 2 years ago when her boyfriend left her and she could no longer afford their apartment. She lives by herself; her 4 year old daughter child was taken by Child Protective Services. She gets an occasional meal at one of the homeless centers, and on really cold nights will sleep in the center, but doesn't like to go there. She panhandles sometimes, but doesn't like how people look at her, or give her a hard time. Most of the time she eats what she can find in dumpsters behind grocery stores and fast food restaurants late at night. She sleeps most of the day because of her night-time foraging.

Ms. Crowley has no medical insurance. She has not had the documentation she needs to apply for Medicaid, and doesn't really have the energy or ability to try to find what she might need.

She has diabetes, but rarely has money for medication. She has been told she should be on insulin, but doesn't have refrigeration so can't store it. When she has had needles they have been stolen. She receives care at one of the community health centers, but really does not like to go there. People stare at her and move away from her because she can't shower regularly. She often doesn't have the gas to make her appointments; she has missed so many appointments the clinic is threatening to kick her out.

She feels terrible most of the time, is depressed and considers suicide sometimes, but doesn't have the energy or gas to go to the mental health center. Her regular physician is not able to prescribe psychiatric medication, and she is not sure she could afford it if he did.

Background

Homelessness is a significant social issue in the USA. It affects people of every race, ethnicity, age, gender, sexual orientation, and geographic location. Homeless patients are members of the medically underserved populations. There are multiple

---

J. Vanderleest
Department of Family and Community Medicine, Arizona AIDS Education and Training Center; Institute for LGBT Studies, University of Arizona, Tucson, AZ, USA

N.J. Johnson and L.P. Johnson (eds.), *The Care of the Uninsured in America*,   153
DOI 10.1007/978-0-387-78309-3_10, © Springer Science+Business Media, LLC 2010

issues faced by those who want to work with these diverse populations and provide appropriate care both culturally and medically. The following is a review of key issues to be considered when providing services to the homeless people.

Defining homelessness is difficult and is fraught with political and societal implications. Historical epidemiologic studies used different definitions. Perhaps because of the varied definitions, data generated from studies have often been discordant. The United States Federal Government, under the McKinney-Vento Act of 1987, has attempted to operationalize homelessness by providing the following definition:

A homeless individual is someone who lacks a fixed, regular, and adequate nighttime residence, or who has a primary night residence that is:

1. A supervised publicly or privately operated shelter designated to provide temporary living accommodations, OR
2. A public/private place that provides a temporary residence for individuals intended to be institutionalized, OR
3. A public/private place not designed for or ordinarily used as regular human sleeping accommodations. (National Coalition for the Homeless 2007a)

While this more standardized definition is helpful, it still remains difficult to get accurate statistics on who and how many are homeless. There are logistical problems in finding people in remote locations, living in motels, cars, caves, etc. or identifying the "hidden homeless," those staying with friends (temporarily doubled up). In addition, political motivations may minimize or exaggerate the number of individuals facing homelessness in any given community.

Demographics

Despite the difficulties noted above, national statistics suggest that 2% of the U.S. population or over 3.5 million people are homeless each year (National Coalition for the Homeless 2007a). Of those individuals, approximately a quarter are considered chronically (long-term or repeatedly) homeless. The majority of homeless are single individuals; however, 41% are families with children (National Coalition for the Homeless 2007a). A snapshot of urban homelessness in 2007 generated from data from 23 cities showed that single men accounted for 67.5%, single women 32.5%, and unaccompanied minors 2% (U.S. Conference of Mayors 2007). Groups of youth disproportionately affected by housing instability include sexual minority and transgender identified youth and those leaving foster care (Cochran et al. 2002). The National Coalition for the Homeless (NCH) estimates that the national homeless population is 42% African American, 30% Caucasian, 13% Hispanic, 4% Native American, and 2% Asian (National Coalition for the Homeless 2007a). Military veterans are disproportionately homeless, accounting for 23–40% of homeless population while they are approximately 10% of the general population (National Coalition for the Homeless 2007a).

Another source suggests that an estimated 637,000 adults are homeless in a given week and 2.1 million adults are homeless over the course of a year in the USA. These figures increase to 842,000 and 3.5 million when children are included. An estimated 55% of homeless people do not have health insurance. Twenty-four percent of the homeless in the USA needed medical attention in the last year and were unable to get it. The majority of the homeless (about 60%) are not eligible for public health insurance in most states because they are not pregnant, disabled, elderly, or do not have dependent children (Robert Wood Johnson Medical School Uninsured in America 2008).

Homelessness occurs for multiple reasons, but the NCH suggests that there are two trends largely responsible for the rise in homelessness over the past 25 years in the USA – increasing poverty and a growing shortage of affordable housing. (National Alliance to End Homelessness 2007a; National Coalition for the Homeless 2007a). Direct causes of homelessness include poverty, lack of affordable housing, low incomes that fail to keep pace with housing costs, and long waiting lists for housing subsidies. In addition, unemployment, personal or family life crises, and reductions in public benefits can lead to financial turmoil and eventually to homelessness. Indirect causes include substance abuse, mental illness, intimate partner violence, pregnancy, prisoner re-entry, and again a lack of needed services to respond to these issues (Gelberg et al. 1997; Kushel et al. 2006; National Coalition for the Homeless 2007b). In the most recent survey by the U.S. Conference of Mayors, over 50% of those surveyed reported that their cities are not meeting the need for providing adequate shelter for homeless persons and that people are turned away some or all of the time (Singer 2003).

In 2008, an estimated 2.2 million foreclosure actions have been initiated in the U.S. The effects of adding potentially millions of Americans, particularly families, to the ranks of the homeless could completely overwhelm an already overburdened system, and further dilute programs for the chronically homeless (Urban Institute 2009).

Health Status

The Institute of Medicine stated that "poor health causes homelessness, and homelessness causes poor health" (Institute of Medicine 1988). It is important to remember that while people who are homeless may have any type of medical or psychiatric illnesses, specific situations unique to homelessness confer health-related risk. Lack of food and/or water, poor hygiene, residing in unsanitary conditions, infestations, sleeping in an upright position, exposure to heat and cold, and extensive walking often in poorly fitting shoes all can cause or worsen a variety of medical problems. Homeless individuals are also exposed to higher levels of health risk through lack of personal security, overcrowded living conditions, and disproportionately high rates of tobacco, alcohol, and drug use. Upper respiratory infections are the most commonly noted diagnoses for adults and children, followed by trauma, skin conditions, and infestations in adults (Kidder et al. 2007; Kushel et al.

2001; Levy and O'Connell 2004; Martens 2001; Singer 2003). In children, immunization delay, iron deficiency, ear disorders, and elevated blood lead are the top five diagnoses. Many homeless people do not receive routine preventive health care, for example, screening for a variety of malignancies (Chau et al. 2002). Chronic medical illness such as heart disease, stroke, hypertension, and COPD also disproportionately affect the homeless. Oral health and lack of dental hygiene can lead to worsened health care outcomes as well (Institute of Medicine 1988). Sexually transmitted infections, including HIV and hepatitis, tuberculin skin test positivity and tuberculosis, mental illness and substance dependence, and abuse are also important health-associated concerns (Kidder et al. 2007; Kushel et al. 2001; Levy and O'Connell 2004; Martens 2001; Singer 2003).

Higher emergency room use and hospitalization rates result from the lack of primary care. Homeless children have twice the hospital admission rate than children who are not homeless. Homeless adults have an admission rate 4–5 times greater than adults who are not homeless (Robert Wood Johnson Medical School Uninsured in America 2008).

Compared to housed, age-matched controls, homeless persons have almost four times the mortality rate with a median age of death from 40 to 47 years (Kushel and Sharad 2007).

There are numerous barriers to medical care for homeless people. One significant point that may be difficult for health providers to understand, is that individuals who are homeless have multiple competing needs, so health care is important on an urgent or emergent basis (Gelberg et al. 1997). This is not to say that there are not homeless men and women who are interested in staying healthy and controlling their chronic illnesses. Another issue for many homeless people is that they have no regular source of care. In one survey, only 16% had consistent care (Gallagher et al. 1997). This is not solely attributable to lack of insurance; mental illness, substance use, any associated cost (e.g., co-pays), and transportation difficulties are also listed as significant barriers.

Homeless people will often state that it is difficult to simply survive or that they are "living in survival mode." For example, fear of leaving a home territory for reasons of personal safety or fear of personal belonging theft can make it more likely for people not to travel to keep appointments (Gelberg et al. 1997). Apprehension of interaction with or reporting to persons of authority including police, immigration or Child Protective Services may make it less likely for people to access care as well. In addition, homeless individuals may have a different time orientation, making it difficult to keep appointments. Finally, patients may feel embarrassed about personal hygiene, or have anxiety about any cost (real or perceived) that can be associated with limited financial resources (Kushel et al. 2006).

Unfortunately, medical facilities and providers themselves may pose multiple barriers to homeless persons seeking to access care (Bonin et al. 2004; Bureau of Primary Health Care 2008a; Gelberg et al. 2000; Montauk 2006). Many homeless individuals are uninsured or underinsured and do not know they are eligible to receive services. Clinics and other medical facilities are often not set up to accommodate unique needs of these populations, including assisting homeless patients who may not have all the documentation required for Medicare or Medicaid enrollment. Health care providers are often not prepared to properly care for homeless individuals given that they lack experience in caring for the homeless and/or lack experience working in non-traditional environments. The medical consequences of residential instability such as lack of address/telephone, place to store/refrigerate meds, or inability to obtain food for medical-specific diets can easily be overlooked by medical providers and can been seen as "patient non-compliance." Poor attitudes about caring for homeless, including inappropriate language and stigmatization can also signal to homeless patients that they are not welcome.

Programs

In order to address the many barriers listed above, strategies to increase services to homeless populations include attention to the where, when and how medical and psychiatric services are delivered. The inclusion of emergency and transitional shelters, domestic violence services, permanent and supportive housing agencies, employment assistance groups, food programs (i.e., food banks and soup kitchens), pre-natal programs, substance use treatment centers, youth-specific agencies, homeless advocacy organizations as well as health care entities are all necessary when designing and provisioning the comprehensive services to improve the health of homeless persons. The concept of a "medical home" or "health home" that meets more than just the medical needs of uninsured or underserved populations will be addressed further in another chapter (Chap. 6). This concept needs to be expanded further to adequately address the needs of the homeless.

McMurray-Avila et al. (2009) provide a list of seven necessary points that providers and agencies must consider when planning to work with or to improve existing services for homeless patients:

- Effective outreach to engage clients in treatment
- Respect for the individuality of each person
- Cultivation of trust and rapport between provider and client
- Flexibility in service including location and hours of service as well as flexibility in treatment approaches
- Attending to the basic survival needs of homeless people and recognizing that until those needs are met, health care may not be an individual's highest priority
- Integrating service provision and case management to coordinate the needed services
- Clinical expertise to address complex clinical problems including access to specialized care
- Knowledge of a range of housing options including programs combining housing with services (Cochran et al. 2002)

Collaborative, community-wide efforts are best suited to effectively address the health care needs of homeless people. The Health Care for the Homeless (HCH) program is a federally funded program that provides support to community-based organization throughout the USA (Bureau of Primary Health Care 2008b). It promotes aggressive community outreach for homeless persons with integrated systems of case management, client advocacy, primary care, mental health, and substance abuse services (Bonin et al. 2004). These locally administered programs are designed to deliver clinical care and assure continuity of care to heterogeneous homeless populations. The HCH Clinician's Network provides clinical and administrative best practices accessible for public use. More about locally funded programs may be found at the HCH Information Resource Center at http://www.bphc.hrsa.gov/hcirc/directory (Bureau of Primary Health Care 2008b).

In 2000, the National Alliance to End Homelessness released a plan to end homelessness in the USA. This plan, often referred to as the "Ten Year Plan to End Homelessness," was adopted by the Federal government and the U.S. Interagency Council on Homelessness. Key points from this include: "....making mainstream programs more accountable for outcomes of their clients, developing and maintaining adequate levels of affordable housing and building infrastructure, and addressing systemic problems that lead to crisis poverty" (National Alliance to End Homelessness 2000, 2007a). In addition, a "Housing First" strategy that recognizes lack of affordable housing as a primary cause of homelessness is also promoted. As of 2007, over 300 communities have undertaken efforts to end homelessness using guidance from these documents (National Alliance to End Homelessness 2007b).

As an example of the type of program that can be developed for the homeless population, the El Rio Community Health Center in Tucson, Arizona provides primary health care, case management, advocacy, and behavioral health services. Over 8,500 of an estimated 12,000 homeless individuals in Tucson, have received services through The Health Education Project (THE Project). In addition, El Rio coordinates with 25 other non-profit and government entities to deliver workforce development and health education classes at shelters and prison sites, in developing the curricula, recruiting volunteer instructors who conduct health education classes for homeless and at-risk persons living in transitional housing or prison. With supporting grants from corporations, foundations and individuals El Rio is also able to provide eyeglasses and transportation (bus passes) to Tucson's homeless population (El Rio Health Center 2008).

The new federal administration has already begun supporting homeless programs through the "recovery plan." Almost $1.6 billion will be made available through Continuum of Care Grants which is awarded competitively to local programs to provide permanent and transitional housing to homeless persons. About $160 million of this money will be provided for Emergency Shelter Grants for the operation of local shelters and to fund related social service and homeless prevention programs, based on a formula to state and local governments to create, improve, and operate emergency shelters for homeless persons (US Department of Housing and Urban Development 2009).

References

Bonin E, Brehove T, Kline S, Misgen M, Post P, Strohlew AJ, Yungman J (2004) Adapting your practice: general recommendations for the care of homeless patients. Nashville TN: Health Care for the Homeless Clinician's Network. www.nhchc.org/Publications/6.1.04GenHomeles sRecsFINAL.pdf. Accessed 2 Apr 2008

Bureau of Primary Health Care (2008a) Principles of practice-a clinical resource guide for health care for the homeless programs. ftp://ftp,hrsa.gov/bphc/docs/1999PALS/PAL99-12.PDF. Accessed 2 Apr 2008

Bureau of Primary Health Care (2008b) Health Care for the Homeless Information Resource. The comprehensive response. http://bphc.hrsa.gov/hchirc/about/copm_respose.htm. Accessed 2 Apr 2008

Chau S, Chin M, Chang J, Luecha A, Cheng E, Schlesinger J, Rao V, Huang D, Maxwell AE, Usatine R, Bastani R, Gelberg L (2002) Cancer risk behaviors and screening rates among homeless adults in Los Angeles County. Cancer Epidemiol Biomarkers Prev 11:431–438

Cochran BN, Stewart AJ, Ginzler JA, Cauce AM (2002) Challenges faced by homeless sexual minorities: comparison of gay, lesbian, bisexual and transgender homeless adolescents with their heterosexual counterparts. Am J Public Health 92:773–777

El Rio Health Center Foundation (2008) http://www.elriofoundation.org/elrio_programs.html. Accessed 31 Mar 2009

Gallagher TC, Andersen RM, Koegel P, Gelberg L (1997) Determinants of regular source of care among homeless adults in Los Angeles. Med Care 35:814–830

Gelberg L, Gallagher TC, Andersen RM, Kogel P (1997) Competing priorities as a barrier to medical care among homeless adults in Los Angeles. Am J Public Health 87:217–220

Gelberg L, Andersen RM, Leake BD (2000) The behavioral model for vulnerable populations: application in medical care use and outcomes for homeless people. Health Serv Res 34:1273–1302

Institute of Medicine. National Academy of Sciences. (1988). Homelessness, health and human needs. National Academy Press, Washington, DC

Kidder DP, Wolfski RJ, Campsmith ML (2007) Health status, health care use medication use and medication adherence among homeless and housed people living with HIV/AIDS. Am J Public Health 97:2238–2245

Kushel MB, Sharad J (2007) Care of the homeless patient, Chapter 24. In: King TE, Wheeler MB (eds) Medical management of vulnerable and underserved patients. McGraw Hill, New York, pp 245–253

Kushel MB, Vittinghoff E, Hass JS (2001) Factors associated with health care utilization of homeless persons. JAMA 285:200–206

Kushel MB, Gupta R, Gee L (2006) Housing instability and food insecurity as Barriers to health care among low income Americans. J Gen Intern Med 21:71–77

Levy BD, O'Connell JJ (2004) Health care for homeless persons. N Engl J Med 350:2329

Martens WH (2001) A review of physical and mental health in homeless persons. Public Health Rev 29:13–33

McMurray-Avila M, Gelberg L, Breakey WR (2009) Balancing act: clinical practices that respond to the needs of homeless people. National Symposium on Homelessness Research, 1998. http://aspe.hhs.gov/progsys/homeless/symposium/8-Clinical.htm Accessed 11 Apr 2009

Montauk SL (2006) The homeless in America: adapting your practice. Am Fam Physician 74:1132–1138

National Alliance to End Homelessness (2000) A plan not an idea: how to end homelessness in ten years. Washington, DC

National Alliance to End Homelessness (2007a) What is a ten year plan to end homelessness? September 2007. www.Endhomelessness.org Accessed 2 Apr 2008

National Alliance to End Homelessness (2007b) Affordable housing shortage. www. Endhomelessness.org. Accessed 2 Apr 2008

National Coalition for the Homeless (2007a) How many people experiencehomelessness? Fact Sheet #2, June. www.Endhomelessness.org. Accessed 2 Apr 2008

National Coalition for the Homeless (2007b) Who is homeless? Fact Sheet# 3, August. www.
    nationalhomeless.org. Accessed 2 Apr 2008
Robert Wood Johnson Medical School Uninsured in America (2008) http://rwjms.umdnj.edu/
    hiphop/promiseclinic/images/homelessness.pdf. Accessed 1 May 2008
Singer J (2003) Taking it to the streets: homelessness, health and health care in the United States.
    J Gen Intern Med 18:964
U.S. Conference of Mayors (2007) Hunger and homelessness survey. A status report on hunger
    and homelessness in America's Cities. A 23 city survey December. www.usmayors.org.
    Accessed 2 Apr 2008
Urban Institute (2009) Children and foreclosures: the economic crisis hits home. A forum cospon-
    sored by the Urban Institute and Chapin Hall at the University of Chicago, March 12. http://
    www.urban.org/events/thursdayschild/Children-and-Foreclosures.cfm. Accessed 30 Mar
    2009
US Department of Housing and Urban Development (2009) Obama administration awards nearly
    $1.6 billion in homeless grants. http://www.hud.gov/news/release.cfm?content=pr09-010.cfm.
    Accessed 31 Mar 2009

Care of Underserved People with Mental Illness

Francisco A. Moreno and Sarah Heron

Introduction

Before delving into a discussion about care of the uninsured and underserved mentally ill population, it is important to reflect on the historical under-representation of the field of mental health as a whole from a medical, political, social, and economic standpoint. The approach to the care of the mentally ill has been an area of debate for centuries, and the evolution of the field of mental health and substance use disorder has often lagged behind other areas of health care and social services. Following an extensive period of institutional care of the mentally ill using therapeutic asylum, a revolutionary movement came to light in the 1960s with the promise of delivering comprehensive community-based mental health services to support the de-institutionalization of the mentally ill. The Community Mental Health Movement was ethically strong and philosophically progressive, yet it was very poorly funded, and services were intermittently dispersed and fragmented. The challenge to implementation grew more daunting as a result of a drastic concurrent increase in our country's population, an epidemic rise in drug and alcohol use disorders, and the worsening medical and social infrastructures. Communities in the United States continue to experience the unfavorable consequences of this movement, while poorly equipped criminal justice systems, and overwhelmed emergency medical and homeless services are left to deal with the results of this tragic legacy.

In an era where a general healthcare care crisis has received little attention, the severe limitation of services for the mentally ill and those affected with substance use disorders is not an exception to the rule. Rather, it has become a sad symbol of the neglect for the needs of this special community which has traditionally received a disproportionately small amount of funding (federal and otherwise), attention to reform and policy, and medical services. This is especially concerning, given the social and moral burden that mental illnesses engender. According to the World

F.A. Moreno (✉) and S. Heron
Psychiatry, University of Arizona, College of Medicine, Tucson, AZ, USA

N.J. Johnson and L.P. Johnson (eds.), *The Care of the Uninsured in America*,
DOI 10.1007/978-0-387-78309-3_11, © Springer Science+Business Media, LLC 2010

Health Organization, "mental disorders collectively account for more than 15% of the overall burden of disease from all causes and are among the most disabling." To put this into more tangible terms, five of the top ten causes of disability worldwide are mental health conditions (Depression #1, Alcohol use #4, Bipolar Disorder #6, Schizophrenia #9, and Obsessive Compulsive Disorder #10) (Murray and Lopez 1996).

Demographics

Current estimates suggest that there are about 47 million uninsured in the United States. On the basis of reports from the National Alliance for the Mentally Ill indicating that more than 25% of the uninsured have a mental illness, addiction disorder, or both, the total number of uninsured mentally ill is likely greater than 12 million.

Lower socioeconomic status as reflected by income, education, and occupation, is strongly correlated with a higher rate of certain mental and addiction disorders. Those in the lowest strata are 2.5 times more likely to have a mental disorder than those in the highest strata. Other underserved mentally ill populations include immigrants, gay and lesbian populations, homeless persons, those in rural communities, and patients at the extremes of age.

About one third of the "poor" mentally ill and one fifth of the "severely mentally ill" are uninsured, and adults with serious mental illnesses die an average of 25 years earlier than those who do not have a mental illness. Two-thirds of the U.S. homeless population are adults with chronic alcoholism, drug addiction, mental illness, or some combination of the three. Additionally, approximately one-fifth of jail, as well as state and federal prison, inmates have a serious mental disorder.

Of those persons with limited or no health insurance coverage, 20% have a major depressive disorder in comparison to a prevalence of 16% in the general population. Similarly, 36% have an anxiety disorder in contrast to 11% of the general population. Treatment rates for depression among the medically uninsured are half that of the insured population and people with mental illness are more likely to lose their medical insurance because of disability or underemployment (DSM-14 2004). The lack of medical care in turn further feeds into this cycle. Adults in a primary care population have a 25% rate of psychiatric disorders, half of which are estimated to remain undiagnosed and untreated (Price-Hanson 2007).

In areas where mental health services are limited, the suicide rate is significantly higher, twice as frequent in some rural areas, especially among men (NHRA 2008). Even given equal insurance coverage, higher mortality is noted for the severely mentally ill when affected with medical problems (Jeste and Unutzer 2001). Care for alcohol, drug, or mental health problems is more likely to occur for patients with Medicaid than for medically uninsured populations. Satisfaction with care for alcohol, drug, or mental health problems is also much higher for those in Medicaid or Medicare than for the medically uninsured (Wells et al. 2002).

Programmatic Issues Affecting Access and Quality of Care

As mentioned above, advances in psychiatric science have led to an exponential growth in our understanding of the underlying basis for mental illness. Progress has also been very apparent in pharmacological and other therapeutic modalities; yet a number of factors impede access to adequate assessment and treatment for patients with mental illnesses of all kinds.

Historically, the care of people with mental illness has been separate from the care of people having general medical problems. Over time, this distinction has influenced the structure of care systems, as well as the flow of funds for services such that an artificial split was created between the health of the brain and of the remainder of the body. Less expensive private insurances exclude mental health and substance abuse treatment altogether, while some Medicaid programs around the country exclude or limit coverage for these services. In other cases publically funded programs around the country limit care to people with general mental health or substance related conditions and resort to focusing only on those with serious mental illness. As a result, uninsured people often do not have access to mental health services unless their condition is very severe.

A 45 y/o patient with severe hepatic failure undergoes an extensive battery of neuropsychological tests in order to assess his appropriateness to receive a liver transplant. The transplant procedure is of course a major ordeal and one that is very costly to the payer of medical services, all of which are covered to support this life saving effort. The said patient becomes agitated and psychotic several days following his stressful surgical procedure. He had received multiple drugs to minimize organ rejection and risk of infection. A psychiatric consult for this patient is requested but not covered, given the separate contract for mental health services to a capitated provider. The well-trained master level clinician provider assigned to psychiatric consults in the area finds himself ill-equipped to deal with this medical psychiatric challenge. The psychosomatic team is consulted and helps resolve the clinical condition in spite of exclusion of their services by the health insurance plan.

Similarly, in several states of the country, patients who are hospitalized and treated for extensive stays in intensive care units, and other rehabilitation services after attempting suicide, are not provided needed psychiatric services during their stays. Even after medical clearance is obtained, a transfer to psychiatric services is not paid for unless the patients remain an imminent threat to themselves or others, and the coverage cannot exceed 72 hours.

Parity

Fortunately in recent times (October 2008), after two decades of pursuit by advocacy groups and allied medical organizations, congress gave final approval to the Paul Wellstone-Pete Domenici Mental Health Parity and Addiction Equity Act of 2008 as part of the Emergency Economic Stabilization Act (HR 1424). This legislation becomes effective 1-year after enactment of the bill. This will mean that group health plans will no longer be able to impose restrictions on inpatient days or outpatient visits nor will they be permitted to require higher deductibles or cost sharing for mental illness or addiction treatment that are not also applied to all other medical-surgical coverage.

In recent years, the marked limitation on services provided by private insurances has led to an overutilization of publically funded agencies which are mandated to provide care for the indigent mentally ill. These community agencies are often so taxed by the demand for services and the overt limitation on resources that they are forced to prioritize crisis stabilization over programs that promote chronic care, recovery, education, and wellness initiatives (http://healthcareforuninsured.org/).

Misinformation and stigma have plagued the political landscape and facilitated a health care culture in which mental health issues have been assigned lower priority and merit than other components of health. This issue, as well as the lack of resources to provide adequate services may have facilitated the drastic workforce shortage in the field. The limited profitability of psychiatric inpatient services, given the lack of payment and constraints on service approvals, has led to a drastic shortage of inpatient unit beds, and private insurers seldom pay for residential and less restrictive environment options along the continuum of care. Too often across our nation, there is nowhere for even the most severe patients with mental illness to receive treatment. They remain for days, at times physically or chemically restrained in emergency department rooms or hallways. These patients may also be incarcerated for longer periods of time in local jails and correctional facilities where horrific abuses have been documented.

Psychiatric care is also costly; hospitalizations in psychiatric units are at least as expensive as admissions to medical-surgical services. In addition most patients with chronic mental illnesses who failed to achieve remission after standard monotherapy require combinations of frequently expensive medications. Fortunately, recent availability of generic antidepressants, anxiolitics, mood stabilizers, and second generation neuroleptics brings significant relief to payers for those patients with condition severe enough to warrant continued treatment. Uninsured persons with less severe disease are still at a disadvantage in accessing and continuing mental health care.

Primary Care Services

The limited access to specialty care may have also influenced a trend towards greater mental health services being expected from and in many cases being provided by primary care and other specialty providers. However, many primary care providers in medical clinics are often uncomfortable – because of training, resources, or time constraints – diagnosing or treating mental disorders such as uncomplicated anxiety and depression, much less more complex problems involving severe mood and thought disorders, or complications with suicide, violence, and substance use disorders (Price-Hanson 2007). Studies of adequacy of care at times point towards inconsistent prescription practices in primary care settings and not surprisingly underutilization of psychotherapy interventions (Duhoux et al. 2009). This suggested that even when uninsured patients do access primary care services, mental health issues are less likely to be addressed.

In response to this concern a number of innovative approaches have been proposed to alleviate this unmet need. One of the more promising new programs is the use of a collaborative mental health model that integrates primary care medical clinics with behavioral health workers to provide basic mental health services in a primary care setting. Many of these programs are based in clinics (often grant or government supported) that serve the medically uninsured, though they may target particular populations such as the elderly or chronically ill (Unützer et al. 2002).

The advantages of such a model are obvious. Basic screening and treatment of mental disorders by primary care medical providers can be developed, implemented, and supported by in-house behavioral health specialists. "Warm hand-offs" of patients from behavioral to medical providers, (or vice versa) can be readily accomplished. When these integrated services can be further combined with community agencies like geriatric or family support programs, these "medical homes" can be the foundation of a very powerful community model (Gallo et al. 2004).

Challenges for the implementation of these programs can be significant including issues related to readiness for change among the providers involved, funding, and patients' acceptance of this approaches. Outcomes of the integrative models need to be assessed carefully, in spite of multiple positive results (Katon et al. 2005); success is not guaranteed (Smith et al. 2001). Moreover, given that this approach is significantly more expensive than standard primary care, the importance of good evaluation is critical.

Physical Access to Care

In certain rural communities, remote Indian reservations, or correctional facilities access to mental health services is an even greater challenge. There are fewer mental health professionals per capita outside urban areas, and traveling clinicians are pricier and less consistently accessible, resulting in care being delivered by less well trained providers (McCabe and Macnee 2002). Stigma and lack of anonymity may be worse in rural communities (Fuller et al. 2004). Rural hospitals are half as likely to provide emergency mental health care as urban hospitals, and not surprisingly, the suicide rate is significantly higher than in urban areas especially among men (NHRA 2008). Rural areas often have larger numbers of uninsured and Medicaid/Medicare patients.

Fortunately, technology-based interventions promise to improve the delivery of care to areas where access is difficult. The use of telemedicine services has been studied and implemented in psychiatry for a number of years. There are several limitations to the use of traditional telemedicine services such as the requirements of dedicated, high-velocity telecommunication lines and electronic equipment for videoconferencing in real time. With the recent extensive use of the internet and wireless broadband access there is now a possibility of using standard webcam equipment to facilitate access to psychiatric assessments and treatments (http://www.solvingdisparities.org/grantees/round2/arizona). Whether these technologic innovations make mental health services more accessible to the uninsured remains an open question at this time.

Literacy

Literacy represents a challenge for patients with general medical conditions; yet, given the general disinformation and misinformation about the meaning of mental illness, its causes, and perceptions of what treatment may be beneficial, mental health literacy represents an even greater obstacle, even more so with the uninsured population. This issue is presently being addressed through comprehensive campaigns geared towards decreasing stigma, facilitating access to resources, and increasing education and support by advocacy and consumer-based associations such as the National Alliance for the Mentally Ill (NAMI), the Depression Bipolar Support Alliance (DBSA) among others; provider networks such as the National Council for Community Behavioral Healthcare; governmental agencies such as The Substance Abuse and Mental Health Services Administration (SAMHSA), The National Institute of Mental Health (NIMH); and many universities and academic institutions worldwide. Other collaborative efforts include massive screening efforts during Mental Health Week, and education by providers at the time of diagnosis or initiation of treatment.

Other Clinical Issues that Further Compromise Access

The further patients with mental illness are from clinical stability, the less likely they will be to seek clinical care. For example, patients with severe obsessive compulsive disorder are likely to keep their condition secret because of shame, anxious patients fear adverse effects of medication, those with severe depression often lack motivation to seek care and maintain treatment compliance, patients with mania have little interest in letting go of the feeling of excitement and euphoria, and patients with paranoia often worry about malicious intentions of caretakers fearing that they may be controlled, sabotaged, or harmed. Delaying diagnosis and treatment contributes to the natural progression of these disorders, which may include a series of complications like greater medical and psychiatric co-morbidities, and violence towards self or others.

Civil Rights and Refusal of Care

Care avoidance or rejection may result in an ethical dilemma often encountered by relatives, caregivers, and providers of the mentally ill. To what extent should patients' autonomy be respected allowing them to make decisions about mental health care in cases when they are not competent to understand their need for treatment, the risks and benefits of proposed interventions, and the consequences of treatment refusal? In America, mentally ill patients have the right to decline care unless it can be legally established that as result of their mental illness they pose an imminent threat to the safety of themselves or others, or have become unable to meet their basic needs including food, shelter, and physical care.

In many states, public sector community agencies responsible for the care of the mentally ill are so inundated with clients that their frequency of contact with individual patients is drastically decreased. This often leads to limited clinical monitoring, poor supervision of compliance with appointments and/or medications, and ultimately decompensation. This in turn results in a greater challenge to patients' participation in the informed consent process, and greater involvement of the court systems with consequent loss of civil liberties.

Criminalization of the Mentally Ill

According to a recent report by the U.S. Department of Justice more than half of all prison and jail inmates have a mental health problem compared with 11% of the general population, yet only one in three prison inmates and one in six jail inmates receive any form of mental health treatment (James and Glaze 2006). These are not trivial emotional adjustments related to detention, but 43% of state prisoners and 54% of jail inmates reported symptoms that met the criteria for mania, and approximately 23% of state prisoners and 30% of jail inmates reported symptoms of major depression. An estimated 15% of state prisoners and 24% of jail inmates reported symptoms that met the criteria for a psychotic disorder. The barriers for mental health care in the "detained" mentally ill are many, including insufficient budget and resource allocation, lack of legislative commitment to divert mentally ill and substance abusing offenders for treatment, lack of self identification, or refusal by the patient to undergo mental health assessment and treatment, among others (Daniel 2007).

The field of forensic psychiatry has evolved significantly, the attention given to people with mental illness in jails and prisons although limited has clearly improved over time, and related professional organizations and advocacy groups continue lobbying to make the advantages of standard psychiatry and substance use disorder treatments available in the community available to detained people.

Mental Illness and the Immigrant

Although mental health issues are taboo in many regions from where immigrants to this country originate; the mental health of immigrants varies drastically depending on many factors like their conditions of migration and their motivating factors. Immigrants are often energetic, dedicated, and focused people pursuing upward mobility. Although the stress of migration and process of acculturation may contribute to worsening of mental illness, an apparent paradox has been observed in the decreased prevalence of mental illness in first generation Mexican immigrants to the U.S. (Vega et al. 1998). Alternatively in certain cases, those seeking asylum because of persecution or civil rights abuses may present with a discrete array of symptoms related to trauma exposure or deprivation.

Independent of the above observations, many immigrants share a number of factors that complicate adequate delivery of services to their community. Issues such as language proficiency, traditional beliefs about mental illness within their culture of origin, and attitudes towards the treatment of mental illnesses are more extensively discussed below. In cases in which legal resident or citizenship status is being processed, patients may not want to generate a record of mental illness as they are required to report if they have a diagnosis or require treatment for mental health on the U.S. immigration application documents. Immigrants also are less likely to have financial solvency or adequate insurance, and are often ineligible for entitlements such as Medicaid or Medicare.

In many communities around the country, immigrants receive attention from faith based, educational, and charitable organizations which provide clinical services, advocacy, and education in many cases delivered by immigrants or providers who are often well tuned to the special needs of these communities.

Cultural Aspects of the Underserved Mentally Ill

Throughout the medical field, the perceptions of health status, causality attribution, and adequacy of intervention play an important role in wellness behaviors and healthcare seeking. Cultural factors are a major determinant of these perspectives, behaviors, and values about health, but have a particular impact in the field of mental health given the multitude of traditional, spiritual, and social misperceptions about psychiatric and substance use disorders.

Ideal mental health care should be culturally congruent and mindful of the following issues among others: language and communication adequacy; congruent interpretation of symptoms, predisposing factors, and outcome expectations; role assignment to the caregiver; and attitudes about involvement of family and other groups. The development of rapport between mental health consumers and providers is also influenced by the perception of cultural congruence.

In an effort to increase the cultural sensitivity of mental health practitioners and take into consideration how socio-cultural differences impact an individual's mental illness and treatment, the cultural formulation was introduced in the DSM-IV. A full description and examples of the cultural formulation are not appropriate for this chapter, but the following vignette illustrates some of the issues addressed in this chapter.

A 27 year old medically uninsured African-American (AA) woman recently attempted suicide. She identified multiple stressors at home and work, many related to her moving to a relatively small town with a significantly smaller AA community. Patient reported a history of chronic depression, which failed to improve after treatment with medication and therapy with a Caucasian therapist with whom she had trouble relating.

The patient was adopted at age three because of the inability of her biological parents to care for her. Her biological mother was Caucasian and her biological father was AA. While the patient identifies herself as "mixed" or "black and white," she says she associates with "blacks". Her adoptive parents are both AA and have two biological sons but she was raised in a predominantly Caucasian community. While the patient described having a clear ethnic identity as biracial, she worried about offending her adoptive family by distinguishing herself from their race.

The patient identified several ways in which her race affected her mental health and psychiatric treatment. First of all, she stated "I was raised to be a strong black woman." From her cultural perspective, seeking help was a sign of weakness and she felt that she should be able to handle these difficult situations independently. Secondly, the patient commented on the importance of her relationship with her mental health provider. She reflected that when her Caucasian therapist told her that her life was "hard," she was uncomfortable with the comment and she questioned the therapist's ability to truly understand and be empathic, given the perceived differences in background. Influenced by the nature of the transference, the patient believed that the therapist was feeling sorry or making excuses to her. The patient felt that she needed a therapist regardless of racial background, who had also "been through something" or "had a hard life" as well.

Although the patient stated that she did not need a therapist who was AA or even a minority, she felt that she was better able to relate and open up to her new AA psychiatrist assuming erroneously a commonality of life experiences and perspective. The bias demonstrated by this patient is often experienced by family members and providers. This issue when addressed properly may facilitate collaboration and favorable outcomes.

Summary

Uninsured and underinsured people with mental illness often go unidentified and untreated, and even those clearly recognized frequently are underserved because of restrictions in coverage by private and public insurances. Factors that influence this phenomenon include the limited comfort and time for mental health care by primary care providers, the short supply of specialist care and inpatient facilities, the restrictions on funding for mental health and substance use disorder treatment, the specific issues in mental health patients who often avoid or refuse care, and the legal systems and social service agencies that are poorly equipped to deal with the extensive demand for services.

In spite of these challenges, a series of policy changes, social awareness, scientific progress, and implementation of novel modalities of care promise to enhance our ability to decrease disparities in mental health care, and enhance the mental health of all Americans.

References

(2004) Diagnostic and statistical manual of mental disorders, 4th ed: DSM-IV. American Psychiatric Association, Washington, DC

Daniel AE (2007) Care of the mentally ill in prisons: challenges and solutions. J Am Acad Psychiatry Law 35(4):406–410

Duhoux A, Fournier L, Nguyen CT, Roberge P, Beveridge R (2009) Guideline concordance of treatment for depressive disorders in Canada. Soc Psychiatry Psychiatr Epidemiol 44(5):385–392

Fuller J, Edwards J, Martinez L, Edwards B, Reid K (2004) Collaboration and local networks for rural and remote primary mental healthcare in South Australia. Health Soc Care Community 12(1):75–84

Gallo JJ, Zubritsky C et al (2004) Primary care clinicians evaluated integrated and referral models of behavioral health care for older adults: results from a multi-site effectiveness trial. Annals of Family Medicine 2(4):305–309

James DJ, Glaze LE (2006) Mental health problems of prison and jail inmates. Department of Justice, Bureau of Justice Statistics Special Report, Washington, DC

Jeste DV, Unutzer J (2001) Improving the delivery of care to the seriously mentally ill. Med Care 39(9):907–909

Katon WJ, Schoenbaum M, Fan MY et al (2005) Cost-effectiveness of improving primary care treatment of late-life depression. Arch Gen Psychiatry 62(12):1313–1320

McCabe S, Macnee CL (2002) Weaving a new safety net of mental health care in rural America: a model of integrated practice. Issues Ment Health Nurs 23(3):263–278

Murray CJL, Lopez AD (eds) (1996) A comprehensive assessment of mortality and disability from diseases, injuries, and risk factors in 1990 and projected to 2020. The Global Burden of Disease. Published by The Harvard School of Public Health on Behalf of the World Health Organization and The World Bank

National Rural Health Association (2008) What's different about rural health? http://www.nrharural.org/about/sub/different.html. Accessed 29 Mar 2008

Price-Hanson DR (2007) The medical treatment of patients with psychiatric illness, Chapter 28. In: King TE, Wheeler MB (eds) Medical management of vulnerable and underserved patients. McGraw Hill, New York, pp 285–295

Smith JL, Rost KM, Nutting PA, Elliott CE (2001) Resolving disparities in antidepressant treatment and quality of life outcomes between uninsured and insured primary care patients with depression. Med Care 39(9):910–922

Unützer J, Katon W, Callahan CM, Williams JW, Hunkeler E, Harpole L, Hoffing M, Della Penna RD, Noël PH, Lin EH, Areán PA, Hegel MT, Tang L, Belin TR, Oishi S, Langston C (2002) IMPACT investigators. Improving mood-promoting access to collaborative treatment. Collaborative care management of late-life depression in the primary care setting: a randomized controlled trial. JAMA 288(22):2836–2845

Vega WA, Kolody B, Aguilar-Gaxiola S, Alderete E, Catalano R, Caraveo-Anduaga J (1998) Lifetime prevalence of DSM-III-R psychiatric disorders among urban and rural Mexican Americans in California. Arch Gen Psychiatry 55:771–778

Wells KB, Sherbourne CD, Sturm R, Young AS, Burnam MA (2002) Alcohol, drug abuse, and mental health care for uninsured and insured adults. Health Serv Res 37(4):1055–1066

Medically Uninsured Older Americans

Lynne Tomasa

Introduction

America is becoming a more diverse nation. Older Americans are increasing in number at a rapid rate, and we are living longer. With these changes come an increasing demand for health care services and the increasing costs of care. This chapter identifies the importance of focusing on our uninsured, and often underinsured, older Americans, and the issues surrounding their access to health insurance coverage. Due to the overall small percentage of uninsured older Americans aged 65 years and above, this population is easily ignored. To appreciate the need for a closer examination, this chapter provides an overview of several issues and topics. The chapter begins with an overview of the changing demographics of America's older adults; identifies the uninsured in this population; provides a review of Medicare Parts A, B, and C; describes the role of Medicare Part D; investigates the issue of health insurance for the group of adults aged 50–64; and concludes with how some states are moving forward in providing expanded health care insurance and access to their uninsured. Older Americans, also referred to here as older adults, are defined in the chapter and in national datasets as persons 65 years and older.

Demographics of Older Americans

The U.S. Census Bureau, the Center for Disease Control's (CDC) National Center on Health Statistics (NCHS), and the Bureau of Labor Statistics are among the several federal agencies that provide important statistics on the changing profile of our older population. The statistics collected from these federal agencies are utilized by the Administration on Aging (AoA), U.S. Department of Health and Human Services (DHHS) in a concise yearly report, *A Profile of Older Americans*

L. Tomasa
Department of Family and Community Medicine, University of Arizona, College of Medicine, Tucson, AZ, USA

N.J. Johnson and L.P. Johnson (eds.), *The Care of the Uninsured in America*,
DOI 10.1007/978-0-387-78309-3_12, © Springer Science+Business Media, LLC 2010

(Fowles et al. 2008). The 2008 AoA report highlights the fact that one in every eight persons living in the United States is over the age of 65. This equals 12.6% of the total population or 37.9 million people in 2007, a 11.2% increase since 1997. The population aged 65 and over is projected to increase to 40 million in 2010, 55 million in 2020, and 72 million in 2030. Americans over age 85 are projected to increase 36% in number, from 4.2 million in 2000 to 5.7 million in 2010. Other pertinent points for our discussion include the fact that in 2007:

- Women reaching age 65 had an average life expectancy of an additional 20.3 years while men had an average life expectancy of an additional 17.4%.
- Minorities represented 19.3% of persons 65 and older.
- Median income was is $14,021 for women and $24,323 for males.
- Approximately 3.6 million older adults, representing 9.7%, had incomes below the federal poverty level.

These statistics indicate a longer life expectancy for Americans, and a growing and more diverse older population. The longer life expectancy may portray overall improved health, but there continue to be inconsistent gains between genders, across age brackets, income levels, and racial and ethnic groups. Despite the longer life expectancy of older Americans, it is still behind that in other industrialized nations, such as Japan, where women aged 65 live 3.2 years longer on average than women in the United States (Federal Interagency Forum on Aging-Related Statistics 2008, p 24). The Federal Interagency Forum on Aging-Related Statistics (Forum), a collaborative effort of 15 Federal agencies made a comprehensive examination of the overall health and well-being of our older population. Their report, *Older Americans 2008: Key Indicators of Well-Being* (http://www. agingstats.gov) includes 38 indicators in the areas of Population, Economics, Health Status, Health Risk and Behaviors, and Health Care. Older Americans use more health care services and cost more than other age groups. Some of the most common chronic conditions reported by Older Americans were hypertension, arthritis, and heart disease. Stroke, cancer, diabetes, and heart disease are among the most costly health conditions (Federal Interagency Forum on Aging-Related Statistics 2008, p 27).

Uninsured Older Americans: Who Are They?

Since 1957, the Center for Disease Control's (CDC) National Center for Health Statistics (NCHS) monitored the health of the nation by compiling important statistical information about health insurance and access to care. The National Health Interview Study (NHIS) is a large-scale household interview survey that is conducted throughout the year on the civilian non-institutionalized U.S. population (http://www.cdc.gov/nchs/nhis.htm). Interviews are conducted with 75,000–100,000 individuals from 35,000 to 40,000 households. The survey content includes a core set of questions that remain constant year-to-year and supplemental questions that are of interest to sponsors. The core questions measure health status and disability, insurance coverage, access to care, use of health services, immunizations, health behaviors, injury, and the ability to perform daily activities. The quarterly updates provide a useful mechanism to relate health insurance coverage to health care utilization and outcomes. Helpful to our discussion and crucial to minimizing errors in reporting, is the fact that beginning in late 2004, two questions were added about Medicare and Medicaid status (Cohen and Martinez 2007).

The NHIS utilizes three measures of the lack of health insurance coverage: *current, intermittent, and long term.* Individuals can be counted in more than one of the three measures, therefore each is not mutually exclusive. For example, *current* includes individuals uninsured at the time of the interview, *intermittent* includes persons uninsured for at least part of the year prior to the interview and can include persons uninsured for more than a year, and *long term* are those who were uninsured for more than a year at the time of the interview. Uninsured is defined as

"not having any private health insurance, Medicare, Medicaid, State Children's Health Insurance Program (SCHIP), state-sponsored or other government-sponsored health plan, or military plan. Uninsured persons also include individuals who had only Indian Health Service coverage or had only a private plan that paid for one type of service such as accidents or dental care." (Martinez et al. 2008)

Mold et al. (2004) published an in-depth analysis on uninsured older adults with his examination of the 2000 NHIS dataset. Mold's analysis is discussed here. In 2000, approximately 1.1% of the older population or 353,754 adults over 65 were uninsured. The sociodemographic characteristics were that the uninsured older adults were more likely to be younger in the age range of 65–74; widowed or never married; and either African American, Asian American, or Hispanic. They were also more likely to have been born in another country. A closer look at the sociodemographic characteristics follows. The age breakdown reflected that 72.3% of the older uninsured Americans were 65–74 years old,, 24.3% were 75–84,, and 3.4% were 85 and older. There were more females (55.5%) than males (44.5%) who were uninsured. Regarding marital status – 40.8% were married, 40.1% were widowed, and the remainder were either separated, or divorced, or had never married. The ethnic breakdown included 64.2% who were non-Hispanic, 35.8% being Hispanic. Of the Hispanic older adults, 66.2% were Mexican or Mexican American; 17.1%, Central or South American; 9.3%, Cuban; 3.9%, Puerto Rican; and others, 1.6%. Looking at race, 60.8% were Caucasian; 16.6% were African American;, 13.4% were Asian or Pacific Islander;, and 9.2% identified as others. African Americans were more likely to be in the younger age group of 65–74. The insurance status of Asian Americans was unrelated to age, sex, marital status, or residence.

Of those over 65 and uninsured, 55.8% were born in a country outside the United States. Of this group, 5.7% had come within the last year; 18.1% within the last 5 years; and the rest had come more than 5 years earlier. Of the older adults who had come to the U.S. more than 5 years earlier, almost 20% had not obtained citizenship. For household income, there was an almost even distribution: 49.6%

had an income of more than or equal to $20,000, and 50.4% had an income less than $20,000. Three-quarters of the uninsured older adults lived in a metropolitan service area.

Mold et al. (2004) also looked at health characteristics and found that uninsured older adults enjoyed slightly better health than those with insurance. Even with this good news, 5–10% reported significant functional impairments. More than 10% did not receive needed care and almost 12% delayed seeking care because of cost. The high cost of health insurance was the reason given by 53.8% of the respondents for seeking delayed care. This accounted for 190,417 older adults. Some of the other reasons given for not having health insurance included: employer does not offer (6.7%), chooses not to have insurance (4.9%), moved from another state or country (4.7%), and never had insurance (3.2%).

The early release of National Health Interview Survey (NHIS) data of January–June 2008 estimated that 14.3% of all persons in America were uninsured. These data were obtained from the Family Core component of the 2008 NHIS estimates, based on household interviews of a sample of civilian non-institutionalized population collected from January through June. For persons 65 and over, 0.7% (standard error of 0.11) were uninsured at the time of the interview; 1.4% (standard error of 0.17) had been intermittently uninsured for at least part of the past year; and 0.6% (standard error of 0.09) were uninsured for more than a year (Martinez et al. 2008, Table 7). According to earlier reports, estimates were generally 0.1–0.3% points lower than the final data (Cohen and Martinez 2007). The standard error of these estimates range from 0.09 to 0.17. These figures were estimates at the time of publication of the report but it reflects that individuals who remain uninsured for longer periods of time may be at higher risk due to lack of access to preventive care.

Alternate data collection methods may show a different picture of our older uninsured population. Gray et al. (2006) looked at the uninsured population in New York City that was 65 years and older. Using a variety of data sources, they focused on individuals discharged from a New York City hospital in 2001. The findings are interesting because 16–20% of the city's 65 and older adults did not have Medicare. This suggested that individuals who lacked Medicare were poor and did not have access to more expensive private insurance. In addition, racial/ethnic groups who experienced high levels of immigration in recent decades were less likely to have Medicare and Social Security. Among immigrants, the country of origin mattered and reflected the waves of immigration. For example, most immigrants who were born in the U.S.S.R., East and Southeast Asia, and the Persian Gulf were on average, 50 and older when they moved to the United States. This did not provide them the opportunity to meet the 40 quarters of employment requirements for receiving Medicare and Social Security benefits. For older New Yorkers, the likelihood of having Medicare increased steadily as one became older. For comparison, 25% of individuals between 65 and 69 did not have Medicare while only 11% of the hospitalized older adults over 85 did not have Medicare. A closer examination of employment opportunities may shed some light.

Despite the small percentage of uninsured older adults, the lack of health insurance also has a major impact on the receipt of preventive health care. Okoro et al. (2005)

used the nationally representative survey data from the Behavioral Risk Factor Surveillance System (BRFSS) to compare uninsured and insured older adults' access to physician care, use of preventive health services, and vaccinations. In their sample, Blacks and Hispanics, those with less than a high school education, the formerly married or the never married, those who were employed, and those who lived in the South had the highest prevalence of not having insurance. Their findings confirmed that uninsured adults 65 and older are less likely to report receiving preventive health services. This study found that 17% had not seen a doctor in the past year because of cost, 37% did not have an annual checkup, and 80% were uninsured for over a year (Okoro et al. 2005).

There are several factors that may impede someone's ability to receive health insurance coverage and benefits. To increase one's chances of receiving health insurance, an individual must be a U.S. citizen or a permanent resident of 5 years or longer,and work or have a spouse who worked where the employer paid Federal Insurance Contribution Act (FICA) taxes for at least 40 calendar quarters. This being the case, it is important to have a broad understanding of Medicare and Medicaid in order to later identify how potential gaps can be minimized.

It is easy to assume that once a person reaches 65 years of age they will obtain Medicare and all of their health care needs will be met. This is not the case. There are several gaps in coverage and individuals living in America continue to be uninsured.

Health Insurance for Older Adults: Medicare and Medicaid

Most Americans 65 and older have health care coverage through Medicare, Medicaid, or private insurance. Medicare was created in 1965 and implemented in 1966 as a federal health insurance program for U.S. citizens or permanent residents 65 years and older. There are no income or asset tests to qualify for Medicare. Since its original design, it has been expanded to provide medical benefits to people under age 65 with permanent disabilities and to individuals of any age with End Stage Renal Disease (ESRD). Individuals with a permanent disability who have been receiving Social Security Disability Income (SSDI) or Railroad Retirement disability payments for 24 months can obtain Medicare. People with ESRD or Lou Gehrig's disease do not have to wait 24 months and can receive Medicare as soon as they receive SSDI payments. Medicare has four parts: Part A, Part B, Part C, and most recently, Part D (The Henry J. Kaiser Family Foundation 2009a)

Medicare Part A helps to pay for part of the inpatient hospital, skilled nursing facility, home health (first 100 days), and hospice care. It is funded by payroll tax contributions paid by employers and workers. To become eligible for Part A benefits, a person or their spouse must have contributed payroll taxes for 10 years or 40 quarters. There are no premiums for people who meet the work and tax requirement. Individuals with less than 30 quarters of payroll tax contributions can voluntarily enroll in Part A coverage by paying a monthly premium if they also sign up for Part B. Individuals must also meet citizenship or residency requirements. The 2009 Part A premium rate is $443, up from $423 in 2008. Individuals who have made contributions toward 30–39 quarters will pay a reduced premium of $233. These premium amounts are adjusted every year (Hoffman et al. 2008).

Medicare Part B helps to pay for physician and outpatient visits, home health visits (after 100 days), and preventive services to maintain one's health. Beneficiaries of Part B pay a monthly premium. Beginning in 2007, individuals with a higher income paid a higher monthly premium. For example, in 2009, individuals with a yearly income of less than $85,000 pay a monthly premium of $96.40 while individuals with a yearly income of more than $213,000 will pay $308.30. Monthly premiums for joint tax returns are adjusted accordingly. Individuals must also pay a yearly Part B deductible of $135 before Medicare starts paying for Part B covered services or items. To complicate things further, there is also a late-enrollment penalty if one does not sign up for Part B when they become eligible to receive benefits (CMS 2008a; The Henry J. Kaiser Family Foundation 2007).

Medicare Part C is a different way of offering Medicare benefits and is referred to as the Medicare Advantage program. Individuals are eligible for Part C if they are entitled to Part A and enrolled in Part B. These Medicare approved plans are private health plans (HMO, PPO, or private fee-for-serve/PFFS) that offer a combination of Part A, Part B, and often Part D (prescription drug) coverage. These plans are managed by private insurance companies who charge different co-payments, co-insurance, or deductibles for medically necessary services. Congress has encouraged enrollment by increasing payments to Medicare private plans in both urban and rural areas. In 2008, 24% of the total Medicare benefit payments went to Part C (CMS 2008b; The Henry J. Kaiser Family Foundation 2007; The Henry J. Kaiser Family Foundation 2009b).

Medicare Part D is a voluntary outpatient prescription drug benefit that went into effect in 2006. Enrollees who participate can choose among 50 or more plans in their states and this number continues to change and increase yearly. Premiums, benefits, covered drugs, and mechanisms to manage utilization can vary significantly across Part D plans and geographic regions (The Henry J. Kaiser Family Foundation 2008a). Selecting an appropriate Medicare Part D is a complicated and intimidating process for many older adults. Online assistance in selecting a plan is available at the Medicare website at http://www.medicare.gov. In 2006, the Medication Management Center was established in the University of Arizona, College of Pharmacy (2007) to assist Medicare D beneficiaries in understanding their medications and selecting an appropriate plan based on individual needs. Individuals can also seek guidance from their local pharmacy.

Older Americans spend a significant portion of their income on prescription medications. Even those who have Medicare Part D can spend thousands of dollars out of pocket for their medications. A further explanation highlights confusing and often misunderstood aspects of Part D coverage. The drug benefit is offered through stand-alone prescription drug plans (PDPs) and Medicare Advantage prescription drug plans (MA-PD). The MA-PD plans are HMOs that pay for all drugs and other

Medicare benefits in one plan. The number of PDPs offered each year varies: in 2006, there were 1,429 plans; in 2008, there were 1,824; and in 2009, there are 1,689 PDPs offered nationwide (excluding the territories) (The Henry J. Kaiser Family Foundation 2008a; The Henry J. Kaiser Family Foundation 2009a).

The PDPs offer a defined standard benefit with a deductible and co-insurance up to an initial coverage limit in total drug costs. Once this limit has been reached, there is a coverage gap, known as the "doughnut hole" where enrollees then pay 100% of their medications. In 2009, enrollees have a $295 deductible and 25% co-insurance up to a limit of $2,700 in total drug costs. During the doughnut hole, enrollees must have spent $4.350 out of pocket (excluding premiums) before they receive assistance again. After the doughnut hole, individuals will pay 5% of the drug cost or a co-payment of $2.40 for generics or $6.00 for brand names for each prescription for the rest of the year. Only 12% of PDPs offered the standard benefit in 2008 and 10% in 2009. Besides the standard benefit, PDPs offer an alternative that is "actuarially equivalent" and can also offer enhanced benefits. To show how complicated it can be for older adults who wish to choose an alternate plan, the majority of these alternate plans charge no deductible; most charge co-payments instead of the 25% co-insurance; and some charge tiered co-payments. In 2009, 75% offer no gap coverage and if it does, the coverage may be limited to generic drugs only (The Henry J. Kaiser Family Foundation 2009a).

The monthly premiums for PDPs vary, and increase each year; they can be influenced by whether the plan pays for costs in the doughnut hole. In 2006, the average monthly PDP premium was $37.43; in 2008 it was $40.02; and in 2009 it is $45.45 (The Henry J. Kaiser Family Foundation 2008a). In 2009, the variation by region ranged from a low of $10.30 in New Mexico (standard benefit plan) to $136.80 per month in New York (PDP with enhanced benefits) (The Henry J. Kaiser Family Foundation 2009a). Overall, less than a quarter of the plans have premiums under $30 per month and the percentage of these plans decreased from 40% 1 year earlier (Hoadley et al. 2008). Enrollees in Medicare Part D who have an income below 150% of poverty ($15,600 for an individual; $21,000 for a couple in 2008) and have limited assets are eligible for assistance through the low-income subsidy program. Despite the availability of drug coverage, it is estimated that one in 10 Medicare age older adults still have no known source of drug coverage (The Henry J. Kaiser Family Foundation 2009a).

For those not eligible for Medicare Part D, there are subsidies and discounts available for seniors, disabled, uninsured, and other persons. The National Conference of State Legislatures (NCSL) tracks the State Pharmaceutical Assistance Programs, referred to as SPAPs, available at: website: http://ncsl.org/PROGRAMS/HEALTH/drugaid.htm. These subsidy programs utilize state funds to pay for a portion of the costs and some states use discounts or bulk purchasing approaches to avoid spending state funds for drug purchases. The first states to authorize programs started in 1975 and by late 2008 at least 42 states had established or authorized some type of SPAP. By June 2008, 32 states had SPAP programs in operation (NCSL 2009 update).

Health care costs for older Americans continue to increase dramatically, especially for prescription drugs. Out-of-pocket health care expenditures place a heavy burden on older adults. The implementation of Medicare Part D in 2006 provided some help to pay for the high cost of drugs. This is a complicated system to understand and access due to the increasing number and variety of benefit plans, the different co-payment structures, the increasing costs of premiums, and the need to access much of the information via the computer and internet. It has also become big business with extensive marketing strategies in place.

In 2004, Medicare paid for 53% of health care costs for Medicare enrollees. The remainder was paid by either private insurers, the individual, or Medicaid. Medicare financed most of the hospital and physician costs as well as short-term institutional, home health, and hospice costs. Even with Medicare, older adults still face significant health care costs. The inflation-adjusted health care costs for older Americans with Medicare increased significantly from 1992 to 2004. Average health care costs varied by age groups, with substantially higher costs at older ages, and by health status. For example, the average annual health care costs for Medicare enrollees for all age groups (65–74, 75–84, 75–84) was $8,644 (in 2004 dollars). This cost increased to $13,052 in 2004 (Federal Interagency Forum on Aging-Related Statistics 2008, pp 56, 117).

The Medicaid program was established to provide health coverage and supportive long-term care services for groups of low-income families, dependent children and their mothers, the older adult population, and people with disabilities. The Center for Medicare and Medicaid Services (CMS) interprets and implements the federal Medicaid statute, and issues regulations for the program. Each State will then determine the eligibility income, types of services provided, the amount and duration of services, and payment structure. The payment structure operates like a vendor program where states may directly pay the providers on a fee-for-service basis or through other prepayment arrangements such as a health maintenance organization (CMS 2005; CMS 2008b; Hoffman et al. 2008). Medicaid does not provide medical assistance for all poor persons unless they are in one of these three eligibility groups: categorically needy, medically needy, and special groups. In order to determine if an individual is covered by one of the three eligibility groups mentioned above, they must refer to their own state or check with Medicare at http://www.medicare.gov or http://www.cms.hhs.gov/medicaid/whooiseligible.asp.

Some people who qualify for Medicare Part A and/or Part B as well as Medicaid are referred to as "dual-eligibles." For these individuals, most of their health care costs are covered. Dual eligible individuals can receive benefits or "Medicare Savings Programs" (MSP) that pay for out-of-pocket medical expenses like deductibles, premiums and other services or supplies not covered or partially covered by Medicare (Medicare and You 2009, and CMS website: http://www.cms.hhs.gov/DualEligible/). Medicaid coverage is also particularly helpful for older adults who need long-term nursing home or home health care.

Despite the government's attempt to cover the majority of older Americans, there continues to be gaps between Medicare and Medicaid health coverage. Another reason to focus on the numbers of uninsured older adults has to do with the cost of care provided to low-income uninsured older adults. Uncompensated care is care not paid for by the uninsured person or an insurance program. Most of the uncompensated care is provided by the health care safety net, an informal network of hospitals, clinics, community health centers, and community-based providers.

DeLia (2006) documented trends in the use of hospital charity care by uninsured older adults in New Jersey from 1999 to 2004. The data from the New Jersey Charity Care Program found that every year between 1999 and 2004 more than 90% of older adults had family incomes below 200% of the federal poverty level, and therefore did not pay anything for hospital services. Older adults typically generated higher costs for inpatient and outpatient services. In New Jersey, the use of charity care by older patients grew much faster than it did for younger patients.

Vulnerable and at Risk: The Near Elderly Adults Age 55–64

The discussion of uninsured older adults is not complete without an examination of adults between the ages of 55 and 64, those not yet Medicare eligible due to age alone. In the literature, this group is referred to as the "near-elderly" and they are a very diverse group. Even if they are shown to have higher rates of health insurance coverage than other age groups, these adults are often faced with challenges that affect their health, their employment status, and access to health care coverage and services. One report prepared by Holahan and the Urban Institute (2004) felt that this population of near-elderly warrants taxpayer support. For many of the near-elderly, decreasing workforce participation, lower incomes, and declining health are often interrelated. Holahan found that the availability of health insurance and the health status of the near-elderly varied by income and retirement status. In general, non-retirees have better health than the ill and disabled but are in worse health than the retired. This finding was found to depend largely on income. For the low-income workforce, the availability of employer-sponsored insurance is low, eligibility for public programs is limited, and private non-group insurance is expensive. The middle-income workforce may have higher rates of employer-sponsored insurance but have less access to public programs. This still leaves many uninsured. The examination of health care access and utilization for the uninsured near-elderly found that they fared considerably worse than those who had private or public insurance, in measures such as the number of doctor visits in a year, having a usual source of care, unmet health needs, and obtaining regular preventive screening exams for women. In other words, the working near-elderly are more likely to be uninsured than their healthier retired peers.

Mere numbers and statistics do not fully portray the realities of adults who are approaching 65 years of age. In 2003, Sered and Fernandopulle spent time traveling and interviewing uninsured men and women between the ages of 55 and 64. The interviews of six adults revealed several problems. The problems included the onset of chronic conditions, the cumulative physical toll of a lifetime of hard work;

slower recovery from accidents, injury, and illness; the double burden of working and caring for an older, disabled, or ill spouse; no longer having the right skills for jobs that come with health benefits; and the loss of a late spouse's income or benefits (Sered and Kaiser Commission on Medicaid and the Uninsured 2004).

Baker and Sudano (2005) utilized the longitudinal Health and Retirement Study (HRS) and tracked a cohort of individuals for the 8 years before they were eligible for Medicare. The final cohort consisted of 6,065 adults between the age 51 and 57 at baseline. Between 1992 and 2002, the factors associated with higher mortality were older age, male sex, worse self-reported overall health, having one or more chronic illness, and being uninsured at baseline. They found that people frequently transitioned between being insured and uninsured during the 1992, 1994, 1996, 1998, and 2000 interviews. Over the 8-year period between 1992 and 2000, almost 25% of the cohort examined was uninsured at least once during the five interview intervals. Their analysis of the HRS data suggested that these individuals were at an increased risk of declining health due to being uninsured before retirement and Medicare eligibility. Multivariate analyses showed that baseline income and having less than a high-school education was associated with being uninsured more than twice during the study period. In addition, African American, Hispanic, and other ethnicities were more likely to be uninsured. This study suggested that examining data on the proportion of people who are uninsured each year may not accurately reflect the magnitude or impact of being uninsured over time or the effects of frequent transitions between being insured and uninsured (Baker and Sudano 2005).

In another study, Baker et al. (2006) analyzed the HRS data for years 1996, 1998, 2000, and 2002. They examined health and mortality data for 2,141 subjects who reached Medicare eligibility during the 1996, 1998, and 2000 HRS interviews and followed them for 2 years. Uninsured individuals before Medicare were more likely to be female, black or Hispanic, and unmarried. This group also had lower income levels, less educational attainment, was in markedly worse health, had worse self-reported overall health, more physical difficulties and a higher prevalence of chronic diseases. These physical and health risks continued during the 2-year period after receiving Medicare coverage. A follow-up observation period when subjects had Medicare coverage for 2–4 years showed that the duration of the period of increased risk appeared limited. Subjects no longer were more likely to have their health deteriorate when compared to subjects who had private insurance (Baker et al. 2006). McWilliams et al. (2007) also examined the longitudinal HRS data and compared health care use and expenditures for previously insured and uninsured individuals at 59 and 60 years of age. Based on self-reported use of health services, previously uninsured individuals used more health services and required more expensive care. For those with cardiovascular disease or diabetes, the use of health services remained high through 72 years of age. Both cardiovascular disease and diabetes are chronic conditions that can benefit from preventive care and ongoing health monitoring, only readily available to those with insurance coverage. Another examination of the costs of being uninsured is West Virginia's analyses of hospital charges based on adult inpatient discharge data. Spencer et al. (2007) compared the insurance status of the near-elderly (50–64) with other adults. The near-elderly represented the second largest group of uninsured discharges and incurred the most in charges. The high cost of care was associated with admissions for emergency conditions, more co-morbidities and complications, and longer hospital stays.

Beginning in 2001, the Institute of Medicine (IOM) published six reports that examined the consequences of maintaining the uninsured in the United States on the basis of families, health care, quality of life, as well as the economic and social impact. When contrasting the health of insured and uninsured adults age 18–64 years of age, the IOM (2002, May) found that working-age Americans were more likely to: "receive too little care and receive it too late; be sicker and die sooner; receive poorer care when they are in the hospital even for acute situations like a motor vehicle crash." Uninsured adults often do not use or have access to preventive services, screening tests and care necessary to prevent or manage chronic diseases; do not have regular access to medications; and receive fewer diagnostic and treatment services after a traumatic injury or heart attack. Another IOM (2002, September) also emphasized that when family members change jobs or retire and become uninsured, this impacts the individual and their family members as well as their economic viability.

Studies consistently highlight the impact of being uninsured on a person's health, economic viability, and family for individuals who are 50–64 years old. Another important issue that requires legislative initiatives and policies has to do with obtaining health insurance at a later age. Monheit et al. (2001) noted that near-elderly workers as a group are unlikely to be able to obtain health insurance once they become uninsured when compared to younger workers. A sub-group at particular risk was near-elderly women with health problems. The additional challenge for near-elderly female when compared to younger or healthier women may reflect that their economic status may be poorer thus making them less able to purchase coverage or have opportunities to job that offer coverage, and the lack of dependent coverage. Another study looked at near-elderly women's health insurance coverage and its impact. This study by Xu et al. (2006) analyzed the HRS data for 2002 for women between the ages of 55 and 64. The results confirmed earlier studies that showed how near-elderly women are a particularly vulnerable group due to reliance on spouse's employer for health coverage, widowhood, or divorce. Insurance coverage significantly affects the access and use of important preventive and ongoing health care services for women aged 55–64 years.

It is not difficult to identify potential consequences of not having ongoing health insurance. The lack of consistent care, preventive health care, and affordable care can lead to poor health outcomes. Poor health outcomes and late diagnosis can lead to more costly hospital admissions and an increased need for health services. The last section will show how several states are trying to expand services to the uninsured in their communities.

Health Care Reform for the Uninsured

The following are examples of how cities are providing care to their uninsured communities. They are not insurance programs but mechanisms to provide necessary health care services to those who cannot afford private insurance or who do not qualify for federal programs like Medicare. The following programs were not designed specifically with the older population in mind but the proposals presented provide a good idea on how states are creatively trying to address the needs of the uninsured who cannot afford to purchase the necessary care.

One way that programs provide health care is through universal access, not coverage. The *Healthy San Francisco* program became the first city in the United States to provide health care access and services to all uninsured residents regardless of their immigration status, employment status, or pre-existing medical conditions. Although geared toward the 18–64 age group, the program does address the issues faced by the near-elderly that were discussed earlier. The program is administered by the San Francisco Department of Public Health and care can be obtained only from the San Francisco General Hospital and the network of 27 participating clinics operated by the San Francisco Community Clinic Consortium. The key feature of this program is the use of medical homes. Enrollees are required to pay quarterly participant fees based on their income. The fees do not exceed 5% of the family income for individuals with income below 500% of the federal poverty level. Individuals whose income falls below the poverty level are not charged. Those with incomes above the poverty level pay point-of-service fees that range from $10 for a primary care visit to $200 per hospital admission. *Healthy San Francisco* is also funded by redirected city funds. The program has at least one controversial aspect. Beginning in January 2008, employers from medium and large firms with more than 20 workers must contribute between $1.17 and $1.76 per hour, per covered worker. There are several ways the employers can satisfy this requirement. Resulting lawsuits have challenged this employer requirement (Kaiser Commission on Medicaid and the Uninsured 2008a).

The Kaiser Commission on Medicaid and the Uninsured tracks states who have enacted or proposed universal health care coverage. None of these plans specifically target our older population but do attempt to provide greater health care coverage for adults. As of November 5, 2008 – Maine, Massachusetts, and Vermont enacted reform plans to achieve near universal health care coverage for its residents. Here are just some of the key features of each plan. Maine's Dirigo Health Reform Act was signed into law in 2003. Dirigo Choice is a voluntary and affordable health plan for individuals, self-employed, and for smaller business with 50 or less employees. Recent reform efforts have focused on individual and employer mandates, reinsurance programs that would lower the community base rate for premiums, and premiums to be based on health status and claims history. Massachusetts mandates that all adults purchase health insurance. The premiums are adjusted based on income levels below the federal poverty level. Vermont's Catamount Health also has premium assistance and requires employers to pay an assessment fee for employees who are not offered a plan, do not take up health care coverage, or are uninsured (Kaiser Commission on Medicaid and the Uninsured 2008b – states). Unfortunately, these three states do not have a large percentage of older adults. Updates on states' legislative efforts to cover the uninsured are updated at http://www.kff.org and http://www.health08.org.

In 2006, California, Florida, New York, Texas, and Pennsylvania had over 1.5 million older adults in each state (Greenberg 2007). Of these states, only California, New York, and Pennsylvania have proposed a universal coverage plan. California's *Stay Healthy California* creates a statewide purchasing pool, includes an individual mandate with exceptions for affordability and hardship, includes subsidies for low and moderate income individuals, and requires employers with 10 or more employees to provide coverage or contribute to the cost of their employees' coverage. New York's plan focuses on expanding coverage to families with children. Pennsylvania's proposed health care reform focused on several individual legislative bills that addressed premium subsidies, insurance mandates for adults, fair share tax on employers, and improving patient safety in hospitals. In New Mexico and Colorado, the population of 65 and older increased by more than 20% between 1996 and 2006. The Colorado Blue Ribbon Commission for Health Care Reform endorsed several recommendations. The recommendations include: mandates that individuals purchase a Minimum Benefit Plan or face a tax penalty, expands eligibility of federal programs up to 205% of the federal poverty level for all uninsured residents, creates an insurance exchange to lower cost, provides premium subsidies to workers, requires employers to establish plans to allow employees to withhold money for health insurance on a pre-tax basis, contains insurance market reforms, and requires health carriers to offer a Minimum Benefit Plan. *Health Insurance New Mexico* includes an individual mandate and an employer mandate for employers with six or more employees, creates larger risk pools, requires commercial health care insurers to spend a percentage of premiums directly on health care, and utilizes electronic claims submission and payments. These plans and proposals are constantly evolving. Many focus on both individual and employer mandates and adjusting premiums depending on income levels (Kaiser Commission on Medicaid and the Uninsured 2008b).

On September 2008, Howard County in Maryland launched the *Healthy Howard* program that provides a health program for uninsured residents in the county who make too much to qualify for state and federal programs but not enough to afford care. This program offers medical benefits for as little as $50 a month and provides as many as six visits a year to primary care providers, free in-patient hospital care, mental health care, discount prescriptions and other services. Enrollees will also have access to coaches that will assist them with personal health plans. The program will be subsidized with county and private foundations as well as physicians who will provide free or reduced fees. Healthy Howard will be open to 2,200 individuals in the first year (Aratani 2008).

Another innovative approach using technology is an internet version of the house call for residents of Hawaii. The Hawaii Medical Service Association (HMSA), the state's Blue Cross-Blue Shield license introduces *American Well* in

January 2009. This service, based in Boston, provides the uninsured and others access to 10-min appointments with doctors for a fee. Enrollee's without insurance pay $45 to use the service and HMSA pays American Well a license fee per member and a transaction fee of approximately $2 for each patient-doctor encounter. In contrast, Hawaii State residents who have HMSA insurance pay $10 to use the service. Patients must log on to the website and services include: an extended appointment for a fee, filing of prescriptions, and electronic medical histories. This service is viewed as a viable option for persons in rural areas, those with transportation issues, and time constraints. Concerns focus around missing important symptoms due to the inability to see or touch the patient (Miller 2009).

Collaborative Efforts Required

Providing health care to our near-elderly and those 65 and over will require a collaborative effort. Policy makers must have a greater awareness and understanding of the limitations of Medicare and Medicaid. Surveys and reports that address insurance status and health status should consistently include adults 65 and older even if their percentage does not have the same magnitude or impact. Community members, program administrators, and government officials must constantly be reminded of our changing demographics and increasing diversity so they can be proactive when designing and advocating for changes in our health care system.

Appendix: Helpful Resources on Aging and Geriatrics

- Medicare and You 2009 (additional helpful numbers available on page 14). Available from: http://www.medicare.gov

  1-800-MEDICARE   1-800-633-4227
  Social Security   1-800-772-1213 (TTY 1-800-)

- *Centers for Medicare and Medicaid Services/DHHS.* CMS Data and Statistics available from: http://www.cms.hhs.gov/home/rsds.asp
- *Geriatrics at Your Fingertips: 2008–2009 10th Online Edition.* A reference to clinical geriatrics on the evaluation and management of diseases and disorders most common to older adults. Updated annually, PDA version available for download. Available from: http://www.geriatricsatyourfingertips.org/
- *American Geriatrics Society.* Not-for-profit organization of health professionals providing leadership and advocacy in patient care, research, professional and public education, and public policy. Available from: http://www.americangeriatrics.org
- *American Gerontological Society.* The nation's largest interdisciplinary organization devoted to research, education, and practice in the field of aging.

There are four sections: Biological Sciences, Health Sciences, Behavioral and Social Sciences, and Social Research, Policy and Practice. Available from: http://www.geron.org
* *Administration on Aging, Department of Health and Human Services.* Available from: http://www.aoa.gov.
* *MEDLINEPlus.* Web resources for the consumer on health, medications, and disease-related topics. Available from: http://www.nlm.nih.gov/medlineplus/
* *Health Finder.* An encyclopedia of health topics, services, and information. Available from: http://healthfinder.gov/

References

Aratani L (2008, September 30) Howard health initiative ready to enroll uninsured. Washington Post.http://www.washingtonpost.com/wp-dyn/content/article/2008/09/29/AR2008092902904.html. Accessed 6 Jan 2009

Baker DW, Sudano JJ (2005) Health insurance coverage during the years preceding Medicare eligibility. Arch Intern Med 165:770–776

Baker DW, Feinglass J, Durazo-Arvizu R et al (2006) Changes in health for the uninsured after reaching age-eligibility for Medicare. J Gen Intern Med 21:1144–1149

CMS/Centers for Medicare and Medicaid Services (2008, Sepember) Medicare and You 2009. www.medicare.gov. Accessed 6 Jan 2009

CMS/Centers for Medicare and Medicaid Services (2008, November) Dual eligibility overview. http://www.cms.hhs.gov/DualEligible/. Accessed 6 Apr 2009

CMS/Centers for Medicare and Medicaid Services/DHHS (2005) Medicaid at a Glance: 2005. http://www.cms.hhs.gov/Medicaid GenInfo/. Accessed 6 Jan 2009

Cohen RA, Martinez ME (June 2007, Corrections August 2007) Health insurance coverage: early release of estimates from the National Health Interview Survey, 2006. National Center for Health Statistics. http://www.cdc.gov/nchs/about/major/nhis/releases.htm. Accessed 6 Jan 2009

DeLia D (2006) Caring for the new uninsured: hospital charity care for older people without coverage. J Am Geriatr Soc 54:1933–1936

Federal Interagency Forum on Aging-Related Statistics (2008, March) Older Americans 2008: key indicators of well-being. Federal Interagency Forum on Aging-Related Statistics Washington, DC: U.S. Government Printing Office. http://www.agingstats.gov/agingstatsdotnet/main_site/default.aspx. Accessed 7 Jan 2009

Fowles DG, Greenberg S, Administration on Aging (AoA), U.S. Department of Health and Human Services (2008). Profile of older Americans: 2008. http://www.aoa.gov/AoARoot/Aging_Statistics/Profile/index.aspx. Accessed 15 Apr 2009

Gray BH, Scheinmann R, Rosenfeld P, Finkelstein R (2006) Aging without Medicare? Evidence from New York City. Inquiry 43(3):211–221

Greenberg A (2007) Agingstats.gov Available at: http://www.aoa.gov/Agingstatsdotnet/Main_Site/Data/Data_2008.aspx. Accessed 4 Ap 1009

Hoadley J, Thompson J, Hargrave E, Cubanski J, Neuman T (2008, November) Medicare Part D, 2009, Data spotlight: premiums. http://www.kff.org/medicare/7835.cfm. Accessed 10 Jan 2009

Hoffman ED, Klees BS, Curtis CA (2008, November) Brief summaries of Medicare & Medicaid Title XVIII and Title XIX of the Social Security Act. Office of the Actuary, Centers for Medicare and Medicaid, DHHS. http://www.cms.hhs.gov/MedicareProgramRatesStats/02_SummaryMedicareMedicaid.asp. Accessed 6 Jan 2009

Holahan J, Kaiser Commission on Medicaid and the Uninsured (2004, July) Health insurance coverage of the near elderly. http://www.kff.org/uninsured/7114.cfm. Accessed 6 Jan 2009

Institute of Medicine (2002, May) Report brief. Care without coverage: too little too late. http://www.iom.edu/CMS/3809/4660/4333/4160.aspx. Accessed 7 Apr 2009

Institute of Medicine (2002, September) Report brief. Health insurance is a family matter. http://www.iom.edu/CMS/4161.aspx. Accessed 7 Apr 2009

Kaiser Commission on Medicaid and the Uninsured (2008, March) Healthy San Francisco. http://www.kff.org/uninsured/7760A.cfm. Accessed 6 Jan 2009

Kaiser Commission on Medicaid and the Uninsured (2008) States moving toward comprehensive health care reform. http://www.kff.org/uninsured/kcmu_statehealthreform.cfm. Accessed 6 Jan 2009

Martinez ME, Cohen RA, Division of Health Interview Statistics, National Center for Health Statistics (2008, December) Health insurance coverage: early release of estimates from the National health Interview Survey, January–June 2008. http://www.cdc.gov/nchs/about/major/nhis/releases.htm. Accessed 6 Jan 2009

McWilliams JM, Meara E, Zaslavsky AM, Ayanian JZ (2007). N Engl J Med 357:143–153

Miller CC (2009, January 6) Doctors will make web calls in Hawaii. The New York Times. http://www.nytimes.com/2009/01/06/technology/internet/06health.htm?_r=2. Accessed 6 Jan 2009

Mold JW, Fryer GE, Thomas CH (2004) Who are the uninsured elderly in the United States? J Am Geriatr Soc 52:601–606

Monheit AC, Vistnes JP, Eisenberg JM (2001) Moving to Medicare: trends in the health insurance status of near-elderly workers, 1987–1996. Health Aff 2:204–213

National Conference of State Legislatures (2009, January 2) State pharmaceutical assistance programs. http://www.ncsl.org/PROGRAMS/HEALTH/drugaid.htm. Accessed 6 Jan 2009

Okoro CA, Young SL, Strine TW et al (2005) Uninsured adults aged 65 years and older; is their health at risk? J Health Care Poor Underserved 16:453–463

Sered S, Kaiser Commission on Medicaid and the Uninsured (2004, August) At the edge: Near-elderly Americans talk about health insurance. http://www.kff.org/uninsured/7127.cfm. Accessed 6 Jan 2009

Spencer DL, Richardson S, McCormick M (2007) Inpatient hospital utilization among the uninsured near elderly: Data and policy implications for West Virginia. Health Serv Res 42(6 Pt II):2442–2457

The Henry J. Kaiser Family Foundation (2007, February) Medicare at a glance fact sheet. http://www.kff.org/medicare/1066.cfm. Accessed 6 Jan 2009

The Henry J. Kaiser Family Foundation (2008, November) Medicare part D prescription drug plan (PDP) availability in 2009. http://www.kff.org/medicare/7426.cfm. Accessed 10 Jan 2009

The Henry J. Kaiser Family Foundation (2008) Medicare at a glance fact sheet. http://www.kff.org/medicare/1066.cfm. Accessed 6 Jan 2009

The Henry J. Kaiser Family Foundation (2008) The Medicare prescription drug benefit. http://www.kff.org/Medicare/7044.cfm. Accessed 6 Jan 2009

The Henry J. Kaiser Family Foundation (2009) Medicare at a glance fact sheet. http://www.kff.org/medicare/1066.cfm. Accessed 6 Jan 2009

The Henry J. Kaiser Family Foundation (2009) Medicare: a primer. http://www.kff.org/Medicare/7615.cfm. Accessed 6 Jan 2009

The University of Arizona, College of Pharmacy (2007) UA pharmacists to train others in patient counseling. http://www.pharmacy.arizona.edu/media/uViewPressRelease.php?releaseID=21. Accessed 10 Jan 2009

Xu X, Patel DA, Vahratian A, Ransom SB (2006) Insurance coverage and health care use among near-elderly women. Womens Health Issues 16:139–148

Direct Caregivers Association: An Option for a Rapidly Growing Aging Population?

Judith B. Clinco

The unmet need of caregivers and community caregiving organizations for our elderly, disabled, and chronically ill population is a crisis not for the future – it's happening right now.

There is evidence of a rapid growth in the current system of long term services, care and support as the population of the United States grows older; the number of people projected to need assistance with the activities of daily living is expected to double from 13 million in 2000 to 27 million in 2050 (Kaye et al. 2006).

The total annual expenditure on long-term care (from consumers, insurance benefits, State governments) is $ 271 billion. For this huge sum, the returns are:

- An unstable workforce – workers who are underpaid, undertrained, and undervalued.
- Long-term care employers who deal with shortages and chronic turnovers of qualified workers.
- Recipients of care receiving substandard care and services.

Who Pays For Long-Term Care?

Government

Medicaid, financed by State revenues that are matched with Federal dollars, is the largest purchaser of direct care services, including home and community based services, group homes, and nursing homes. Medicaid is available for people with very low income, or minimal assets, and for those who meet strict medical guidelines. Public funds pay for 70% of long-term care according to the Georgetown University Long-Term Care Financing Project (Institute for the Future of Aging 2007).

J.B. Clinco
CEO, Catalina In-Home Services, Inc, Tucson, AZ, USA

N.J. Johnson and L.P. Johnson (eds.), *The Care of the Uninsured in America*,
DOI 10.1007/978-0-387-78309-3_13, © Springer Science+Business Media, LLC 2010

Those who meet the income threshold but have assets, are required to liquidate the assets and spend it all on care, before the government benefit commences. Those who wish to transfer their assets to beneficiaries, have not only to deal with the tax consequences, but they also need to do so at least 5 years prior to applying for this Medicaid benefit. For every $10,000 transferred within 60 months of applying for the benefit, the beginning of the benefit will be delayed according to each State's standards. Care can be provided in the recipient's home, if the cost does not exceed facility care. There is a major national trend toward financing home and community-based care with Medicaid. This is mainly because the vast majority of care recipients prefer to live at home, and also because it is usually less expensive than institutional care.

In the past, Medicaid usually paid home care agencies directly. With the new movement toward consumer-directed care, States are aggressively switching to a model in which care dollars are given directly to the family members or to the care recipients, to hire and supervise their own home care workers.

Insurance

Long-Term Care insurance is purchased by those with the financial resources to pay the premiums, or by those who work for employers who offer this benefit to their employees, and sometimes their parents. The beneficiary of a long-term care policy must not only meet the insurance company's health criteria, but also decide in advance, on the basis of the amount of the premium he/she wishes to pay, the amount of coverage he/she will receive. This amount is either a daily benefit, or a lump sum that is made available to purchase care. The policy customer decides the duration of the care: either a specific number of years or for life. Some policies have a built-in increase in benefits tied to the inflation rate; others provide a fixed benefit.

At one time, insurance companies made no delay in the provision of benefits, and policies could be used for acute situations, such as recovery from a hip fracture. Today, policies have a 90-day elimination clause, requiring out-of-pocket provision of necessary services until the benefit becomes activated. Therefore, the insurance companies provide benefits only for chronic conditions. Some people may die during the "elimination period," therefore never being able to access the benefit. Many purchasers of Long Term Care policies do not understand this. If they have purchased such a policy and do not have the cash saved to pay for 90 days of out-of-pocket care, they will become financial burdens on their families.

Although earlier Long-Term-Care policies specified the location of care (home, adult care home, or nursing home), contemporary policies are written to provide benefits throughout the continuum of long term care venues. Also, the trend in disbursement of home care benefits is to provide the funds for hiring caregivers privately, utilizing a professional agency for services, or paying family caregivers.

Paying Privately

Most people believe that Medicare will pay for long term care. Usually they are quite surprised to discover, when they're too sick to purchase a Long-Term-Care policy and their income excludes them from Medicare, that long term care will be a personal expense. Nursing Home care may cost as much as $70,000 per year; Assisted Living can cost $2,800–$8,400 per month. The price range of agency-provided home care is approximately $17–$28 per hour; hiring someone privately may cost $7–$15 per hour (depending on geographic location).

There is an income level that disqualifies people from receiving Medicaid, but which is insufficient to purchase private care and medication, along with food and housing. This income range is where most aging baby boomers will be found. The average baby boomer has approximately $100,000 in assets. This is an income level that disqualifies people from receiving Medicaid, but which is insufficient to purchase private care and medication, along with food and housing. Clearly, this is insufficient for long term care.

By 2030, there will be 71 million American older adults accounting for roughly 20% of the U.S. population. The nation's health care spending is projected to increase by 25% because of these demographic shifts (CDC 2007).

In addition to the aging population, there is also an increasing proportion of long term care recipients who are young and permanently disabled, including tens of thousands of injured military veterans. This reflects advances in medical care, trauma care, and pharmaceuticals.

To date, there has been no governmental leadership or national conversation regarding this crisis. There is no discussion about the source of funds to pay for long term care, or about the governmental policy of impoverishing citizens in order for them to be eligible for Medicaid.

Other Sources of Care and Support

Family Caregivers

Informal caregivers are the backbone of support for an aging population. "Informal caregivers provide the majority of long-term care services in the U.S. In 2000, there were 22 million unpaid informal caregivers aiding 14 million elderly persons in the U.S. These numbers are projected to increase to approximately 40 million individuals caring for approximately 28 million Americans in 2050. The value of informal care-giving goes far beyond nurturing and social support that enables people who need care to remain in their homes. Economic estimates based on 2003 data find that not only do informal caregivers – family, friends and volunteers – supplement the health care workforce and provide the majority of long-term care services in the U.S., in 2003 they provided services with an estimated market value of $257 billion (Citizens Workgroup on the Long-Term Care Workforce 2005)."

Although informal caregivers are the primary agents of direct long-term care, a simple extrapolation from today's data does not take into account two important factors:

1. The increase of divorce among the baby boomers means that fewer spouses will be available to provide care.
2. The decrease in the average number of children among the baby boomers means less likelihood that children will be available to provide care and support.

This means an even greater reliance on paid, professional direct care.

Today, there are approximately 34 million informal caregivers. About three fourths of all elders who receive care at home rely exclusively on paid or unpaid spouses and children who are generally between the ages of 45 and 64, two-thirds of whom are women. Almost all states provide pay for family caregivers through Medicaid's Home and Community-Based Waiver Program or another state program (Institute for the Future of Aging Services 2007).

Volunteers

It is clear that there will not be sufficient money to pay for caregivers as the nation's population ages. Volunteer caregivers through churches or secular organizations (such as neighborhood associations) will be an essential component of the caregiving continuum. Programs such as the Minnesota Live-At-Home Block Nursing Program and the Boston Beacon Village Program are successful examples of mobilizing neighborhoods to assist individuals in continuing to be an active part of community life despite progressive physical frailty.

The Old Fort Lowell Neighborhood Live-At-Home Program

In 1997, the author started a neighborhood 501(c)3 program for volunteer support services, based on the Minnesota Live-At-Home Block Nursing Program. Our neighborhood has a higher-than-average proportion of elderly residents who live in their own homes. The intent of the program is to support people living at home independently as long as possible.

The Old Fort Lowell Neighborhood Live-At-Home Program has a volunteer Board of Directors composed of retired business and professional people, and one part-time paid staff member, a retired Social Worker who lives in the neighborhood. She recruits and trains neighborhood volunteers, meets with prospective clients and stays in communication with neighbors who are being served, schedules the volunteers, maintains the data files, and creates a volunteer/client newsletter. The most requested service is transportation to doctors and shopping centers. The Program also provides daily wellness calls, companionship visits, yard work, and minor home repairs. Services are provided on a long-term or short-term basis. We sponsor two annual social events for volunteers and clients, and offer a health lecture series open to everyone in the neighborhood.

The average cost for running the program is $21,000 per year, which pays the staff salary, cell phone, postage, and insurance. The neighborhood raises the money for the program by hosting an annual communal yard sale, our "Flea Market." We also send an annual fundraising appeal letter to all neighborhood residents.

This program has been so successful that it has been replicated in numerous neighborhoods and homeowner associations throughout Tucson, thus greatly increasing the city's active direct care workforce.

Creating a Qualified Long-Term-Care Workforce

Of all professional direct care workers:

1. 20% are licensed professionals, including physicians, nurse practitioners, nursing home and assisted living administrators, other home health and community service agency directors, chief executive officers, registered nurses (RNs), licensed practical and vocational nurses (LPNs/LVNs)
2. 80% of hands-on care is provided by Professional Direct Care Workers, approximately 1.85 million employees (facility-based and home care settings), including home health aides, nursing aides, orderlies, attendants, and personal and home-care aides, as well as privately hired direct care workers (US Bureau of Labor Statistics 2000).

Estimating the size of the privately hired home direct care workforce is particularly difficult. In 2006, the paraprofessional workforce consisted of:

- 1,391,430 nurse aides, orderlies and attendants, largely employed in nursing homes;
- 663,280 home health aides, a slight majority of whom work in home-based care settings; and
- 566,860 personal care and home care aides, two-thirds of whom work in home-based services. The majority of these direct care workers are employed in long-term care settings.
- Women make up about 90% of the paraprofessional workforce. About 50% are racial or ethnic minorities, including 33% who are African American and 15% who are either Hispanic or other persons of color.
- Between now and 2015, [...] the native-born population aged 25–54, the pool of individuals from which both paid and family caregivers have largely come – will not increase at all.
- The average wages for Direct Care Workers are $17,000–$19,000 per year (Institute for the Future of Aging Services 2007).

One in four direct care workers employed in nursing homes, and two in five employed in home care agencies, also lack health insurance. Nursing home workers are twice as likely to be uninsured as hospital personnel. High injury rates may make them especially vulnerable without adequate insurance coverage (Paraprofessional Health Care Institute 2006).

Not only is the number of qualified direct care workers decreasing with respect to the demand, turnover in employment is higher than in the fast-food industry. According to the Department of Labor, direct care work is one of the four fastest growing industries in the U.S., yet it is listed as one of the ten worst jobs.

Turnover rates range between 40 and 100% annually (2003 American Health Care Association Workforce Report).

[...] the most important reason direct care workers stay in their jobs is the relationships they have with the older adults in their care. Turnover and job dissatisfaction is clearly linked to poor pay and benefits (PHI 2004). [...] Direct care workers whose work is valued and appreciated by their supervisors, and who are listened to and encouraged to participate in care planning decisions, have higher levels of job satisfaction and are more likely to stay in their jobs (Citizens Workgroup on the Long-Term Care Workforce 2005).

Other reasons for which direct care workers leave this industry include poor working conditions, inadequate staffing which leads to excessive and dangerous work loads, poor training, the second highest worker injury rate (truck drivers are first), and insufficient wages, usually less than $12.00 per hour.

Training the Direct Care Workforce

To become a Certified Nursing Assistant or Home Health Aide, individuals are required to have less than 2 weeks of training. Home Care Aides are not subject to Federal training requirements, and few states require training for them (Institute for the Future of Aging 2007).

Our experience as a private duty home care employer for 26 years has shown that 2 weeks of training is simply not sufficient for an individual to qualify as a competent, trained worker. In Arizona, dog grooming requires 600 hours of training, while manicurists and pedicurists require 650 hours of training. We have found that 200 hours of training is the minimum for assuring a high standard of care.

Despite the dissatisfaction with being poorly trained, the lack of training requirements means that individuals who need a job can get one right away. Although increased training may lead to increased wages, higher quality care, and opportunities for advancement, States and the federal government have not allocated funds for training, other than the money available for Nursing Homes to train Certified Nursing Assistants.

The majority of people who seek entry into Direct Care are economically and educationally disadvantaged. Even if adequate training dollars were available, prospective trainees require stipends for their cost of living while being trained. Structuring these stipends as loans requiring repayment after starting employment would be a considerable hardship. Government funding to support these people during their caregiver education should be mandatory.

With more training comes higher wages, which means that facilities, home care agencies, and consumers will require higher rates of reimbursement.

An Innovative Training Model

In 2000, responding to the already critical shortage of qualified direct care workers, eight long-term care employers, including home, residential, and facility based companies, for-profit and not-for-profit, came together to create a solution. They founded The Direct CareGiver Association (DCGA), a 501(c)3 company whose exclusive mission is to recruit, screen, and train prospective direct care workers through a combination of private, corporate, foundation, and government funding. All dues-paying employer members of the DCGA are eager to hire graduates of this 200 hours training program, often offering wages higher than the community standard for this work ($9.00 to $12.00 per hour). In addition to caregiving skills, training includes cooking, time management, stress management, communication skills, team building, working with supervisors, and strategies and coaching for becoming a reliable and desirable employee. The DCGA has a high success rate among its graduates: 87% graduation rate, almost all of whom sought work in this industry and were hired. Many graduates report moving upwards, achieving further education and higher levels of health care employment, thus demonstrating that direct care work is truly the first step on a health-career path for motivated individuals.

The cost of tuition is approximately $3,000, and the DCGA has the philosophy that no student will go into debt to become a direct care worker. The average self-pay student pays approximately 10% of the total cost, which includes supplies (e.g., nursing shoes, gait belt, blood pressure cuff, watch, stethoscope, the fee to cover the state certification exam).

Since 2001, the DCGA has developed positive relationships with government funders such as the County One-Stop Program. Our industry now has representation on The Pima County Workforce Investment Board. Students meeting DCGA and One-Stop, VocRehab, or DES criteria have their entire tuition paid by government job-training dollars.

The DCGA also brings in grants from foundations, as well as donor funding from concerned citizens.

Through community outreach such as Op-Ed articles, presentations in community organizations, television features, Tucson's local citizens have become increasingly aware of the DCGA, its work, and the problems which the DCGA addresses.

Unlike nursing home-based training funded by the government, or assisted-living or home-care agency in-house training funded by employers, the DCGA brings additional training dollars to support its longer-than-state-mandates program. And unlike community college-based training, the DCGA does not require a high school or GED diploma, thus providing opportunities for a vastly underserved population.

The private for-profit or not-for-profit employer can spend up to $4,000 to recruit, screen, and train an individual who may not stay on the job. Given the low profit margin in the service industry, this is an intolerable burden. When budgets are cut and cash flow is diminished, training is often the first expense to be cut. The DCGA has not only taken over the training burden, it also demands quality, dedication, and skills from its graduates, assuring employers that their clients will be well served. If the employer–employee relationship doesn't work out, both parties can find a better situation without the employer having lost significant resources.

The DCGA is a win–win solution to the direct care worker shortage. Workers receive better training, employers know they're hiring very well trained workers, and consumers benefit from better care. Well-trained direct care workers are more able to recognize subtle changes and imminent health crises in their clients, leading to reduced rates of hospitalization or institutionalization. This reduces the total cost of long-term care, making more money available for direct care worker wages and benefits. Better training, better wages and benefits, and more respect from employers means that more individuals will be attracted to this work, will stay longer, and solve the nationwide crisis.

In other words, the DCGA model is a money-saving bargain in health care.

References

Centers for Disease Control and Prevention (2007) The State of Aging and Health in America 2007 Report. Centers for Disease Control and Prevention. Available at: http://www.cdc.gov/aging/saha.htm. Accessed 11 Apr, 2009

Citizen's Workgroup on the Long-Term Care Workforce (2005) Will anyone care? Leading the paradigm shift in developing Arizona's direct care workforce. Available at: http://www.ahcccs.us/Contracting/BiddersLibrary/ALTCS/Reference/CWGReport_Final_June2005.pdf. Accessed 11 April, 2009

Kaye HS et al. (2006) Supply and demand: coming trends foretell a shortage of these workers, reversing recent gains. Health Aff 25(4) 1113–1120

Institute for the Future of Aging Services (2007) The long-term care workforce: can the crisis be fixed? American Association of Homes and Services for the Aging. Available at: http://www.aahsa.org/uploadedFiles/resources/Advocacy/Policy_Statements/LTC%20workforce.pdf. Accessed 11 Apr, 2009

Paraprofessional Health Care Institute (2006) Who are direct-care workers? Available at: http://www.directcareclearinghouse.org/download/NCDCW%20Fact%20Sheet-1.pdf. Accessed 11 Apr, 2009

US Bureau of Labor Statistics (2000) The U.S. direct care workforce – overview. Available at:https://egov.azdes.gov/CMS400Min/uploadedFiles/DAAS/direct_care_workforce_united_states.pdf. Accessed 11 Apr, 2009

The Rural Uninsured

Lane P. Johnson

Carmen Gonzales is a 63 year-old who has been sent home to her rural community of about 1,500 residents from an urban hospital following surgery and chemotherapy for colon cancer. She has metastasis of the cancer to the liver and throughout the peritoneum. No further treatment is being considered. She has only one daughter, a single mom who lives with her three children in an urban community 75 miles away. She tries to visit Ms. Gonzales regularly but, with her job and family responsibilities, cannot come down to the community except on weekends. Ms. Gonzales has no other family. She lives in a small house with her 76 year-old husband, who has barely been able to care of himself in her absence. The community has a part-time clinic staffed 3 days a week by a traveling nurse practitioner. The county health department provides Well Child and Preventive Services at a monthly clinic only. There is a small general store, but no drug store or pharmacy. Ms. Gonzales and her husband retired to the community about twelve years back. They have kept to themselves and have not been active in church or social activities, and have not made many friends. Ms. Gonzales is currently able to take care of herself, cook light meals, bathe and dress, but she is getting progressively weaker. The pain is getting worse and she is requiring increased amounts of narcotic medication to control it.

Introduction

One of the more important considerations regarding healthcare in rural areas is to recognize that rural areas and rural populations in the United States are not homogenous. There are vast geographic, demographic, ethnic, cultural, political, and economic differences among rural areas and rural residents. While it is necessary in a book such as this to look at rural populations collectively, these differences must also be considered. There are more than 15 different definitions of "rural" currently used for federal programs. The two most commonly used by the Census

L.P. Johnson
Arizona Health Sciences Center,
Tucson, AZ, USA
e-mail: lpj@email.arizona.edu

N.J. Johnson and L.P. Johnson (eds.), *The Care of the Uninsured in America*,
DOI 10.1007/978-0-387-78309-3_14, © Springer Science+Business Media, LLC 2010

Bureau, and the Office of Management and Budget, result in defining very different locations and populations (Coburn et al. 2008).

None of the definitions is entirely satisfactory. "Rural" definitions can include differing geographic locations, such as county or community, population size, distance from urban center, among other characteristics that vary considerably across the United States. In eastern states, for example, there may be a number of small communities relatively close together and near an urban center defined as rural. In western states, very small communities with minimal health resources may be many miles, and hours of travel time, apart from each other, much less an urban center. A federal designation of "Frontier" is given to those areas with a population density of less than six people per square mile. There is little consistency among rural populations in demographic characteristics as well, including age, gender, ethnicity, economic status or education.

In the introductory chapter, a number of features of rural vs urban populations were described; rural populations, in general, are older, poorer, and less healthy. They are also less likely to have health insurance, or are more likely to go without insurance for longer periods of time.

Compounding the difficulties for rural populations is a significantly lower level and quantity of health services. From primary care providers to specialists, from clinics to hospitals to tertiary care services, rural populations have fewer, if any, options. There are fewer dental, pharmacy, mental health, home health, or hospice services. In general, demographic disparities, health status, and level of health services, all worsen with increasing distance from urban centers.

Another important consideration is that health care services may provide a significant economic base for many small communities. A weakening local economy leads to a vicious downward spiral where fewer services mean less financial support. This further erodes the ability of the community to provide health services, leading to an economic, human resource, and intellectual exodus of some of the brightest, economically able, and most involved of the community's population. Approximately, 500 rural hospitals have closed in the United States over the last 30 years (National Rural Health Association 2009).

Over the last two decades there has been at least a tacit recognition of some of the difficulties rural communities face in providing health care services. A number of federal, state, and local programs have been developed to enhance payments to rural providers, to encourage and support more rural health care providers, to improve the financial stability of rural hospitals and institutions, and to develop innovative technologic programs to improve care. These issues will be explored further in this chapter.

Demographics

In the United States, rural residents make up 20% of the total population. Eighteen percent of the rural population is over 65 years of age, compared with 15% in urban areas. This figure is considered to reflect younger adult rural residents seeking better economic opportunities elsewhere, an option not available to the poor, rural elderly. Rural populations tend to have a greater representation of ethnic minorities, and tend to have lower educational levels than urban populations (National Rural Health Association 2009). This is thought to reflect the agricultural economic base of many rural areas.

Economically, rural residents fare much worse than urban residents. Across the United States, the per capita income of rural residents (1996) was $19,000 compared to $26,000 for urban residents. Correspondingly, the percentage of rural residents living below 100% of the poverty level is 14% compared to 11% of urban residents. While about 22% of the U.S. population lives in rural areas, 31% are food stamp beneficiaries Almost 25% of rural children live in poverty (National Rural Health Association 2009). Economic conditions for rural residents are often more tenuous due to a greater dependence on a single industry (i.e., agriculture, mining, logging, manufacturing, or tourism) subject to the vagaries of the economic climate, as well as more self-employment, small businesses, and part-time or seasonal jobs. The lack of availability of private health insurance in rural areas is also related to these issues.

Health Status

The health statistics of rural areas reflect a younger population with increased mortality at higher risk from accidents, injuries, chronic diseases, high-risk behaviors, and mental illness, with poorer access to health care and ancillary services.

The death rate for males aged 1–24 in rural areas is 80/100,000 compared to 60/100,000 in urban areas. The death rate for females aged 1–24 in rural areas is 40/100,000 compared to 30/100,000 in urban areas. Rural residents have higher rates of hypertension, cerebro-vascular disease, and are significantly more likely to die after a heart attack. Following a heart attack, they are less likely to receive appropriate treatment (National Rural Health Association 2009). Hospitalization rates are higher for rural residents, while length of stay is shorter. These figures, coupled with decreased availability of health care providers and facilities suggest that rural residents may seek hospital care for issues that could have been treated as an outpatient, due to lack of health insurance (National Center for Health Statistics 2001).

While only 1/3 of motor vehicle accidents occur on rural roads, they account for 2/3 of fatalities from motor vehicle accidents. Not only are rural residents more likely to die in motor vehicle accidents, they are twice as likely to die from other unintentional injuries, and are at significantly higher risk of death by gunshot. Less access and decreased availability of emergency communication leads to longer times to initiate emergency services. Distances from first responders and primary facilities, availability of basic emergency care, and lack of advanced trauma services also contribute to the increased mortality from injuries. Average response times for EMS arrival in rural areas is 18 minutes, at least 8 minutes greater than in urban areas. About 60–90% of first responders in rural areas are volunteers (National Rural Health Association 2009).

Chronic illnesses are more prevalent in rural areas. Rural residents are less likely to follow up on recommended treatments due to economic, transportation, distance, and other issues in accessing care (National Rural Health Association 2009). Type II diabetes rates among rural adults, for example, are also greater than in urban areas. Rural residents with diabetes are also less likely to receive appropriate treatment and monitoring (DeDoncker 2008).

While national outcomes have not demonstrated significant differences in infant mortality between Metropolitan and Not-Metropolitan Counties (1996–1998), analyses of several state studies have shown increased infant mortality, neonatal mortality, lower birth weights, shorter gestations, lower Apgar scores, longer hospital stays, higher costs, fewer prenatal visits, and greater distances traveled for delivery than urban women or women living in rural areas adjacent to urban areas (Peck and Alexander 2003). This lack of consistency of perinatal data on a national level underlines the significant variability among rural areas and populations in the United States.

Based on parental perceptions, children in rural areas are as likely to be seen in very good or excellent health as their city counterparts. However, rural children are less likely to have preventive visits, are less likely to be breast-fed for six months after birth, and are more likely to live with a smoker in the house (U.S. Department of Health and Human Services 2005).

In contrast to children, the percentage of adults who describe health status as only fair/poor is 28% among rural residents compared to 21% of urban residents. Obese men over the age of 18 years comprise 22% of rural populations compared to 18% of urban populations. Adolescent smoking rates are 18% in rural areas, and 11% in urban areas. Forty percent of rural 12th graders reported using alcohol while driving compared to 25% of their urban counterparts (National Rural Health Association 2009).

Despite the prevailing perception that rural life is more laid-back, the suicide rate is nearly twice as high in rural vs urban areas. It is particularly higher among men and children; the rate among women is rapidly increasing towards that of men. There are fewer mental health professionals per capita in rural areas. Rural hospitals are only half as likely to provide emergency mental health care (National Rural Health Association 2009).

Rural residents are significantly less likely to receive preventive care, even when statistics are adjusted for demographic, health insurance status, and availability of health facilities. They were less likely to have a routine medical check, or to be evaluated for hypertension, cholesterol, pap smear, mammogram, or screening for colorectal cancer. The disparity increased for populations further away from urban centers (Casey et al. 2000).

Rural residents are less likely to receive routine dental care: about 50% of rural adults in comparison with about 70% of their urban counterparts during the preceding year. Dental caries is the most common chronic disease suffered by children (National Center for Health Statistics 2001). Almost 50% of seniors in non-metropolitan areas have lost all their natural teeth (National Rural Health Association 2009).

Health Services

Health insurance: Rural residents are more likely to be employed part-time by small employers, be self-employed, or be employed in agricultural occupations where they are less likely to be provided health insurance. Per capita earnings are much less in rural areas. The percentage of rural residents covered by any commercial insurance is 64% compared to 68% of urban residents. Even those rural residents who have health insurance (i.e., 31% rural vs. 45% of urban Medicare recipients) are less likely to have prescription drug coverage (National Rural Health Association 2009).

Medicaid, one of the major government insurance programs, covers fewer poor rural residents. Only 45% of the rural poor are covered by Medicaid, compared to 49% of the urban poor. Fewer Medicare and commercial insurance vendors are willing to offer rural products due to high costs of administering services. Choices for health insurance for rural populations are fewer, if they exist at all, and generally with higher premiums or co-pays, that price many rural residents out of the insurance market.

Health care institutions and providers: As described above, almost 500 rural hospitals have closed over the past 30 years. Reasons for this include the initial rollout of Medicare prospective payments to hospitals based on Diagnostic Related Groups (DRGs), an increased percentage of non-reimbursed or poorly reimbursed care due to the lack of commercial insurance, causing less ability for clinics and institutions to make up these losses by better reimbursement from commercial plans. The smaller size of rural hospitals and distance from urban centers requires them to pay more for goods and services than larger urban facilities (Rural Assistance Center 2009a). Seventeen percent of rural hospitals had an average 3-year negative total margin of profit (National Rural Health Association 2009; Morris 2009).

While 20% of the U.S. population lives in rural areas, only 11% of physicians and 10% of medical specialists work in rural areas. Rural primary care providers are most frequently family practice physicians or generalists with a broad scope of practice. Mid-level practitioners (physician assistants or nurse practitioners) have filled in gaps in many rural areas in the last few decades, but current trends suggest that mid-level practitioners are also moving toward the more urban sites.

Rural providers generally have not only an increased scope of practice, but also an increased call for responsibility, fewer options for time off, vacation, or continuing education. That there may be fewer opportunities socially, economically, and educationally for their families can be burdensome as well. Rural providers who are serving under a contractual obligation may feel that they are there under duress, and not fully commit to practice, or leave as soon as their obligation has ended. Financial incentives such as loan repayment that support working in a medically underserved area does not necessarily mean that providers are serving medically uninsured patients.

For specialists, especially in surgical fields, the decreasing size and scope of rural hospitals makes it more difficult to provide surgical services. Surgery requires a higher level of staffing, facilities, and equipment that necessitate a larger investment and ongoing support. Obstetrical services are also more difficult to provide, not only in terms of increased need for facilities and staffing, but also the rapidly increasing costs associated with obstetrical malpractice that are forcing many rural obstetric practices to close, including those that rely on family practice physicians to provide prenatal, labor, and delivery services (National Opinion Research Center 2009).

Rural obstetrical programs are particularly threatened. The added expense of an obstetrical facility and low volume, added to the issues of soaring malpractice costs, and fewer providers have caused many rural hospitals to discontinue providing obstetrical services. The effect of this is added to the burden of poor pregnant women having to travel longer distances for prenatal care as well as delivery, contributing to an increased likelihood for a high-risk delivery (Zhao 2007).

Nurses are also in short supply in rural areas, though the small number of beds and patients in rural facilities may make the nursing to patient ratios appear greater. Rural nurses also need to be able to perform a broader scope of practice; yet in general their training and certification are less than urban nurses performing similar functions (National Center for Frontier Communities 2004).

Significant disparities exist in the pharmaceutical distribution system as well. Fewer rural residents can afford medication, due both to lower income and less insurance coverage. Pharmacies, an important health and economic resource in many rural communities, are becoming fewer and farther between, as private pharmacies cannot afford to stay open and there is insufficient financial incentive for chains to come in. Without health care providers, there is no source for prescriptions. More rural pharmacists are reaching retirement age and there are fewer students to replace them. On-line and mail order have not achieved the affordability to help in supplanting the loss of rural pharmacy and pharmacists (The National Advisory Committee on Rural Health and Human Services 2006).

There are only 40/100,000 dentists in rural areas compared to 60/100,000 in urban areas. Many state Medicaid plans do not provide dental care. Many dentists do not accept Medicaid dental patients. The shortage of dentists is further exacerbated by large numbers of dentists reaching retirement age, and fewer students being admitted to dental schools (National Center for Health Statistics 2001).

The paucity of trained health care professional exists across the health care spectrum, including health care administrators, nursing supervisors, radiology and laboratory technicians, nutritionists, physical and occupational specialists, behavioral health workers at all levels, patient care technicians, paramedics, and other skilled help professionals. Lower pay, more difficult working conditions and hours, reliance upon less skilled personnel and fewer opportunities for improved pay or advancement conspire to entice rural health care professionals to pursue other options or move to other locations.

Programs

Local service organizations: The self-sufficiency and taking care of one another ethic that is frequently a part of rural community is often the backbone of service provision. Churches, in particular, often serve as the developer and support of clinical and ancillary support services, such as transportation, supplies, clothing, and other services for uninsured rural residents. While there may be at least a theoretical concern about proselytizing in contrast to providing service as an expression of spirituality; as well as historical or cultural schisms that may exist between religious organizations in a community, the financial, organizational, and political abilities of religious organizations must be an important consideration.

Rural health programs: There are a number of federal and state programs that support rural health services and providers. A fact sheet of rural health programs sponsored by the Health Resources Services Administration HRSA can be viewed at http://www.hrsa.gov/medicaidprimer/rural_health_part3only.htm (Health Resources and Services Administration 2009). Some of these programs will be highlighted below.

Increased payment for Medicare to rural hospitals: Medicare represents the largest payer for virtually all hospitals, and the viability of rural facilities have been especially sensitive to the Medicare payment structure. Until 1987 rural hospitals were penalized for their smaller size, as they received no differential for payment through Medicare, although the role this played in the actual closing of rural hospitals has been questioned (Associated Press 1990). Since then, rural hospitals have received increased payment in comparison to urban hospitals.

The critical access hospital (CAH) program further attempts to shore up rural hospitals by optimizing efficiency of the smallest hospitals by limiting the numbers of beds, intensive care, and surgical services. Hospitals can receive up to 100% of cost-reimbursement from Medicare for agreeing to adhere to these guidelines; there are currently almost 1,300 rural hospitals participating in this program (Rural Assistance Center 2009a). Since rural hospital are less able to "dump" patients, and rural patients go on and off insurance more frequently and for longer periods than in urban areas, increased support for these facilities becomes even more critical.

Another old idea being revived is the collaboration of Rural and Urban hospitals. In the past these collaborations were seen primarily as a way to capture patients from rural areas for a specific hospital, but recent collaborations have tried to be innovative in looking at shared services and supporting rural areas with part-time or innovative programs in delivering health care and ancillary services. Some of these are further delineated below (Morris 2009).

Health care clinics and providers: There are a disproportionately smaller number of providers and specialists in rural areas, although pay for rural providers is not necessarily less. As with facilities, the expectation to provide services regardless of the ability to pay becomes more important (and more difficult) in a rural setting.

Federally-funded health centers can receive grants under Section 330 of the Public Health Service Act. Federally-qualified health centers (FQHCs) are discussed in greater detail in other chapters. In addition, community-based health care providers that meet federal grant requirements can gain FQHC status as "look-alikes". Under the Balanced Budget Act (BBA), look-alike clinics can also receive reasonable cost-based reimbursement from Medicaid (Health Resources and Services Administration 2009). The ability of Federally-Qualified Health Centers to provide malpractice coverage under the Federal Torts Claims Act (FTCA) has been a critical component for rural providers, especially in providing obstetric services.

Rural Health Clinics (RHCs) are certified to receive special Medicare and Medicaid reimbursement; they can be for profit or not for profit, public or private. They can be attached to a hospital, nursing home or home health agency that is already a Medicare-certified provider. Reimbursement is handled through the provider associated with the RHC. RHCs are expected to use a team of physicians and mid-level practitioners such as nurse practitioners, physician assistants, and certified nurse mid-wives. The clinic must be staffed at least 50% of the time with a mid-level practitioner (Rural Assistance Center 2009b). A comparison of the Rural Health Clinic and the Federally-Qualified Health Center Programs can be found at http://www.ask.hrsa.gov/downloads/fqhc-rhccomparison.pdf.

Over 50% of the public health departments are rural and small. There is significant variation in the governance structure, funding and services provided by rural health departments. Many are providers of last resort and, as such end up providing much preventive care including well child, women's preventive care, and school health services, as well as traditional communicable disease and environmental programs. The most successful programs have strong community collaborations with local governmental institutions, hospitals, and referral providers to develop programs to share scare resources (Wellever 2006).

The use of mid-level providers (nurse practitioners and physician assistants) is greater in rural areas. State and federal scholarship and loan repayment programs also help entice health professionals to consider working in underserved areas. The National Health Service Corp has been instrumental in helping to provide both scholarship and loan repayment facilities from a variety of health care specialties (primary care, mid-levels, dentists, mental health professionals) in some of the most remote practice sites (http://nhsc.bhpr.hrsa.gov/about/). The J1 visa program allows Foreign Medical Graduates in the U.S. to work in rural or urban medically underserved areas. Thirty slots are given to each state. This has also been an important source of medical providers for some of the rural areas (Rural Assistance Center 2009c).

Other important efforts are recruiting and supporting rural students in health professions; development of health personnel training programs in rural areas or by telemedicine, locum tenens programs to support time away for rural providers, and improved model of continuing medical and health professional education that recognizes the situation and needs of rural providers.

Innovative rural practice models: A number of specialties, such as surgery, cardiology, gastroenterology, dermatology, psychiatry, and even oncology can be increasingly found on a part-time or itinerant basis in rural areas. While a full range of diagnostic and treatment modalities may not be offered, part-time basic specialty services may help the local population avoid long distance travel. Technologic interventions such as telemedicine, used increasingly for a surprising array of services, including dermatology and psychiatry, further extend the urban-based health care services to rural areas. While these programs may not directly support uninsured patients, supporting the fragile fragmented health care infrastructure in rural areas is an important part of the overall picture.

Conclusions

Populations living in rural areas in the United States are generally older, poorer, and more ill, though there is a wide diversity in what is defined as rural and between the different populations. Increased burden of disease include great mortality among the young, worse outcomes due to accidents and trauma, more chronic disease, and less preventive care. Poorer economies in rural areas are related to fewer people on insurance, fewer health care and ancillary providers and institutions, and a greater strain on existing resources. While a number of state and federal programs are directed at supporting rural health providers and institutions, economic and geographic realities continue to make the provision of rural health services problematic, and even more so for residents without insurance.

References

Associated Press (1990) Medicare cleared in hospital closings. Available at http://query.nytimes.com/gst/fullpage.html?res=9C0CE0D6143CF935A35754C0 A966958260. Accessed 3 Jan 2009

Casey MM, Call KT, Klinger J (2000) The influence of rural residence on the use of preventive health care services. University of Minnesota Rural Health Research Center; Working Paper #34. Available at http://www.hpm.umn.edu/rhrc/pdfs/wpaper/working%20paper%20034.pdf. Accessed 3 Jan 2009

Coburn AF, Mackinney AC, McBride TC, Mueller KJ, Slifkin RT, Wakefield MK (2008) Choosing rural definitions: implications for health policy, Issue Brief #2, Rural Policy Research Institute Health Panel. Available at: http://www.rupri.org/Forms/RuralDefinitionsBrief.pdf. Accessed 3 Jan 2009

DeDoncker M (2008) Study: Diabetes more prevalent in rural population. *PatriotLedger.com*. Posted December 16, 2008. Available at http://www.patriotledger.com/lifestyle/health_and_beauty/x415881436/Study- Diabetes-more-prevalent-in-rural-population. Accessed 3 Jan 2009

Health Resources and Services Administration (2009) Available at http://www.hrsa.gov/medicaidprimer/rural_health_part3only.htm. Accessed 3 Jan 2009

Morris T (2009) Rural health policy issues and challenges, presentation given in the scholar seminar series at the Mel and Enid Zuckerman Arizona College of Public Health, Tucson, AZ, 4 March 2009

National Center for Frontier Communities (2004) Addressing the nursing shortage: impacts and innovations in Frontier America. Available at http://www.frontierus.org/nursing.htm. Accessed 4 Jan 2009

National Center for Health Statistics (2001) Health, United States 2001 with Urban and Rural Health Chartbook Hyattsville Maryland: 2001. Available at http://www.cdc.gov/nchs/data/hus/hus01.pdf. Accessed 3 Jan 2009

National Opinion Research Center (2009) Declining access to hospital-based obstetric services in rural areas: causes and impact. Available at http://www.norc.org/projects/Declining+Access+to+Hospital-based+Obstetric+Services.htm. Accessed 19 Jan 2009

National Rural Health Association (2009) What's different about rural health? Available at http://www.ruralhealthweb.org/go/left/about-rural-health/what-s- different-about-rural-health-care. Accessed 3 Jan 2009

Peck J, Alexander K (2003) Maternal, infant, and child health in rural areas. rural healthy people 2010: a companion document to healthy people 2010. Volume 1. College Station, TX: The Texas A&M University System Health Science Center, School of Rural Public Health, Southwest Rural Health Research Center. Available at http://www.srph.tamhsc.edu/centers/rhp2010/07Volume1MIC.htm. Accessed 3 Jan 2009

Rural Assistance Center (2009a) Critical access hospitals. Available at http://www.raconline.org/info_guides/hospitals/cah.php. Accessed 3 Jan 2009

Rural Assistance Center (2009b). Rural health disparities. Available at http://www.raconline.org/info_guides/disparities/. Accessed 3 Jan 2009

Rural Assistance Center (2009c). Rural Health clinics. Available at http://www.raconline.org/info_guides/clinics/rhcfaq.php#whatis. Accessed 25 Jan 2009

Rural Assistance Center (2009d). J-1 visa waiver. Available at http://www.raconline.org/info_guides/hc_providers/j1visa.php. Accessed 25 Jan 2009

The National Advisory Committee on Rural Health and Human Services (2006) The 2006 report to the secretary: rural health and human service issues. U.S. Department of Health and Human Services. Available at http://ruralcommittee.hrsa.gov/NAC06AReport.htm. Accessed 19 Jan 2009

U.S. Department of Health and Human Services, Health Resources and Services Administration, Maternal and Child Health Bureau (2005) The National Survey of Children's Health 2003. Rockville, MD: U.S. Department of Health and Human Services, 2005. Available at http://www.mchb.hrsa.gov/ruralhealth/index.htm. Accessed 3 Jan 2009

Wellever A (2006) Local public health at the crossroads: the structure of health departments in rural areas (issue brief). Kansas Health Institute. Available at http://www.khi.org/resources/Other/40-0601HealthDeptStructureHRSABrief.pdf. Accessed 25 Jan 2009

Zhao L (2007) Why are fewer hospitals in the delivery business? Rural Health Research Gateway. Available at http://www.ruralhealthresearch.org/projects/100002057/. Accessed 25 Jan 2009

Dental Care for the Uninsured

Lane P. Johnson

Ms. Smith was enjoying substituting for the regular fourth grade teacher who was off on medical leave. If only, she could figure out Michael's behavior. A quiet and generally cooperative 10 year old – except for the paper spitball problems. No sooner would she start writing on the whiteboard or working with another student, and there would be a complaint about Michael and the spitballs from the girls sitting around him. Ms. Smith had asked him to stop for three days so far without success.

Finally, the next morning, Ms. Smith asked Michael to come and talk with her. She asked: why do you continue to throw the wet spitballs around your desk after I've asked you not to? Michael looked embarrassed but said: "my teeth hurt really bad and chewing on the paper helps make them hurt less." Ms. Smith thanked Michael and called his mother to check on when he had last been to the dentist. He had never been due to the dentist due to the expense. Ms. Smith was able to make arrangements with the community sliding fee scale dental clinic to see Michael and take care of the caries in his teeth.

Sheila was at the community health center for her first visit with the obstetrician. She was excited to find herself pregnant as was her husband. Both of them were 25 years old and anxious to start a family. Fortunately, Sheila was able to qualify for the Prenatal Package at the health center.

During her assessment, Dr. Rios asked her about her last dental cleaning and check-up. Sheila looked confused, but replied that her teeth were fine, but she had never been to the dentist before. In fact, no members of her family went to the dentist on a regular basis. They had no dental insurance and only sought out dental care if someone had a toothache that did not go away. Dr. Rios took the opportunity to talk with her about the risk of prematurity and gestational diabetes in mothers with poor or no oral health care. Dr. Rios referred her to the county health department's prenatal dental program to assure that she would have her teeth cleaned as well as would receive education on caring for the needed oral health of her unborn child as well.

L.P. Johnson
Arizona Health Sciences Center,
Tucson, AZ, USA
e-mail: lpj@email.arizona.edu

N.J. Johnson and L.P. Johnson (eds.), *The Care of the Uninsured in America*,
DOI 10.1007/978-0-387-78309-3_15, © Springer Science+Business Media, LLC 2010

Introduction

"You are not healthy without good oral health."

-Former US Surgeon General C. Everett Koop

"Ancient thinkers considered the mouth as "a sacred gate to the temple of the body" – a gate that permanently needs attention, vigilance, and care. Any worsening of the oral ecology implies worsening of the functioning of the body that negatively affects human health and the perception of quality of life (Inglehart and Bagramian 2002)."

Poor oral health has been called *The Silent Epidemic.* "People seem to think oral health – nice, shiny white teeth – is a luxury. It's not. We need to make it a national priority.... There's a lot of pain. There's is a lot of disfigurement. People can't even get jobs if they have bad teeth. No one is going to hire a person who has to hold a hand over their mouth when they talk because the teeth are so bad." So speaks Marcia Brand of the Federal Health Resources and Services Administration, Office of Rural Health Policy (NCSL 2007).

...West Virginia Delegate Barbara Evans Fleischauer concurs. "During our evaluation of welfare reform, we asked people who had difficulties getting jobs why they had problems. Twenty-one percent said it was because of their teeth. I thought it was heartbreaking, a sad problem and one people don't seem to take very seriously (NCSL 2007)."

Poor oral health leads to pain and discomfort, difficulty with eating and maintaining good nutrition, and can lead to, or be a complication of, more serious systemic disease. It can be an important factor in maintaining a positive self image and better interpersonal relationships.

In 2004, U.S. health spending was about $963.9 billion, with dental care accounting for 7.5%. While 47 million Americans lack health insurance, a staggering 108 million lack dental insurance (RAC 2009).

This chapter will discuss how specific populations of Americans are affected by poor oral health, the consequences that they have to suffer, and the programs that are being, or have been developed to address the oral health needs of uninsured Americans.

Demographics

Children

Children in lower income families are less likely to have had a dental visit in the last year, and are twice as likely to have untreated cavities when compared with children in higher income families. Eighty percent of tooth decay is found in 25% of children from low income families. Low income, immigrant, and minority populations are at greater risk for poor oral health (CDF 2007; Chin 2008).

While dental coverage under Medicaid is available for children to some degree in all the states, there is no guarantee that they will receive dental services. In 1 year, only 18% of the Medicaid-covered children received preventive dentistry services. A major factor is the limited number of dentists treating the Medicaid population (CDF 2007). Dentists do not participate because of low reimbursement rates, difficult administrative requirements, and patient failure to keep appointments (from 30 to 50%) (NCSL 2007).

The use of dental sealants in children is a low-cost, effective way to help prevent cavities. This is a plastic material applied onto the teeth; the sealant forms a hard coating that protects against decay. Only 3% of children under 8 in low income families, and less than 25% of children overall, have received dental sealants (NCSL 2007).

Ethnic Groups

Black, Hispanic, and American Indians, and Alaskan Natives (AI/AN) generally have poorer oral health than other racial and ethnic groups in America (PHS 2000). In every age group, children and adolescents, adults, and older Americans, Black and Hispanics have higher rates of tooth decay, destructive peridontal disease, or tooth loss compared to the white population (CDHP 2009).

AI/AN Preschoolers aged 2–4 years have over five times the rate of dental decay of all American children. In children aged 6–17 years, 38% of Latinos and 28% of African American children have untreated dental caries, compared to 19% of the white population (NACHC 2007).

Rural Americans

Problems with lack of insurance, low Medicaid reimbursement, geographic distribution of dentists, transportation issues, lack of fluoridation are the major factors that contribute to poor oral health. Children and senior citizens are at highest risk. Most rural dentists are old and approaching retirement age (RAC 2009).

Older Americans

The good news is that more people are keeping their natural teeth now than ever before. But the prevalence of periodontal disease increases with age; from about 6% of persons 25–34 years to 41% of those 65 and older. Nearly 1/3 of persons over 65 years have untreated dental caries, and despite improvements 44% of elderly adults no longer have their natural teeth.

Dental insurance for older Americans (if they ever had it) usually stops at retirement; Medicare does not pay for routine care, only limited services deemed to be "medically necessary," such as overt weight loss or chronic infection are covered. Only 22% of older Americans are covered by dental insurance; only 10% of dental expenses for older Americans are paid by insurance, 79% are paid out of pocket (RAC 2009; Vargas et al. 2009).

It should not be surprising that the unmet dental needs of older persons living below the poverty line are three times greater than those of persons at or above the poverty line, and they are more likely to have untreated cavities (Vargas et al. 2009).

Dental needs of older Americans are more complex and expensive, and may require specialized dental skills. As older Americans are the fastest growing segment of the population, the decreasing dentist to population ratio will more likely affect the older American's access to dental services (Vargas et al. 2009).

Dental Personnel

In the United States, over 2,000 counties or parts of counties have been designated Dental Health Professions Shortage Areas, indicating a lack of dental providers. Fewer than half of these areas have a safety net provider (Sliding scale dental clinic or services provided by an FQHC.) (NACHC 2007).

Dentists are in short supply, and the problem is getting worse. The National Health Service Corps is able to fill only one out of every three vacant dentist positions in underserved areas. Seven dental schools have closed between 1986 and 2001. The dental workforce peaked at 59.5 per 100,000 in 1990, and has been declining since then; it is projected to drop to 52.7 per 100,000 by 2020. Thirty five percent of dentists are over 55. The number of dentists retiring is expected to be greater than the number entering the field by 2014. There is also a shortage of dental hygienists (NCLS 2007; Valachovic 2002; Chin 2008).

Dental personnel of minority background are in even shorter supply. The African-American population represented 12.3% of the U.S. population in 2000, but only 2% of practicing dentists, 3% of dental hygienists, and 4.2% of dental school faculty are African-American. Hispanics made up 12.5% of the U.S. population in 2000, but only 4% of dentists, 1% of hygienists, and 4.8% of dental faculty were Hispanics. The difference is even more striking in California, where the Hispanic population makes up 32.4% of the population, and only 4.6% of dentists are Hispanics (CDHP 2009).

Health Status

Tooth decay and pain interfere with the daily activities of 4–5 million children and adolescents a year (NCSL 2007). One of the most common chronic diseases in children is tooth decay. Fifty percent of children have cavities by the first grade, and 80%, by the time they finish high school. Untreated dental disease in children can cause pain, swelling, and infection. The pain can lead to poor concentration and malnourishment. It can also lead to social isolation due to appearance and discomfort (CDF 2007).

Problems in the mouth can signal problems in other parts of the body. Bone loss in the lower jaw can precede skeletal bone loss in osteoporosis. The first signs of HIV infection may be mouth lesions (CDC 2000). Furthermore, gum infections can be a significant complication of diabetes, can be a factor for an increased rate of heart disease, stroke, pneumonia, and endocarditis. In pregnancy, gum infections may be related to preterm, low birth weight babies, and gestational diabetes (CDC 2000).

Edentulous (total loss of teeth) people have greater difficulty chewing, which leads to eating fewer raw vegetables, salads, and fresh fruit (Vargas et al. 2009).

Smoking is associated with a vastly increased risk of gum disease and oral cancer. Many medications can lead to decreased salivary flow, which can result in dry mouth, and increase the risk of cavities and soft tissue problems, as well as make dentures more uncomfortable. Some of these classes of medication include diuretics, antihistimines, antidepressants, and antipsychotics (Vargas et al. 2009).

Oral cancer increases with age; more than half of the 8,000 deaths each year occur in the 65 years and older age group. More older persons die from oral cancer than from skin cancer (Vargas et al. 2009).

Dental Programs

Dental and oral health conditions are among the most preventable of chronic diseases in the American population. The Surgeon General's report on oral health in 2000 stated:

> "…safe and effective disease prevention measures exist that everyone can adopt to improve oral health and prevent disease. These measures include daily oral hygiene procedures and other lifestyle behaviors, community programs such as community water fluoridation and tobacco cessation programs, and provider-based interventions such as the placement of dental sealants and examinations for common oral and pharyngeal cancers (PHS 2000)."

Perhaps the two simplest and most cost-effective population-based approaches to poor oral health are fluoridation of community water supplies and dental sealant programs (NCSL 2007). The safety and efficacy of fluoridation of the water supply has been overwhelmingly demonstrated, but nonetheless, fluoridation remains a lightning rod for generally conservative political activists to rage against government intervention. An assessment of water fluoridation community by community in the U.S. is available at: http://apps.nccd.cdc.gov/MWF/Index.asp.

As discussed above, dental sealant programs are extremely cost-effective methods of decreasing dental caries in children, but they are greatly underutilized. Use of personnel other than dentists to apply this technology will be necessary to make any significant inroads in the effective utilization of dental sealants in the United States.

Fluoride varnish is another oral health preventive technology with great potential. Fluoride varnish is a coating that is painted on the baby teeth of children from

0 to 5 years old and can reduce and stop dental cavities by up to 70%. Fluoride applied as a varnish adheres to the tooth surface for a much longer time and helps prevent decay at a better rate than standard application techniques, and it seems better tolerated by younger children. This is also an application technique that does not require a dentist. Even medical assistants and WIC workers have been trained to use this technique with their patients and clients (Deming 2008).

Medicaid

Medicaid covers dental care programs for children, but the level of care varies by state. A state-by-state assessment of CHIP care can be found at: http://medicaid-benefits.kff.org/ (KFF 2009). In addition, Medicaid in some states covers "medically necessary" dental procedures for adults, such as pulling teeth or treating infections, but often does not cover restorative dental services or dentures.

State Dental Programs

State dental programs, recognizing the shortcomings of the Medicaid system, have been implementing changes to improve the Medicaid reimbursement and decrease administrative burdens. Utah, for example, used state funds to offer urban dentists a 20% increase in reimbursement if they took more than 100 Medicaid patients a year. Rural dentists received a 20% increase for all Medicaid patients. The state also expanded the number of dental clinics provided by the state, and developed a dental case management system, as well as a preventive education program. Other states, including Kentucky, North Carolina, Arizona, New Mexico, and Minnesota are in the process of developing similar programs, though the recent economic downturn has put many of these efforts in jeopardy (NCSL 2007).

Integration of Medical and Dental Care in Schools

School-based programs by nurse practitioners have been developed to include oral screening and early referral for restorative services. Programs have expanded to include oral hygiene education, fluoride varnish application, and nutrition (Heuer 2007).

Mobile Dental Programs

A number of states, including Arizona, Colorado, Nevada, Maine, and Illinois have been using dental mobile units, particularly for rural areas. One program sponsored by the non-profit Oral Health Association, is the Smiles Across America program. Others include Healthy Kids and Seniors, and the Miles of Smiles program (NCSL 2007).

Mobile-based dental services can offer preventive care. School-based programs including sealant programs are one set of services. These programs can also include visits to nursing homes and assistance for living communities, as well as the home-bound and disabled, in addition to patients without insurance.

Mobile-based programs are complicated and expensive. High voltage electricity, running water, waste disposal, and living on the road are among the hurdles these programs face in providing services that otherwise might not be available (NCSL 2007).

Community Health Centers

Federally-Qualified Community Health Centers, "Look-Alike" Community Health Centers without direct federal funding, and faith-based Community Health Centers are the mainstays of the "Safety Net" for oral health serving large numbers of low income, minority, and rural Americans on a sliding scale and regardless of their ability to pay. In 2005, 73% of existing federally-funded health centers provided oral health services onsite. In addition, federal guidelines require all new federally-funded health centers to provide oral health care services. Dental visits make up 10% of all visits to health centers. In 2005, federally-funded health centers had 2.3 million patients with 5.6 million visits, an increase of over 75% since 2000 (NACHC 2007). Under the new Federal administration, significant expansion of the Community Health Center program is expected to take place.

Perinatal Programs for Oral Health

The need for oral health care during the perinatal period has been recognized and is being increasingly promoted by maternal and child health advocates. Difficulty in eating can compromise nutritional status and lead to increased risk of poor birth outcomes, including preterm labor, low birth weight, and gestational diabetes (NMCOHRC 2008).

Lack of knowledge of the association of poor oral health to birth outcomes, fear of risk of dental procedures during pregnancy, as well as lack of oral health insurance coverage are among the reasons for not seeking oral health care during the perinatal period. While this effort is still in its early stages, many providers of maternal and child health services are recognizing the need to ally with dental providers to provide oral health services. National guidelines are in the process of being developed (NMCOHRC 2008). Community health centers providing dental services are particularly able to lead the effort in improving perinatal oral health care.

Primary Care Programs

United Community Health Center Pediatric Dental Program

Even though primary care providers are not generally trained in dental evaluation, treatment, or prevention, a small scale program can be developed even without a dentist on staff. In the mid 1990s, United Community Health Center, a consortium of three small rural clinics in southern Arizona developed a program in collaboration with El Rio Neighborhood Heath Center, a FQHC with a sliding scale dental program. The program had three components:

(1) Assessment of Severity and Referral: Primary care providers evaluated the pediatric patients for caries and periodontal inflammation. Patients with no or few small caries were given routine referral to the El Rio Dental Clinic. Patients with more severe problems were referred urgently. Referred patients were then put into the clinic recall system to make sure they followed up with the dentist.
(2) Ms. Floss and Mr. Toothbrush. A simple health education assessment and training was developed to teach the medical assistants to provide dental health education to the patient and parents. Documentation of the education effort in the medical chart allowed quality improvement assessment. A copy of the Education/Screening Assessment can be found in Fig. 1.
(3) Fluoride Assessment and Supplement. The wells and municipal water supplies were measured area wide by the State Water Safety office for a variety of substances, including fluoride. From this, providers could assess the fluoride content and provide supplementation if warranted.

Family Practice Resident Physicians in Rural Maine are learning to lance oral abscesses, pull teeth, and perform other basic dental skills. Maine has an extreme shortage of dentists (a ratio of 1:2,300 dentists to people compared to 1:1,600 nationally), but a 1:640 physician to patient ratio. Family practice residents learn the dental procedures during their training; about 2/3 stay in Maine to practice, many in rural areas. Although not seen as a replacement for dental care, it provides the physicians an opportunity to triage and refer, as well as offer preventive dental advice (Zezima 2009).

Volunteer Dental Programs

Despite the national shortage of dental personnel, there is still a significant ethic for volunteering among practicing and retired dentists and hygienists. Many volunteer at community health centers or other community organizations sponsoring dental clinics. Others provide free or discounted services to indigent or poor patients referred by community-based organizations. There is a national Dental Volunteer program, which links dental volunteers to opportunities across the United States and across the world: www.dentalvolunteer.com.

Age	Dental Education/Screening
Prenatal	Brushing, flossing, pregnancy gingivitis, bottle caries, fluoride
0-2 years	Teething bottle caries, finger sucking, parent helps with teeth cleaning, brushing, flossing, first trip to dentist (age 3), dental trauma, fluoride
2-4 years	Finger sucking, brushing, flossing regular dental visits, dental trauma, fluoride
4-6 years	Brushing, flossing regular dental visits, dental trauma, fluoride
6-8 years	Brushing, flossing regular dental visits, dental trauma, fluoride
8-10 years	Brushing, flossing regular dental visits, dental trauma, fluoride
10-12 years	Brushing, flossing regular dental visits, dental trauma, fluoride
12-16 years	Brushing, flossing regular dental visits, dental trauma, fluoride

Nursing Assistant should judge the patient/parent level of understanding and motivation and indicate in chart as follows: Excellent; Good; Adequate; Poor (Notify Provider)

United Community Health Center
Sahuarita, Arizona

Fig. 1 Dental disease prevention tracking form guidelines

AT Still Dental School

A refreshing effort in training dentists to care for underserved patients comes from the Arizona School of Dentistry and Oral Health (ASDOH), a school of A.T. Still University, founded in 2003 with the "fundamental aim of identifying applicants with strong community service backgrounds, integrating and emphasizing community and public health principles into the curriculum and graduating dentists with a unique understanding of, and desire to serve communities in need." The Dental School collaborates with Community Health Centers for clinical experience, selecting and directing students to a dental career caring for underserved populations. Specifics of the program can be found at: www.atsu.edu/asdoh/about/index.htm.

Advanced Dental Hygiene Practitioner

Advanced Dental Hygiene Practitioner (ADHP) is a category of practitioner who is the dental equivalent of a Nurse Practitioner, and would, under specific supervision and circumstances, be able to provide diagnostic, preventive, restorative, and therapeutic services beyond traditional dental hygiene activities (Rural Assistance Center 2009).

The National Health Service Corp (NHSC) Scholarship and Loan Repayment Program has programs for qualified general dentists and registered clinical dental hygienists at qualified sites. More information can be found at: http://nhsc.bhpr. hrsa.gov/index.asp. A very limited number of J-1 Visa waivers for foreign-educated dentists may be available if the home country does not object, and there is no U.S. Government education funding. Further information on the process (which is different from the J-1 Visa program for physicians) may be found at: http://travel.state. gov/visa/temp/info/info_1288.html.

References

Centers for Disease Control and Prevention (CDC) (2000) Links between oral and general health. Oral health resources fact sheet. Available at: www.cdc.gov/oralhealth/factsheets/sgr2000-fs4. htm. Retrieved 16 Feb 2006

Children's Defense Fund (CDF) (2007) Child Health: Oral Health. Available at: www.childrens-defense.org/site/PageServer?pagename=childhealth_oralhealth. Retrieved 2 Feb 2007

Children's Dental Health Project (CDHP) (2009) Fact sheet. Racial and ethnic disparities in oral health. Available at: www.cdhp.org/downloads/Disparityfactsheet.pdf. Retrieved 2 May 2009

Chin C (2008) Pediatric oral health in the primary care setting. Available at: http://74.125.95.132/search?q=cache:DKDp3RUaFCEJ:www.aapcho.org/altruesite/files/ aapcho/Presentations/20th_Anniversary_Conference/RedefiningWellness/Courtney%252 0Chinn. pdf + FQHC + and + oral + health&cd = 18&hl = en&ct = clnk&gl = us&client = firefox-a. Retrieved 26 Apr 2009

Deming S (2008) Varnish! Michigan: A fluoride varnish program. Michigan Rural Health Quarterly 15:2. Available at: http://www.mcrh.msu.edu/MCRH_News/spring_08.pdf#page=9. Retrieved 2 May 2009

Heuer S (2007) Integrated medical and dental health in primary care. J Spec Pediatr Nurs (JSPN) 12(1):61–65

Inglehart MR, Bagramian RA (eds) (2002) Oral health-related quality of life, Quintessence Publishing Co, Inc, Carol Stream, IL, pp 111–121

Kaiser Family Foundation (KFF) (2009) Medicaid benefits: online data base. Available at: http:// medicaidbenefits.kff.org/. Retrieved 25 Apr 2009

National Association of Community Health Centers (NACHC) (2007) Health Centers' Role in Addressing the Oral Health Needs of the Medically Underserved. Available at: http://www. nachc.org/client/documents/research/Oral%20Health%20Report%20FINAL.pdf. Retrieved 2 May 2009

National Conference of State Legislatures (NCSL) (2007) Where have all the dentists gone? Rural Health Brief. Available at: www.raconline.org/info_guides/dental/dentalfaq.php#Medicaid. Retrieved 26 Apr 2009

National Maternal and Child Oral Health Resource Center (NMCOHRC) (2008) Access to oral health care during the perinatal period: A policy brief Available at:http://www.cdph.ca.gov/ HealthInfo/healthyliving/childfamily/Documents/MO-OHP-PerinatalBrief9-08.pdf Accessed 18 Sept 1009

Public Health Service (PHS) (2000) Oral health in America: A Report of the Surgeon General. Available at: www.nidr.nih.gov/sgr/sgrohweb/home.htm. Retrieved 26 Apr 2009

Rural Assistance Center (2009) Dental Health. Available at: http://www.raconline.org/info_ guides/dental/. Retrieved 25 Apr 2009

Valachovic RW (2002) Dental workforce trends and children. Ambul Pediatr 2:S154–S156

Vargas CM, Kramarow EA, Yellowitz JA (2009) The oral health of older Americans. Centers Dis Control Prev. Available at: www.cdc.gov/nchs/data/ahcd/agingtrends/03oral.pdf. Retrieved 26 Apr 2009

Zezima K (2009) Short of dentists, Maine adds teeth to doctors' training. NY Times. Available at: http://www.nytimes.com/2009/03/03/us/03dentist.html?em. Retrieved 26 Apr 2009

Other Resources

Dental Health. Rural Assistance Center: http://www.raconline.org/info_guides/dental/. This is a fairly comprehensive list of dental programs, funding and resources for both rural and urban populations

Guide to Children's Dental Care in Medicaid, CMS-HHS: http://www.cms.hhs.gov/MedicaidEarlyPeriodicScrn/downloads/EPSDTDentalGuide.pdf

National Maternal and Child Oral Health Resource Center (NMCOHRC) (2008) Access to oral health care during the perinatal period: A policy brief. Available at: http:www.cdph.ca.gov/HealthInfo/healthyliving/childfamily/Documents/MO-OHP-PerinatalBrief9-08.pdf. Accessed 18 Sept 1009

Oral Health Resource Bulletins from the National Maternal and Child Oral Health Center: http://www.mchoralhealth.org/materials/multiples/interchange.html

The Safety Net Dental Clinic Manual: http://www.dentalclinicmanual.com/. This document provides information on how to start and support a dental clinic for the indigent and uninsured

Uninsured Children at School

Fran Bartholomeaux and Nancy J. Johnson

Ten-year old Jack appeared at the school nurse's office with a complaint of "being sick." His teacher indicated that Jack was a new student of just over 2 weeks and had been having some trouble adjusting as well as not paying attention in class. The nurse noticed that Jack did not have a jacket on, despite the cold weather, and was rather quiet and unable to make eye contact with the nurse. He had no objective symptoms of illness. In addition, the nurse saw that there was no contact number for Jack's parents. Jack rested for the rest of the afternoon, and his older sister tracked him down at the end of the day. She mentioned that they had just moved to the town with their grandparents, and led Jack out of the nurse's office.

The next week, Jack appeared again at the nurse's office early in the morning, without a jacket or long pants. The nurse offered Jack a coat from her supply, along with a long pair of pants for the day, and breakfast. At the end of the day, the nurse joined Jack and his sister for the walk home. Their neighborhood was on the out-skirts of an urban area, but walkable from the small elementary school. The nurse discovered that Jack's grandparents had moved to the new town with the promise of jobs that did not materialize. Consequently, the family of four was living in a tent trailer without sufficient food, heat, and the needed medication that Jack took for his attention disorder. The entire family was without health insurance.

The nurse prioritized healthcare and safety; she assisted the family with housing resources, a social worker, and eligibility applications for health care for the children. Jack's grandparents did not think the children would be eligible for health insurance as the family owned their tent trailer and had a small pension and savings account as well. In addition, as they were new to the community, they were unaware of where to seek help.

Jack and his family were able to take advantage of the school-based health center for their healthcare needs on a sliding scale basis as their eligibility application for SCHIP was in process. The grandparents continued to apply for jobs, still surprised that their luck could change so abruptly with their relocation to a new town leaving them without resources for their grandchildren.

F. Bartholomeaux (✉) and N.J. Johnson
College of Nursing and Health Sciences, Grand Canyon University, Tucson, AZ, USA

N.J. Johnson and L.P. Johnson (eds.), *The Care of the Uninsured in America*,
DOI 10.1007/978-0-387-78309-3_16, © Springer Science+Business Media, LLC 2010

Overview

In 2007, over eight million children in our country were uninsured (11%), as illustrated in Figs. 1 and 2. Historically in 2003, the number of uninsured children under age 17 was as low as 5% in Minnesota and as high as 23% in Texas (Annie E. Casey Foundation 2005). Although most states were ready to expand and cover more

Number of Uninsured – Children

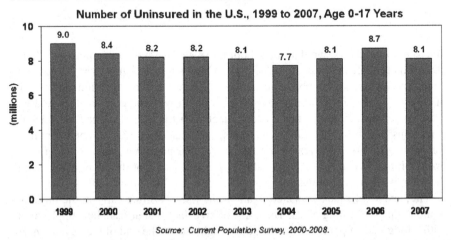

Fig. 1 Number of uninsured children

Percent of Uninsured – Children

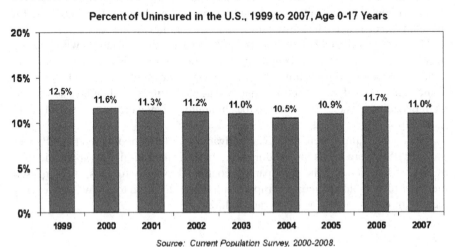

Fig. 2 Percent of uninsured children

uninsured children, the federal government implemented the Medicaid citizenship requirements and a directive from the Centers for Medicare and Medicaid (CMS) limiting state expansions.

Nearly 30% of uninsured children in the United States live in poverty and are part of immigrant families with at least one non-citizen parent (Parker and Teitelbaum 2003). The State Health Assistance Data Center reports 29.1% of uninsured children living in immigrant families (Fig. 3). The Personal Responsibility and Work Opportunity Reconciliation Act of 1996 (Medicaid Citizenship Requirement) prohibited the states from providing Medicaid coverage to legal immigrants during their first 5 years in the United States, which led to this documented increase. In addition, the Children's Health Insurance Program (SCHIP) has not been available to undocumented immigrants. These policy decisions have led to an increase in the number of uninsured children nationally.

However, on February 4, 2009, the Children's Health Insurance Program Reauthorization Act (CHIPRA) was signed into law reauthorizing and expanding the current state of Children's Health Insurance Program to cover eleven million children. This reauthorization should help reach more children needing health insurance (National Association of Community Health Centers 2009). The Children's Defense Fund has identified priorities for America's children, one of them being access to comprehensive health, and mental health coverage and services as evidenced by the nearly nine million uninsured children and the children's health status indicators in the United States, representative of one of the worst in the industrialized world (http://www.childrensdefense.org 2009).

Percent of Uninsured – Children in Poverty

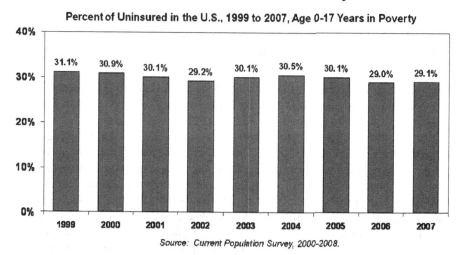

Fig. 3 Percent of uninsured children in poverty

Children's Health Insurance Program

The State Children's Health Insurance Program (SCHIP) was created in 1997 and currently covers over seven million low income children in our country (Peterson 2008). SCHIP was designed to provide health care coverage for children in working families with incomes too high to qualify for Medicaid, but too low to afford or have access to employer-sponsored health insurance plans. In 2007, the United States still reported approximately 8.7 million children without health insurance (DeNavas-Walt et al. 2008).

As mentioned, the Children's Health Insurance Program was reauthorized and expanded in February 2009 to cover eleven million children. This reauthorization act (CHIPRA) also includes several policy changes for covering uninsured children. CHIPRA creates a prospective payment system (PPS) for federally-qualified health centers that matches the reimbursement laws for Medicaid. In addition, it covers about 4.1 million additional children and allows states to provide medical and dental coverage for legal immigrant children and pregnant women, without waiting for 5 years as was required by the previous legislation. CHIPRA also calls for interstate collaboration on providing continuity of care as eligibility changes for children and adults. Dental benefits are a part of the CHIPRA and allow federally-qualified health centers to contract with private practice dental providers to improve timely access to care. Lastly, CHIPRA creates many grant programs to help fund outreach and eligibility activities, childhood obesity programs, and quality and health information technology projects. All these components for the Children's Health Insurance Program Reauthorization should help to not only decrease the number of uninsured children in the United States, but also help address the growing concerns regarding the incidence of childhood obesity, asthma, and diabetes.

Who Are the Uninsured Children?

More than half of the children in the United States have health insurance through their parents' employment, and over 25% are currently covered by Medicaid and SCHIP, our safety net programs for children. This represents one of every four children receiving health care coverage from government-funded programs. However, the approximately 16.8% who are still uninsured, represent about ten million children who are most likely eligible for these state or governmental programs. Seventy-five percent of these uninsured children are Hispanic or White, with the largest group (37.8%) aged 13–18 years (SHADAC 2007). We also find that the largest number of uninsured children live at 200% or more of the federal poverty level, representing 37.9% of uninsured children. This group represents children from working poor families. The collapse of the SCHIP reauthorization process had caused the numbers to grow.

Currently, the economic downturn, decreased work hours, and available insurance benefits have impacted the number of uninsured children. In addition, the rising healthcare costs also threaten to create an even larger number of uninsured children in the coming years.

The coverage of children is essential because without preventive health care, our children are much more likely to have undiagnosed and untreated illnesses, to miss school, and underperform academically. From a positive viewpoint, the ability to insure all children in our country is an achievable goal. The barriers which are presented are many, but with the collaboration of government, health care professionals, and school systems, all children could be insured in our country. Currently, a number of states have made progress in insuring more children, while others have hit barriers such as funding, availability of healthcare providers, and knowledge of eligibility by the target population of families.

Health insurance is the single most important attribute in determining whether or not a child will have access to health care. Children with health insurance are more likely to be immunized, receive well child check-ups, and get prompt treatment for common childhood illnesses, such as upper respiratory and ear infections. Also, children who have insurance are more likely to have a "medical home" or a primary care provider for ongoing anticipatory guidance, counseling and preventive care. Kaiser Foundation Commission on Medicare and Medicaid (http://www.kff.org/healthreform/7980.cfm 2009) documents better quality of care for children once they are insured. For example, children with asthma enrolled in New York's Medicaid/SCHIP program had fewer asthma attacks and lower rates of emergency room visits and hospitalizations compared to when they were uninsured. Other studies (Levine and Schanzenbach 2009) found that children enrolled in SCHIP had improved school attendance, greater ability to pay attention in class, better reading scores, and more active participation in school activities.

Although health insurance is a key variable in access to health care, health care for children is a very broad concept. Children must have access to medical and dental care, but they also need access to health education, disease prevention services, and mental health services that are culturally and linguistically appropriate for the child as well as his/her family, and cater to his special interests or literacy needs.

While their numbers are nearly nine million in the United States, most uninsured children are members of low and middle income working families. Kuhlthau et al. (2004) identified that the children with the lowest access to primary care providers were those from families with incomes between 125% and 200% of the federal poverty level, even though they would qualify for Medicaid and SCHIP. In addition, many low income or middle income families do not enroll their children unless the child is ill or in need of medical care. This results in children not having access to the needed preventive care. In 2007, The Kaiser Survey of California's Health Coverage reported that nearly 75% of low income working families with an uninsured child, and 45% of middle income families, did not have access to the employer-provided health insurance. The study also revealed that most parents wanted their child insured and would like to be able to insure themselves as well. This data supports the assumption that the most likely to be successful approach covering all of our nation's children would be to expand the Medicaid and SCHIP programs in terms of their eligibility requirements. The other opportunity is to ensure that parents know about the Medicaid and SCHIP programs, and about where to seek enrollment assistance.

As of 2009 with the Children's Health Insurance Program reauthorized, 44 states including the District of Columbia had Medicaid and/or SCHIP income eligibility levels at or above 200% of the federal poverty line. Other states have made higher income families eligible as well, because middle class families cannot afford employer-sponsored insurance or have access to employer health insurance, and are forced to leave their children uninsured. DeVoe et al. (2008) did a full year cross-sectional analysis of children and adolescents younger than 19 years, which resulted in a sample size of roughly 39,000 children whose parents were insured. Approximately 3% of these children were uninsured, with the most frequent predictors of uninsured status identified as having low income or middle class income. Parents who had public insurance coverage for themselves had a higher rate of having their children insured compared to those parents with private insurance. Another interesting variable is that public children's health insurance such as Medicaid or SCHIP results in less out of pocket costs and financial hardships for parents in comparison to private insurance coverage for children. Upon comparison, parents of children with private insurance reported a 3% increase in delaying or foregoing care due to cost over the parents of children insured via Medicaid or SCHIP. This is also true in parents' reports of problems in paying children's medical bills. The parents of children insured privately reported 17% more problems in paying bills than the parents of children insured through Medicaid or SCHIP (http://www.kff. org/healthreform/7980.cfm). Hence, the argument is strengthened for expanding the range of income eligibility for SCHIP.

Barriers to Insuring Children

Another barrier for uninsured children has been the actual process of eligibility which can be complicated and difficult to access. The (http://www.kff.org/ healthreform/7980.cfm) reported that 70% of low income Hispanic parents with an uninsured child did not know how to enroll their child and 40% of low income non-Hispanic parents reported the same. The study also reported an average of 50% of parents who did not think or know whether their child would be eligible and did not know where to get the information from (Kaiser 2008). However, nearly all states have eliminated the face-to-face interview process and the asset test for children, in addition to reducing the documents necessary for verification. Other strategies and their prevalence to simplify enrollment and renewal are growing across the United States. Some of these strategies include school and community-based enrollment, online enrollment, annual enrollment telethons, and reaching out with education to middle income families who may not be aware of the assistance available.

When the whole family can obtain coverage, we see children's enrollment increase (http://www.kff.org/healthreform/7980.cfm). However, in many states, the parent's eligibility level is much higher than those established for children, and represents another barrier. For example, a parent working full time at the federal minimum wage ($1.092 per month) does not qualify for Medicaid, even though he/she may not have access to employer-sponsored insurance. Also, some adults who are receiving unemployment benefits may not qualify for Medicaid. However, in both these scenarios, their children most likely qualify for SCHIP. This disparity in eligibility between children and their parents can result in some children being left uninsured.

The barriers to insuring children are diverse and include financial, transportation, knowledge, cultural, social, eligibility criteria, geographic, and time away from work to complete application and/or renewal processes. The perceived stigma of Medicaid may prevent some families from enrolling their children in Medicaid or SCHIP. In addition, the monthly premium for SCHIP may be a constraint for some families who have healthy children and may not be able to justify a monthly premium with other budgetary needs.

Collaborative partnerships in our communities, with schools as hub, can help address some of these barriers.

Enrolling Uninsured Children Through Partnerships and Collaborations

The recognition of these barriers and the need for ongoing outreach resulted in a governmental interagency task force organized in 1999. The task force included the Departments of Agriculture, Education, Housing and Urban Development, Health and Human Services, Interior, Labor, and Treasury along with the Social Security Administration. This task force elected to provide resources to help with aggressive community outreach to improve the enrollment rates of eligible children in Medicaid and SCHIP (http://www.insurekidsnow.gov 2009). The Robert Wood Johnson Foundation also provided more outreach support and enrollment assistance through their Covering Kids Project (http://www.coveringkids.org 2009).

The Kaiser Commission on Medicaid and the Uninsured (2008) also reported that low income families with children relied on many different sources, for information on assistance for their children. The most often cited were word of mouth, the mass media, and health care providers. Schools were also cited by families with school-going children.

Many communities are working with their local schools to ensure that all children are insured. In Stamford, Connecticut, a community with a population of about 115,000, an outreach effort called "Every Child Matters" was initiated in 2000 and required all parents and guardians to identify their child's health insurance status as part of annual school enrollment. The school nurses then follow up with each family with an uninsured child by mail and then by phone to explain the state's health care coverage for children. The families are offered help with application completion and the enrollment process. "Every Child Matters" has been a success since the schools already collect immunization data, emergency information, allergies, and other sorts of data from families. It allows the schools to leverage their relationships of trust with the families as a source of reliable information regarding health care. Over the first 8 years of the "Every Child Matters" program, the school system has successfully connected over 2,250 children to affordable health care coverage. This community advocates healthcare coverage for all children.

In California, state legislation passed the "Express Lane Eligibility" program, where children who are eligible for the school lunch program can be enrolled in California's Medi-Cal program. This program has been successful in more than 70 California schools and has led to the development of similar programs in other states including New Jersey, North Carolina, Illinois, Massachusetts, and Washington.

In Pennsylvania, approximately 96% of all children have health insurance. Pennsylvania was one of the first states to establish the Children's Health Insurance Program (CHIP) in 1992. Today, about 1.17 million or about two out of every five children in Pennsylvania are enrolled in the Medicaid Assistance program or "CHIP." Both programs are funded with contributions from the state and federal funds. Pennsylvania has created a three-tier CHIP program. Free CHIP allows a family of four to earn up to $42,400 per year and currently has approximately 151, 000 children enrolled. About 22,000 children are enrolled in Low-Cost CHIP which allows a family of four to earn between $42,400 and $63,600 per year. Lastly, approximately 1,500 children are enrolled in the At-Cost CHIP program in which a family of four can earn greater than $63,600 and still qualify. Free CHIP is free of charge to children who qualify. Families enrolled in Low-Cost CHIP pay co-pays and a partial premium. Lastly, the families with children in At-Cost CHIP pay the state's cost for coverage; therefore, no public funds are used. In order to qualify for Low-Cost and At-Cost CHIP programs, parents must document that the child has been uninsured for 6 months or greater, demonstrate they have lost insurance due to a job loss, or have a child less than 2 years of age. In March 2007, when Pennsylvania began the Cover All Kids CHIP expansion, over 20,000 more uninsured children were added to the program with most of them coming from lower income levels (60%) rather than the higher income levels that opponents of the expansion predicted. The expansion of CHIP illustrated that more children are enrolled when eligibility is less confusing to families.

The Children's Defense Fund in Houston, Texas collaborated with the local school districts to promote a 100% campaign to enroll all eligible Houston children in low-cost health coverage in 2007. It was a year-long campaign that was launched after the Texas legislature approved policy changes to simplify the application process for Medicaid and CHIP. This policy changed the application process from every 6 months to every 12 months, allowed the children to receive care without the previous 90 day waiting period and child expenses were allowed to be counted when assessing income. The legislature was hopeful of decreasing the number of uninsured children in Texas which was 1.4 million, the highest in the nation. It was estimated that half of these children were eligible for CHIP or Medicaid. Outreach workers were funded to be in the schools, hospitals, and many community events. An extensive media campaign of billboards, banners, public service announcements, and city-wide family events helped to enroll over 176,000 children in their first year (http://www.childrens-defense.org). Other states including Arkansas, New York, Rhode Island, and Washington have sought to replicate the program after the "best practice" recognition received from both the American Association of School Administrators and the America's Promise Alliance.

Nevada currently ranks 49th in terms of uninsured children (16.8%) and has worked in collaboration with their school districts to simplify enrollment for eligible children as well as communicate with many families who are unaware. The outreach efforts in Nevada have been targeted toward the Hispanic community, with bilingual education and enrollment help sessions at the various school districts as well as offering enrollment at various Boys and Girls Club locations and WIC clinics. Families have been told that if their child is receiving reduced or free lunch through the schools, they most likely qualify (http://www.nvckf.org 2008).

Upon review of these school-based or community collaboratives with schools focused on decreasing the number of uninsured children, some best practices and/or recommendations surface. They include ensuring ongoing sources of funding and volunteers to support outreach efforts for Medicaid and/or CHIP enrollment for eligible children, and creating more partnerships with schools and school nurses to assure sustainability of efforts such as education, outreach, and ongoing assistance with the application and renewal processes.

The Role of the School

Our community schools play a large and influential role with parents on an ongoing basis. Once children reach school age or preschool age, parents seek the school system not only for education, but also for help with basic family needs such as housing, food, social support, athletic activities, and parental education. Schools have been demonstrated to be a community gathering place, where families go for information, assistance, and socialization. The future may lead to continued expansion of the role of school in the community. Schools have the capacity to be the hub of health activities and resources for low income and uninsured children and families. In addition, the school nurse plays a multifaceted role in the care of children; ranging from direct care to health education, counseling and advocacy. The teacher and/or the school nurse, at times, are the first to identify the uninsured or underserved children in the school. This supports the success observed in previously described state programs with their school-based outreach and enrollment programs for Medicaid and Children's Health Insurance Programs. However, currently the number of uninsured sick and needy children coming to school is proving a challenge not only to school nurses, but to educators as well.

School-Based Health Centers

Since the early 1990s, school-based health centers have been developing and evolving across the country. Not only do these centers provide easy access to care with less waiting times for children and families, but they are also well positioned to become "medical homes" for uninsured children. The school nurse as well as teachers and parents are available to collaborate on the child's health and its impact on their academic progress and success with the school-based clinic providers. The school-based clinics are aggressive in enrolling uninsured children in any programs for which they may qualify and can assist the parents with the application process and eligibility guidelines. Lastly, the school-based clinics operate on a sliding fee scale, making it an affordable resource for the entire school community.

School-based health centers have expanded tremendously in the past decade and most recently, in 2002, were the focus of a study to assess the growth as well as the local policies associated with the school-based health center expansion (http://www.healthinschools.org 2005). All 50 states and the District of Columbia participated in this study documenting a total of 1,498 school-based health centers providing in-school health care for children. This represents a 650% increase in the number of centers since 1990. These school-based health centers are funded by various sources such as grants, private foundations, and state government all of which have allowed for this rapid growth. Sixty-one percent of the school-based centers are urban, with 27% rural and 12% in suburban communities. They are represented in elementary schools, as well as middle and high schools. The school-based centers are staffed with a multidisciplinary team of nurse practitioners, physicians, mental health workers, and others. Some use telemedicine or webcams for interactive care and more than 50% are open 5 days per week.

Most of the surveyed school-based centers reported that some components of their funding were based on the number of uninsured children for whom the care was provided. Some of the barriers to care documented by the respondents included transportation, working parents, lack of parent involvement, and the shortage of community primary care, and specialty care providers willing to take a sliding fee scale for children and families. The school-based clinics were able to help address these barriers with the easy access to care at the school site for not only the uninsured children, but also other family members.

The school-based clinics also have been able to help mobilize and leverage community resources for needed specialty care and services. For example, one school-based clinic in New Prairie, Wisconsin has engaged the local Lions Club to help pay for glasses for children in need. The school has funds to pay for only two children needing glasses, but with the Lions Club support, they have been able to help more children , thereby improving the school performance. The sliding fee scale helps families keep up with well child visits and immunizations for their children in addition to acute care visits. Other program components of the school-based health centers included nutrition, pregnancy prevention, prevention of HIV and other sexually transmitted diseases, conflict resolution, and other health education topics;

therefore, providing access to needed preventive information commonly unavailable for uninsured families and children.

At Palm Beach Lakes High School in West Palm Beach, Florida, the school board elected to provide $400,000 in partnership with the state health department to start their school-based clinic staffed by a nurse practitioner in 2006. The team also includes a social worker and a medical assistant. The catalysts for the new school-based clinic were teachers and staff driving children home, needing to pay for needed prescriptions for children and seeing sick children repeatedly going home and not getting the care they needed. Currently, more than 420 parents have provided consent to have their children treated at the school-based clinic on a sliding fee scale basis for primary care (http://www.edline.net 2009).

School-based clinics frequently provide services for low income, uninsured, and children with special needs. One such example is the Sunnyside School District in Tucson, Arizona and their Teenage Parent Program. The Teenage Parent Program (TAPP) collaborates with the local federally-qualified community health center, El Rio Health Center to provide a registered nurse, who is also a certified nurse mid-wife to provide health care for the TAPP students. The health program encourages students to choose healthy lifestyles and habits, teaches health promotion activities, coordinates health care referrals to WIC, childbirth classes and other needed services, and addresses urgent health problems (http://www.sunnysideud.k12/az.us 2009). Longitudinal data for these pregnant teens show a very low incidence of second pregnancies along with a high percentage of high school completion rates (Novak 2009).

The Health Care Safety Net Act which was passed in October 2008 (http://www.healthinschools.org 2005) authorizing continuation of funds for community health centers and the National Health Service Corps program also identified school-based clinics. Funds were identified for completion of a national study on school-based health centers and their effectiveness. The law requires the Comptroller General to complete a study by the end of 2010 regarding the health impact of school-based clinics on the student population. The methodology must include an analysis of the impact of federal funding on the school-based centers, the cost savings to other programs by delivering services in the school setting, and the impact on rural and underserved areas of our communities. This study should add to the body of knowledge regarding the benefits of school-based care for low income and uninsured children.

The School Nurse and the Uninsured Child

The population of school children presents as a very complex group for the school nurse. First of all, children attend school to learn and complete an education. However, there are many other expectations for the school from the community, the government, and the parents as to what the child will receive at school. As noted, school-based clinics are growing at a rapid rate across the nation and are sometimes considered a community expectation as well. Regardless of whether the school is a public, charter, or private school, the parents, especially in underserved populations, look to the nurse, faculty, and staff for guidance. Therefore, school nurses need to be flexible and open to creating a diverse role based on the needs of the children and their families. School nurses are an important link between education and health care. Sick or injured children are unable to learn effectively in the classroom and also impact the learning of their classmates. The school nurse is the first and the frontline health care provider for these underserved and at risk children.

Many school nurses work in a collaborative model that involves the teacher, school nurse, school psychologist, and other healthcare professionals either in school-based clinics or the community. School nurses not only provide the mandated services such as screenings, immunization management, and direct care services for acute illnesses and injuries of school children, but also serve as the educational resource for parents and educators. Many school nurses are the chief connection between chronically ill underinsured and uninsured children and the health care system. For example, children in school who have asthma and diabetes interact daily with the school nurse for medication administration, collaboration on treatment plans with primary care providers, and parental education to achieve optimal health for the chronically ill child.

Some schools have collaborative relationships with mobile health clinics that come regularly to the school. The school nurse makes the appointments and coordinates the continuity of care and follow up treatment for the child. These visiting clinics are able to see all children in need despite their financial or eligibility status and can also assist with applications for public insurance coverage. In addition, school nurses may be the first to identify neglect, abuse, and mental issues in the family. Access to resources for uninsured children is a crucial tool for the school nurse.

These roles of the school nurse build trusting relationships with children and families. School nurses are best positioned to continue to lead aggressive outreach campaigns and education to reach uninsured children as well as partner with other community leaders. School nurses should include the following best practices in their programs to reach and provide access to care for uninsured children:

- Identify students without health insurance and mail letters or make personal contacts to inform parents and/or guardians of the resource availability and the process.
- Ensure that free and reduced lunch forms include health insurance eligibility information and consent to share information.
- Provide information on "back to school" nights in culturally, linguistically and literacy-appropriate methods.
- Link all SCHIP information with school registration forms, athletic physical forms, report card mailings, etc.
- Write articles for school and district newsletters, and continue to update parents about SCHIP.
- Collaborate with community groups to provide financial incentives to enroll uninsured children (Council of Chief State School Officers 2001).

Best Practices for Schools Working with Uninsured Children

1. Create systems which query medical and dental insurance status of all students. Consider school registration paperwork, athletic/sports registration processes, etc.
2. Identify children without coverage and initiate written and/or verbal contact with the parents or guardians.
3. Create a "toolkit" of all community resources materials including Medicaid and SCHIP materials and lists of needed documentation for the eligibility process.. Include locations for eligibility assessment and application assistance as well as providers.
4. Assure all materials are culturally, linguistically and literacy appropriate for your school population. Develop additional resources for cultural brokering, interpretation, family support, etc in your community.
5. Identify and keep current a list of community physicians and providers who accept Medicaid/SCHIP and also offer a sliding fee scale. Use this resource list to help families create a "medical home" for their children.
6. Provide ongoing health education and promotional activities at school activities and events to further the knowledge level of families.
7. Send school nurses, faculty and staff to community meetings and organizations to build relationships and offer resources.
8. Create annual outreach events to enroll eligible children and build recall systems to assure that coverage is continued.
9. Maintain relationships with elected officials and local healthcare organizations to assure programs are funded and promoted to ensure the health of community children.

Fig. 4 Best practices for schools working with uninsured children

School nurses should be advocates for streamlining and simplifying the eligibility process for uninsured children in their communities. Currently, only two states allow school nurses to enroll students in SCHIP (Council of Chief State School Officers 2001). In addition, school nurses can navigate the application process, coordinate care resources, case manage, and provide the much needed preventive care and health education for the uninsured and underserved children in our schools. Uninsured children are many times first identified in school settings where school nurses can advocate for access to health insurance as well as assist with the establishment of a medical home for continuity of care (Fig. 4).

References

Annie E. Casey Foundation (2005) Kids count: state level data. http://www.aecf.org/kidscount/sld/compare. Accessed 26 Feb 2008

Council of Chief State School Officers (2001) Building bridges to healthy kids and better students. Council of Chief State School Officers, Washington, D.C

DeNavas-Walt C, Proctor BD, Smith JC (2008) Income, poverty and health insurance coverage in the United States: 2007. US Census Bureau, Washington, D.C

Devoe JE, Tillotson C, Wallace LS (2008) Uninsured children and adolescents with insured parents. J Am Med Assoc 300(16):1904–1913

Kuhlthau K, Nyman RM, Ferris TG, Beal AC, Perrin JM (2004) Correlates of use of specialty care. Pediatrics 113(1):249–255

Levine P, Schanzenbach D (2009) The impact of children's public health insurance expansions on educational outcomes. National Bureau of Economic Research (NBER), MA

National Association of Community Health Centers (2009) Reauthorization of SCHIP. http://www.nacc.org. Accessed 1 Mar 2009

Novak B (2009) Interview March 20, 2009: teenage parent program. Tucson, Az

Parker E, Teitelbaum M (2003) Percentage of immigrant children without health insurance is on the rise. *Children's Defense Fund Analysis of March 2002, Current Population Date*. Available at: http://cdf.childrensdefense.org/site/DocServer/ichia_report_111303.pdf?docID=524 Accessed 28 Sept 2009

Peterson CL FY (2008) Federal SCHIP Financing Congressional Research Service, January 9, 2008. Available at: http://openers.com/documents/R40129/ Accessed 28 Sept 2009

SHADAC (2009) Current population survey annual social and economic supplement, 2008. Maximizing Enrollment of Kids. Available at: http://shadac.org/publications

http://www.childrensdefense.org (2009) Priorities for America's children

http://www.coveringkids.org (2009) Robert Wood Johnson Foundation: covering the uninsured: children

http://www.edline.net (2009) West Palm Beach high school: school based clinic

http://www.healthinschools.org (2005) 2002 State survey of school-based health center initiatives. http://www.healthinschools.org/static/sbhcs/narrativeo2.aspx

http://www.insurekidsnow.org (2009) Children eligible for free or low cost health insurance U.S. department of health and human services

http://www.sunnysideud.k12.az (2009) Teenage parent program. Retrieved 1 Mar 2009 http://www.sunnysideud.k.12.az.us/district/teenage-parent-program

http://www.kff.org (2009) Kaiser Foundation Commission on Medicare and Medicaid. Available at: http:www.kff.org/healthreform/7980.cfm

http://www.kff.org (2007) Kaiser Commission Survey of California health coverage

http://www.nvckf.org (2008) Insuring Nevada's children. Accessed 1 Mar 2009

Building Community Collaborations Around Care for the Uninsured

Nancy J. Johnson

The local hospital convened a group of community stakeholders as part of their strategic planning process to address access to healthcare for the estimated one million uninsured in the county. The participants included area hospitals, the county health department, healthcare professionals, community health centers, local governmental officials, business owners, legislators, local advocacy groups and many health and human services organizations including the food bank, women's shelter, and job advocacy groups. Their day-long process consisted of an update on current reality in terms of the numbers of uninsured, the demographics, utilization of the local healthcare system, economic impact, and health status. Community readiness was assessed as well as assets identified for use in future work. Logic models were developed, which identified a lack of coordinated care for the uninsured, the lack of a collaborative health information system, and a need for services in two specific areas of the community. Over the next 24 months, the community collaborative initiated a shared information system for the uninsured to track healthcare service utilization and the care received, recruited volunteer physicians and nurse practitioners to provide primary care services at two health-department-sponsored locations, and began the process of case managing uninsured individuals with chronic diseases. The collaborative continues to meet every month to monitor progress, add additional community partners, and seek long-term sustainable systems to care for the uninsured in their community.

Introduction

Probably in every community, some uninsured individuals face the struggle of seeking medical, dental, or health care in systems that are fragmented and lack coordination. Simply referring an uninsured individual to a community resource does not assure access to the needed care, services, or follow up. At the local community level, many opportunities are available to build collaborations around the care of the uninsured and underserved. These collaborations can provide access to care as well as the coordination of care. Health status and outcomes can be positively impacted for the uninsured. However, building sustainable as well as comprehensive

N.J. Johnson
El Rio Community Health Center, Tucson, AZ, USA

N.J. Johnson and L.P. Johnson (eds.), *The Care of the Uninsured in America*,
DOI 10.1007/978-0-387-78309-3_17, © Springer Science+Business Media, LLC 2010

collaborations in communities is challenging work requiring thoughtful consideration of many community variables as well as some innovative leadership.

What Do We Mean by Community Collaboration?

Collaboration in the community can be defined as working together in an organized manner for the improvement of an aspect of community life. The word collaboration implies building partnerships, collecting data, seeking advice, and reaching consensus on actions to be taken. Collaboration is perceived as a higher level of problem solving where all possibilities are considered and potential consequences analyzed prior to taking action. Community collaborations are easily brought to mind with neighborhood coalitions, advocacy groups, school-community partnerships, business organizations, and government-initiated task forces. Some collaborations may be short lived, dissolving when their purpose has been achieved. These community collaborations are easier to create and lead with an end point in mind. However, community collaborations with an ongoing mission and purpose are more difficult to sustain in terms of membership, productivity, and leadership. London (1995) defines collaborations in two forms. The first form is collaborations designed to problem solve and disband when the work is accomplished. The second form is collaborations designed to develop shared visions for creating systems and solutions to problems. Therefore, community collaborations focusing on the care of the uninsured within their respective purview can be initially productive in identifying problems and shared visions for success, but are difficult to "hardwire" into community minds for ongoing action.

Collaboration requires inclusiveness, diversity, involvement of community leadership and tolerance for differences in beliefs, values, opinions, and organizational missions. Collaboration and effective collaborative thinking in the community is a high-level skill. For collaborative participants, it requires going outside their professional/personal or organizational mission to think collectively. For example, healthcare providers must consider transportation and housing implications in the care of the uninsured, while the food bank representatives must appreciate the challenges in generating funds for needed medications.

The components of community collaboration include analysis of a situation, diagnosis of the problem, and identification of a direction, which forms the mission and vision. Other components that then follow include a strategy to achieve the mission and vision, a timeframe for its accomplishment, and details on how the work will be measured and evaluated (London 1995).

As mentioned earlier, effective leadership is critical for community collaborations to be sustained and successful. The necessary style of leadership is defined as transformational and facilitative as well as creating synergy among the group, rather than determining the direction for the group (Svara 1994). Finley (1994) defines collaborative leadership as a process that results in a relationship rather than as a function of a position, forming a new culture for community work to occur.

Collaborative leadership involves fostering discussion and deliberation among community members to achieve the desired mission. Although community collaboration is the modality for creating ongoing coordinated care systems for the uninsured in communities, collaborations do have their limitations. Collaborations are time-consuming groups and work best with small numbers. As the numbers involved in a collaborative grow, the challenges of consensus, decision making, and action steps are more difficult. Sustainability of any collaborative is continual work, which is best served by ongoing engagement of collaborative members, as well as the ongoing recruitment of additional community stakeholders with essential roles identified.

The Process of Building Community Collaboration

Putnam (2000) discusses the decrease in community memberships over the past two decades, and the challenge this presents to building community collaboration. Putnam uses the term "social capital" to describe the community groups, memberships, and coalitions which work to promote community improvement. This "social capital" is essential for successful community collaboration and must be built by leaders desirous of improving community health and care for the uninsured. New methods of building "social capital" in our present communities may be through electronic methods such as online social and professional networking websites, local businesses, fitness facilities, and community groups of shared interests. The size of the community may also impact the amount of "social capital" in place to help create and sustain coordinated care systems for the uninsured. Smaller and/or rural communities may have more access to social capital as well as better insight as to the big picture for the community.

The initial step of building a community collaboration around access to care for the uninsured is to identify who are the stakeholders. This initial group of stakeholders must be convened by the leader for discussion and formation of the collaborative. When thinking about creating a local community collaboration for this purpose, the first group of stakeholders will need to reach clarity around what defines health as their first action. The health of the community is not simply about the provision of health care services. The health of the community may include the environment, the educational system, the safety of the neighborhoods, the availability of affordable housing, public transportation as well as many other attributes which communities uniquely identify and prioritize as characteristics needed for optimal health. When considering the uninsured population, these characteristics of healthy communities such as food, transportation, safety, and shelter may be the priorities over the establishment of additional healthcare locations or clinics. Data are also collected and shared with the initial group of stakeholders regarding the uninsured in the community. Data may include the numbers of uninsured, the demographics, the geography, and the current community resources for support and care for the uninsured. Based upon these data and clarity around what defines health in the community, the initial stakeholders will identify other representatives and/or organizations to invite to join the beginning work of the collaboration.

Some candidates who may join a collaborative on caring for the uninsured would be individuals who are uninsured, Medicaid providers, safety net providers, community hospitals, health care clinics, community food banks, governmental officials, shelters, public health departments, and healthcare professionals. For healthcare professionals, being present and active in the community will help guide the community efforts to provide access to care that is the right place, the right time, and the right price for the uninsured population.

Community collaborations around the care for the uninsured recognize that the uninsured frequently have little or no access to preventive care, utilize the emergency room for primary care needs, have little follow up care, poor management of chronic conditions, and frequently cannot afford prescription medications. Seeking health care is frequently competing with assuring stable housing, food for the family, and employment.

The uninsured are usually lost within the existing healthcare system, are sporadic users of the system, and lack coordination of care. Thus, the mission and vision for the community collaboration is established – to establish a locally designed and coordinated system to care for the uninsured.

The first step is in building community engagement around improving the care of the uninsured. Some community collaboratives begin with the completion of a community readiness assessment which can be directed toward the issue of concern (Triethnic Center 2008). A community readiness assessment consists of studying the current community efforts such as activities, policies, and existing programs for the uninsured. Community current knowledge is investigated along with existing leadership and the community's attitude about caring for the uninsured.

The second working assignment of many community collaborations, if readiness is verified, is a needs assessment. Although the beginning gathering of the stakeholders identifies preliminary data about the uninsured and the current community resources to establish a mission and vision, there is a need to validate the real needs of the uninsured population in the community. One example of a traditional community health assessment is the North Carolina Division of Public Office of Healthy Carolinians (2008). They define a community health assessment as the process by which community members gain an understanding of the health, issues, concerns, and health care systems of their community by studying information on the community assets, strengths, resources, and needs. Usually this assessment results in a report shared with the community collaboration. For a community collaboration working to create a coordinated system of care for the uninsured, a report on the community would help identify the needs of the population, the current resources, other potential partners and opportunities to leverage funds and/or other activities in place in the community. The University of Kansas has created a "Community Toolbox" which identifies a checklist for a good community needs assessment. This checklist includes:

- Makeup and history of the community for context within which to collect data on current concerns.

- What kind of information best describes your community in terms of demographics, geography, politics, community groups, etc.
- Variety of data collection methods such as interviews, observation, focus groups, data analysis, etc.
- List of questions based on discussions with community members, leaders, and healthcare professionals.
- Illustrate the issues of concern and the priority issues.
- Identify barriers or resistance to solving the priority issue.
- Possible solutions and alternatives included.
- Community indicators for measurement (emergency room visits, uninsured children enrolled in care, immunization rates, prenatal care, etc).
- Resources in the community that address the priority issue (http://ctb.ku.edu/tools/assesscommunity/narrativeoutline.jsp 2008).

McKnight (1995) was one of the first to identify the importance of including community assets in community health assessments. Frequently needs and deficits are identified, without the recognition of the gifts that the target population and the community can bring to the solution or revised system. Asset-based community development focuses on the belief that neighborhoods and communities are built by focusing on the strengths and capabilities of the citizens and associations that call the community "home." It is a place-based approach that focuses on the assets of a geographic area can be mobilized to build community. For example, the community collaboration focusing on building a coordinated care system for the uninsured, may identify that there are a variety of healthcare providers geographically located in a neighborhood with many uninsured, who are willing to rotate after hours sliding fee care for the uninsured, hopefully leading to a decrease in nonurgent emergency room visits. Other assets may be local neighborhood centers where meals could be provided, eligibility applications could be completed, and employment assistance provided, removing the barriers of transportation for people seeking assistance. These would be examples of asset-based community development. The three facets of asset based community development include: identify, ask, and connect to create change.

Another source of data for the community needs assessment for the uninsured is available through city and county governments. Many cities and counties identify and monitor areas of high stress based on socioeconomic indicators. These geographic areas may be the focus of support for improving health status for the uninsured. For example, some indicators which may lead to high stress include high percentages of minor or elder populations in an area, linguistic isolation, poverty status, unemployment, and neighborhood instability (City of Tucson 2008).

Other community collaboratives have created and executed "town hall meetings" to complete community health assessments about the care of the uninsured – as well as various other healthcare topics. Facilitative leaders gather data from a wide representation of stakeholders with discussion questions, surveys, and presentations. The results are used to follow up on identified new stakeholders and to educate other community members on the uninsured population (Arizona Town Hall 2008).

From the report of a community health assessment, a community collaborative can develop their strategic plan and goals. Prior to this point in time, the work has been relatively straightforward and achievable for most community collaboratives. Once the collaborative begins the process of goal setting, challenges begin. This is the work in which priorities must be determined, methods must be identified, and accountability must be assigned. The work in actually creating resources, reformatting existing patterns and relationships, and collecting needed measurement and evaluation data is the difficult work in creating change. The stakeholders may support the work and changes in process, but barriers and conflicts can be identified within the collaborative, with the uninsured patient, resource allocation, ethics, policy, the existing health care system, and the community.

Some strategies for conflict management and catalyzing change in the community around the care of the uninsured can be found in Senge's (1990) work on dialogue. The art of dialogue requires "suspending" one's assumptions about a situation and opening one's mind to new ways of looking at relationships, processes or systems. This sort of communication in community collaboratives allows the various stakeholders to begin to see other participants as colleagues and work to create new methods to work together and manage the care of the community's uninsured. Comfort is developed in addressing trade-offs, compromises, and building consensus. The process of dialogue also allows and supports deliberation as a method of problem solving. The use of dialogue may lead to the most innovative methods in which to improve the fragmented healthcare delivery system for the uninsured.

Creating Community Models of Care for the Uninsured

Community collaboratives have a team ready to create and modify models of community care for the uninsured based upon their stakeholders' expertise and the completed community needs assessment. However, at times, the knowledge and current data collected do not reflect the root cause of the inability for the uninsured to receive preventive, routine, and acute care in a coordinated fashion. One tool to assist community collaboratives with their strategies and goal development is the use of the logic model. Logic models are used in many differing ways and formats, but essentially, the logic model approach to planning asks the community collaborative to look for the root causes of a problem. On the surface, we see the problem of the uninsured lacking access to preventive and routine care and may do a "knee jerk" reaction to identify the goals and initiate problem solving. Without really addressing the question of "why" with a problem, the collaborative cannot identify the root causes upon which the goals should focus.

Renger and Titcomb (2002) identify a logic model as a visual method to ascertain the antecedent conditions to a problem of interest. Applying this to the problem of the uninsured receiving fragmented and uncoordinated health care services allows the community collaborative to identify the "why's" of the problem and focus their goals on addressing the causes. Figure 1 provides a sample logic model for addressing the lack of coordination and fragmentation of the care for the uninsured. Most logic models are continually evolving as program interventions uncover other root causes related to the problem under scrutiny.

The goals for the community collaborative should focus on addressing the root causes of the problem in managing the care of the uninsured. As the sample logic model illustrates, the root causes include current community hospital culture, no case/disease management systems, no information systems, no outcome measures, and organizational self-interest. These are the areas upon which the community collaborative would focus. It is important to note that opening more sources for care is not a current root cause in this scenario, which may have been the "knee jerk" reaction solution for the community collaborative without thoughtful consideration of the antecedent conditions.

Referencing the logic model illustration, some of the key areas of focus for this community collaborative in improving coordination of care for the uninsured might be:

- Developing a community-wide case management program for the uninsured with chronic diseases,
- Assessing and implementing a shared information system for care management of the uninsured,

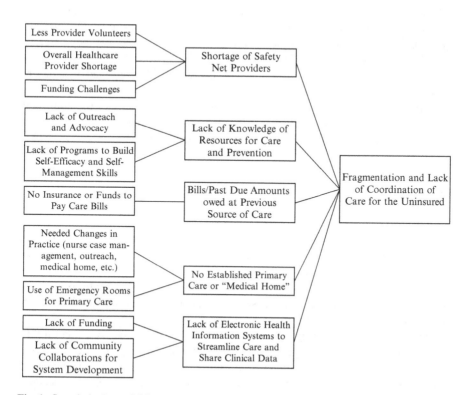

Fig. 1 Sample logic model for care of the uninsured

- Recruitment of volunteer healthcare professionals to assist with care for the uninsured,
- Working with local emergency rooms for direct referrals of the uninsured.

Again, the logic model drives the goals and evaluation focuses on the improvement of the "root causes" identified.

Keeping Community Collaboratives Working

As discussed previously, sustaining the work of community collaboratives is a daunting challenge. Leadership must be consistent and facilitative of all community participants. Roles for the community participants must be clear, identifications of needed resources (stakeholders, organizations, funding, policy, etc.) must be ongoing, and frequent presentations of data analysis crucial. Ongoing recruitment of new collaborative members is essential and the celebration of improvements imperative. Although community collaboratives around the care of the uninsured have no immediate completion of their mission and work, the endpoint is still seen as the decline of disparities of care and access to care for all community members.

Many lessons are learned through community engagement and collaborations. Some of these lessons include knowing that, when we commit to saying "yes" to one strategy, we say "no" to another, communities will support what they perceive to be of value, early successes will energize your collaborative, and ongoing community stories, presentations, and media coverage will keep stakeholders engaged. In addition, the consistent work in building coordination of care for the uninsured in communities will improve health status, provide insight into other related stresses the uninsured face, and bring forth best practices – both financial and quality – in building local systems to optimize the health of all community members.

Working Community Collaboratives

Many examples are available for review across the United States. Many communities have determined that the chance of improving health status for the uninsured in their communities lies with local problem solving and innovative care models. Ownership of the issue is most likely to help with long-term sustainability of community collaboratives. Figure 2 illustrates a sample model of a community collaboration focusing on care coordination of the uninsured.

Project Access is an integrated system which was initiated as a community collaboration in 1996 in the Buncombe County, North Carolina. The collaborative worked to bring together hospitals, free clinics, pharmacies, and physicians to provide coordination of care for approximately 15,000 uninsured and low income individuals annually. The collaborative developed a centralized database to manage volunteer physician commitments and patient referrals. All patient financial screening

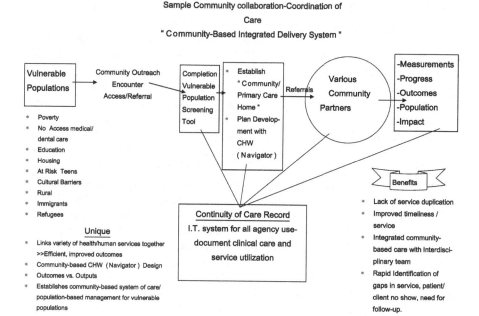

Fig. 2 Sample model for community collaboration

is centralized as well as physician and hospital in kind charity care. The outcomes achieved by the collaboration include a reduced emergency room utilization rate from 28% to 8% for nonemergent visits with 80% of patients reporting improved health status.

Project Access reports reduced hospital charity care, and over $5 million in services donated by the hospitals and private physicians. Lessons learned by the collaborative include the importance of identification, recruitment and nurturing of physician champions, organizing community events to gain momentum, identifying community-based financing and existing assets that may be untapped or underutilized, and providing online systems of managing patients and monitoring data. Project Access has been replicated in twelve other communities across the country (Project Access 2008).

Another example of a successful community collaboration is illustrated in Chatham County, Georgia. As community hospitals identified the gaps in the safety net, the collaborative was initiated when the County Commission allocated $3 million for community care of the uninsured and underinsured. The Commission realized that many others needed to be involved if health status was to improve for the uninsured community. They developed a Safety Net Planning Council in 2004 comprising nonprofit, corporate, county, health and human services organizations that completed a comprehensive needs assessment. This needs assessment report identified that at any point in time, approximately 44,000 individuals are uninsured with most located in the downtown areas. The report also identified the complexity and difficulty in utilizing the community's health care system. A Care Navigator Program was initiated using case managers and a web-based electronic information network (Pathways) to assign medical homes for the uninsured, with the priority focus on those with chronic diseases. Pathways assures coordination of care and services for the uninsured.

The collaborative also created the Community Health Mission which is composed of 54 volunteer physicians who provide care and catalyze additional community partnerships to assure affordable services for the uninsured. The ongoing measures assessed by this community collaboration include assessment in emergency room use, increase in the safety net capacity, improved access to low-cost prescription medications, and decrease in the average cost of care. Challenges and potential barriers that the Safety Net Planning Council has had to address include competing interests, political environment related to health care issues in relationship to other competing governmental priorities, expanding needs, and working with a diverse uninsured community (Healthcare Georgia Foundation 2008).

Integrated Care Collaboration (ICC) is a third example of a community collaborative working successfully and long term to address healthcare coordination for the uninsured. An Ascension Health affiliate, the ICC was formed in 1997 with nine partners in Travis County, Texas. Today, ICC has 24 partners representing three different counties. The ICC is structured as a nonprofit regional collaborative established to develop joint projects to improve access to affordable health care for the uninsured as well as to improve the quality of care.

This partnership began with the creation of their mission, vision, and values which has been invaluable in making decisions and identifying priorities. ICC has built the I-Care system to provide common eligibility screening and outreach as well as share health data for clinical and demographic information for providers of care. This sustainable health information exchange has allowed ICC to be able to track patients through various healthcare providers and services, identify gaps in services for the uninsured, and track real savings in healthcare expenditures. ICC was successful in placing an initiative on the ballot for creating a Healthcare District that was approved and provides a funding stream for the care of the uninsured in 2004. The successful community collaboration of ICC and ongoing work was instrumental in the successful ballot initiative (ICC 2006).

Summary

Successful community collaborations around care for the uninsured include the ability to overcome barriers, maximize resources to expand services and care, partner with many others in the community, engage and empower the uninsured patient, collect and share data, reach out to various members/organizations in the community, and continually address new and/or evolving issues. Community collaboration helps us all get on the same page in terms of improving the existing health care system in caring for the uninsured.

References

Arizona Town Hall (2008) Ninetieth proceedings. Prescott, Arizona

City of Tucson (2008) Neighborhood stress elements. Personal Interview, Sr. Janet Smith. 16 Apr 2008

Community Readiness Assessment (2008) Triethnic Center. Available at: http://www.trienthnic-center.colostate.edu/communityreadiness. Retrieved 25 Jan 2008

Finley NE (1994) Spinning the leadership relationships into the twenty-first century. J Leadersh Organ Stud 5(1):51–61

Georgia Health Foundation (2008) Safety Net Planning Council. Available at: http://www.health-caregeorgia.org. Retrieved 1 May 2008

Integrated Care Collaboration (2006) Available at: http://www.icc-centex.org. Retrieved 15 Feb 2008

Kansas University (2008) Community tool box. Available at: http://ctb.ku.edu/tools/assess-community/narrativeoutline.jsp. Retrieved 24 Apr 2008

London S (1995) Collaboration and community. Pew partnership for civic change. Available at: http://www.scottlondon.com/reports/ppcc.html. Retrieved 5 Jan 2009

McKnight J (1995) The careless society. BasicBooks, New York

North Carolina Division of Public Office of Healthy Carolinians (2008) Community assessment guide book. Available at: http://nciph.sph.unc.edu. Retrieved 6 Apr 2008

Project Access (2008) Project access: Buncombe County Medical Society. Available at: http://www.cjaonline.net/communities/NC_Ashevill.html. Retrieved 15 Aug 2008

Putnam RD (2000) Bowling alone: The collapse and revival of American community. Simon and Schuster, New York

Renger R, Titcomb A (2002) A three-step approach to teaching logic models. Am J Eval 23(4):493–503

Senge P (1990) The fifth discipline: The art and practice of the learning organization. Doubleday, New York

Svara JH (1994) Facilitative leadership in local government: Lessons from mayors and chairpersons. Jossey-Bass, San Francisco

Information Technology and Medically Uninsured

Theresa Cullen

Overview

The uninsured are an invisible face in America. Their health care needs are great and are met by a patchwork of venues scattered throughout their communities. Access to health information technology may appear to be unnecessary, given the overwhelming needs of individual patients. In fact, health information technology (HIT) represents one possible way to increase quality care to this patient population.

HIT is in a unique role to help the uninsured improve their health care outcomes. HIT is used as an enabler to assist in improving access to care as well as the elimination of health inequities. HIT can be designed to increase quality and contribute to cost containment in defined populations, such as the uninsured.

HIT systems have been traditionally developed to capture billing and administrative costs and workload data. The current HIT systems, while secondarily designed to improve outcomes, are primarily driven by these revenue generation concerns. Since the uninsured may lack access to routine care, these HIT systems were not originally designed to address the issues that may confront this population – issues that may not be easily captured by standard code sets and that do not contribute to billing. Since the traditional EHR (electronic health record) is usually driven by practice management outcomes, including increased revenue and charge capture with a focus on the delivery of care that can be captured by standard code sets such as Evaluation/Management, ICD 9, V, and CPT codes, there may not be any connection between the available EHR systems and the needs of the uninsured. Since the uninsured primarily reflect a patient population with decreased access to care due to fiscal reasons, systems that are designed to increase charges may not be supportive of the interventions needed in these populations.

In addition, health status determinants may include a broad range of factors beyond those routinely addressed in modern patient- and provider-centric health care delivery systems. Health status can reflect, among other factors, personal and family genetics, lifestyle choices, environment, behavioral issues, social and political challenges,

T. Cullen
Office of Information Technology for Indian Health Service (IHS), Washington, DC, USA

N.J. Johnson and L.P. Johnson (eds.), *The Care of the Uninsured in America*,
DOI 10.1007/978-0-387-78309-3_18, © Springer Science+Business Media, LLC 2010

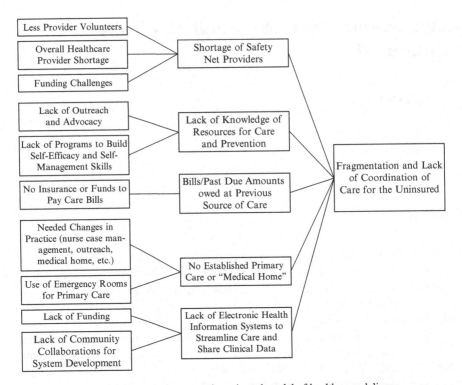

Fig. 1 Comprehensive integrated-community-oriented model of health care delivery

and community attributes, such as the normalization of obesity. The uninsured are at risk to experience these factors to a higher degree than other populations.

Health inequities within the uninsured population reflect the limitations of the traditional medical model of delivering health care to certain populations. Current health IT systems support the traditional model of health care delivery by ensuring that the data for the individual patient are the only data that providers routinely see during a patient encounter. HIT is in a unique position to expedite the development of a new paradigm of health care delivery. HIT solutions may facilitate the development and support for integrated health care delivery teams. This approach requires novel clinical information displays, as well as viewing the patient within the context of their family, community, and population. This chapter presents some of the salient features that must be considered in this shift to a comprehensive, integrated-community-oriented model of health care delivery, a model that should improve access and outcome for the uninsured (Gibbons 2008) (Fig. 1).

Provider Prospective

Health information technology systems have been traditionally designed to record, aggregate, and display health data to help facilitate the provider perspective of care, as well as capture and assist in the financial billing and practice management process. These traditional health record systems (synonymous with the traditional SOAP – subjective, objective, assessment, and plan note of recording patient data in a structured format) reflect the provider perspective. The majority of HIT systems are designed to facilitate this form of data recording. The integration of this historical medical approach to the delivery of care has resulted in HIT systems that are easier for clinicians to adopt; these systems are also easier to integrate into traditional models of health care delivery.

This provider-centric delivery models support the medical model with little attention to other factors that affect health status. Failure to focus attention on non-traditional determinants of health such as ethnicity, sexual orientation, disability, education, nutrition, family concerns, literacy, communication styles, community concerns, and patient goal setting result in a decreased ability to effect changes in health status outcomes. These variables are more likely to be of import to the uninsured patient.

Patient Perspective

The recent attention to personal health records has resulted from the need to include the patient's perspective in health decision making. Personal health records, such as the Veterans Health Administration HealtheVet (the gateway to veterans' health benefits and services), Microsoft Health Vault, Google Personal Health Record, and other public and private solutions are designed to help individual patients' record health data, as well as navigate the health care system. However, the primary focus in the area of personal health records has been the recording of significant health information into an internet-based solution that is controlled by the patient.

The CDC Healthy People 2010 goal to increase access to the internet independent of societal factors is still lagging in certain communities – among them the uninsured. 2003 Census data and the 2004 Nielsen/NetRatings show 54.7–75% of Americans can access the internet from home (US Census, April 8, 2008). Uninsured populations are least likely to benefit from these solutions, since their access to the internet is more limited than this; recent data from American Indian/ Alaska Native screening indicate that internet access in rural areas is usually less than 20% These differences reflect fiscal access as well as electronic literacy problems - issues that contribute to health disparities in certain populations. Decisions about access to personal health records for the uninsured must be attentive to the choice of appropriate technology. In many cases, paper-based personal health records may be the solution for years to come.

Additional pertinent patient factors COULD be included in electronic health records (EHR); for instance, the setting of a patient goal could be recorded in a robust EHR, allowing the provider to recall the goal at the next visit. Since there are clear data supporting a causal relationship between patient activation, patient goal setting, and patient outcome, this functionality is critical to achieving improved quality of care as well as improved individual outcomes. However, a patient's ability to goal set can be limited by many factors, including personal and family crisis, communication concerns, health literacy, mistrust of the health care system, patient preferences, and understanding of the relative importance of specific goals. Uninsured patients are at risk to experience one or many of these issues, resulting in a decreased ability to become activated in their health partnership. Technological recognition of these factors can help assist in addressing them, resulting in improved health care delivery to the uninsured.

Community Perspective

Community perspectives are critical in health care delivery. However, certain subpopulations become invisible from the community perspective. The uninsured are more likely to lack a visible "community face." The uninsured, facing additional difficulties in accessing care, are prone to interact with the health care system on a less frequent basis. As a result, when they do present for care, the health care system should provide "one-stop shopping" that can positively impact their health outcomes.

Electronic records that aggregate data into a longitudinal community health record can assist in this comprehensive delivery of care. Systems that can be used to recognize certain at risk situations, such as fluoride levels in certain communities, known exposure to carcinogens based on historical demographic patterns, and early outbreak recognition, can facilitate the expansion of "what is your chief complaint today" to "what are the other factors that can be addressed to make an impact on your long-term health outcome."

Population Perspective

Finally, the identification of specific populations, defined by a myriad number of individual and combined factors, is critical to improving health status. Once a population is defined, in this case, the uninsured, health information technology can be employed to help track the individual care, the community, and the population. Tracking of population-based health outcomes, determined by an attribute of uninsured, can help identify the critical factors that impact the health status of this population. Ideally, this data aggregation can assist in determining the impact of individual interventions as well as community endeavors on health care outcomes (Fig. 2).

Appropriate Technology

Health information technology solutions abound, including electronic medical records, disease-specific registries, and telemedicine. The current national focus on health information technology has resulted in the recognition of the need to share standardized data in a standard format in a bidirectional fashion with multiple

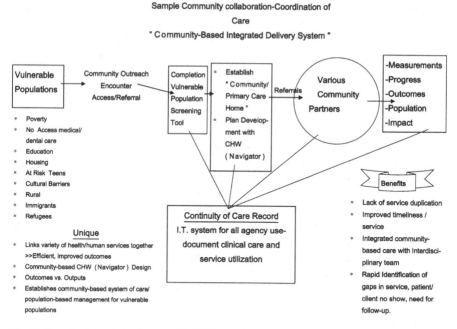

Fig. 2 Data for determining impact of individual and community interventions on health outcomes

health care delivery systems in order to develop a continuity of care record. The uninsured, usually lacking a medical home, are addressed infrequently in this discussion. Technology that is appropriate to the needs of the uninsured may be different from the technological needs of those individuals with traditional and longitudinal sources of access to health care. The following section delineates some specific topics that should be addressed by the health care delivery system interested in implementing HIT into their care delivery model.

Requirements Process

Ensuring that appropriate technological solutions are obtained in specific situations starts with a requirements process. End users including providers, board members, and, in some unique cases, patients should be involved in this process. The initial requirements process should focus on the identification of appropriate technology for the current health care delivery system. For instance, the requirements process must pay attention to the business process. If the homeless clinic takes place in a different place and with different staff each week, then the technology must be portable, quickly understandable, and easy to use for some period of time until there is additional stability in the health care delivery model.

The requirements process is at best laborious; however, the capturing of appropriately specific and granular attributes for a health IT system is essential to the successful integration of HIT into the care delivery model. For instance, stating that the system will include family history is helpful but inadequate. In this case, specifically listing the data sets that are critical to the capture of family history is essential to ensure that the system that is eventually utilized can record what is needed.

Data Field Requirements

Traditional determinants of health and diagnoses of disease are usually accompanied by an appropriate ICD 9, CPT, or V code. However, nontraditional determinants of health are as important as traditional elements to the health outcomes for uninsured populations. For instance, screening for domestic violence is critical in appropriate assessment of health status, yet there is no standard code for screening of this situation. In addition, other fields that may impact health status (health literacy, cultural impact, family composition, adverse childhood events, patient activation, including goal setting and goal met/ not met, as well as refusals of care) are lacking in current standards. The standards development organizations are gradually addressing these areas. In the mean time, it is essential that the requirements process identify those areas that are critical to the assessment and delivery of care of the uninsured, and strive to include those fields in the HIT system. These fields should be included in a standard fashion in the HIT system, even if they are not associated with specific standard codes. As long as the HIT system requires that they be entered in a standard format, they can be retrieved for future analysis and evaluation.

Example American Indian/Alaska Native women are involved in incidents of domestic violence at a higher rate than any other ethnic group. However, there is no standard way to record if screening for intimate partner violence occurred, and the result of that screening. Due to the population-based clinical need, Indian Health Service developed a standard way to record screening and results, as well as reports, for intimate partner violence in their HIT system. As a result, screening rates for domestic violence throughout the Indian Health System have increased form less than 10% to almost 35% in a 4-year period.

Bidirectional Sharing of Health Information

The recognition of the need for bidirectional sharing of health information has existed for over the last two decades. Regional Health Information Exchanges (RHIO) and Health Information Exchanges (HIE) are groups of organizations with business and clinical commitments to improving the quality, safety, and efficiency of healthcare delivery. While many projects have attempted to achieve this result, there are few situations where this has actually occurred. Indianapolis is considered one of the best examples of a results-driven business model that has thrived in producing and supporting a regional health information exchange that accomplishes the sharing of appropriate personal health information among identified stakeholders

(McDonald, et al., 2005). The Office of the National Coordinator at DHHS has recently awarded grants to address this issue through the development of a Nationwide Health Information Exchange (NHIN); there is a complementary federal effort to ensure that federal agencies that deliver direct health care, or are reliant on the receipt of that health information for their business process, are also developing bidirectional health information abilities. (Agencies currently include Veterans Administration, Department of Defense, Indian Health Service, and the Social Security Administration.) In addition, the Public Health Information Network (PHIN), under the auspices of the Center for Disease Control, recently awarded regional grants to increase the bidirectional sharing of public health information.

The uninsured are poised to benefit to a large extent if and when the health care facility that delivers their care becomes part of an HIE. This would accomplish the goal of a semilongitudinal health record, and eliminate a degree of the redundancy and inefficiencies in a health care system that only cares for people in a sporadic fashion.

However, the concept of the HIE still begs the question of the need for a medical home for the uninsured.

Example The Nationwide Health Information Network is designed to help facilitate bidirectional standards-based sharing between health care facilities. The Office of the National Coordinator, Department of Health and Human Services, awarded nine contracts to regional health information exchanges to begin trial implementations of data sharing in 2008.

Clinical Decision Support

The need for clinical decision support (CDS) tools is crucial to improving health decision making as well as health outcomes. CDS tools run the gamut from prompts to record patient demographic data, health reminders about patients with diabetes receiving appropriate eye care, women in certain age groups receiving mammography reminders, reminders to start controller medications on certain asthmatic groups, to artificial intelligence that can help guide complicated decision making. The development of bundled disease quality measures, as well as bundled clinical decision support reminders, is reflective of the advances being made in the area of decision support appropriate requirements can help identify the critical components for individual situations. For instance, HIV clinics may benefit from robust HIV reminders about quality of care, while a general clinic caring for the uninsured may have a limited need for these specific clinical prompts.

Registries

Registries of specific patient populations, defined by specific attributes, have proven useful to improving the quality of care delivered to patients. Registries can be either stand alone, partially integrated into EHR solution, or fully integrated into the electronic health record. Fully integrated registries tend to be the most efficient; these registries, or population-based patient lists, are developed passively based on information already in the HIT system. However, in the best cases, patients populate these lists after there has been human review of the "patient candidate" for inclusion in the list. This human intervention helps ensure that the specific reasons that prompted for inclusion of the patient (diagnosis, medication, lab test, etc.) are accurate. Consequently, these integrated patient registries are more likely to be kept up to date, and include pertinent and timely information in their database.

Stand alone registries have been used to track and improve quality of care for the past two decades. These registries tend to be effective when the EHR is not integrated into the registry and when the registry is a specific disease-based registry.

However, integrated HIT systems that can flag a patient as a possible candidate for enrollment in specific registries at the time of visit can decrease missed opportunities for intervention for patients as well as their families and communities. In the future, registry functions integrated at the point of care will have the best impact on patient outcomes.

Example Health Resources and Systems Administration (HRSA), an operating division within the Department of Health and Human Services, has been involved with disease specific collaboratives in conjunction with the Institute for Healthcare Improvement (IHI). Since 1998, two-third of community health centers have been involved in one or more disease-specific collaborative. These disease-specific collaboratives are designed to improve care and outcomes to patients with specific diseases. Collaborative sites have shown improvements in measures of prevention and screening, using new delivery models as well as disease-specific registries to monitor and evaluate outcomes for involved patients (Landon et al. 2007).

Population Health

In order to improve health status and help eliminate health inequities, information technology must be able to provide clinical users with a fully integrated tool that can manage any patient within the context of his or her population health constructs. Failure to recognize pertinent population characteristics and their impact on individuals hinders our ability to affect the health status of the individual as well as his or her population.

Electronic health records that automatically generate clinical quality reports at the beginning of each day for each scheduled clinic can help a provider identify individual patient needs as well as troubleshoot potential areas of population and community interventions. Bidirectional immunization data sharing with states has helped increase immunization coverage in many communities through the appropriate reporting and sending of immunization records to care providers. The uninsured are particularly at risk in this situation, with the knowledge that many uninsured patients receive immunizations in any available venue. The ability to share immunization data at a state level means that individual providers can query the state immunization registry to input and receive data on the patients that they are seeing. Practically, this means that the failure to have your own immunization record is mitigated, at least within a state, by these state immunization registries.

Example By the age of 2, at least 20% of the children in the US have seen more than one healthcare provider, resulting in scattered paper medical records in their parents' home.

Immunization information systems (IIS) help families and providers share and consolidate immunization information into one reliable source. They can save money by ensuring that children get only the vaccines they need and reducing the time needed for providers to gather and review immunization records. Immunization information systems share confidential, computerized vaccination histories with appropriately authorized health care providers (http://www.cdc.gov/vaccines/programs/iis/default.htm, 2008).

Public Health

The inclusion of public health reporting requirements is essential, especially in vulnerable populations. The ability to automatically share data with the public health departments in a bidirectional fashion does not occur in most counties and states; however, there is a need for the point of care provider to share appropriate public health data with the appropriate public health department. As more public health jurisdictions develop the capacity to bidirectional share data from their public health laboratories with appropriate providers, passive and automatic sharing of public health data will occur. HIT systems should be geared to ensure that data collection occurs in a standard fashion that will facilitate this sharing as appropriate reporting agencies develop this capacity.

Security

Patients expect that their personal health information will be secure with access limited to those with a need to know. Uninsured patients require the same attention to security within health information systems and health information exchanges.

Barriers

Barriers to successful implementations of HIT solutions, be they telemedicine, bidirectional data sharing, or the implementation of electronic health records, are numerous. However, the major factor that predicts success in any information technology solution is the commitment of leadership and administration. This factor is essential when addressing the care of the uninsured. Administrative commitment is critical to the implementation of any health information technology solution; uninsured populations are in an even more vulnerable situation. Information technology is an expensive investment that must be borne by the health care delivery system at this time; the uninsured may receive care in practices that are unable to bear the cost of the IT investment. In addition, sharing of data in a bidirectional format requires additional fiscal and human resources that may be beyond the scope of a practice.

AHRQ (Agency for Health Research and Quality; http://www.ahrq.gov) has funded the National Resource Center for HIT health information technology programs to assist in the provision of guidance to individual sites that are seeking to integrate and develop HIT solutions. Much of their work can be utilized by programs seeking additional information and/ or solutions to the provision of HIT to their practices (http://www.ahrq.gov, 2008).

In addition, HRSA (Health Resource and Service Administration; http://www. hrsa.gov) has made funds available for practices to evaluate and invest in health IT resources; their HIT technology is committed to (http://www.hrsa.gov, 2008):

- Develop a strategy and supportive policy that leverages the power of health information technology and telehealth to meet the needs of people who are uninsured, underserved, and/or have special needs.
- Identify, disseminate, and provide technical assistance to health centers and other HRSA grantees in adopting model practices and technologies.
- Disseminate appropriate information technology advances, such as electronic medical records systems or provider networks.
- Promote grantee health information technology advances and innovations as models.
- Work collaboratively with foundations, national organizations, the private sector, and other Government agencies to help HRSA grantees adopt health information technology.
- Ensure that HRSA health information technology policy and programs are coordinated with those of other U.S. Department of Health and Human Services components.

Future

The current administration (April 2009) has jumpstarted the expansion of the HIT process by allocating $19.5 billion to the further development of the Health Information Technology system in the US headed by David Blumenthal from Harvard's Institute of Health Technology (Rubenstein 2009)

To improve health status and health inequities, information technology must be able to provide clinical users with a fully integrated tool that can manage any patient within the context of his or her health and physical, environmental and community/ population health constructs. This requires a unique set of information when caring for the uninsured; the ability to share data in a timely and secure manner is critical to creating a continuity of care record for the uninsured. In addition, this record must be available at the time of care, with appropriate and adequate information to help facilitate quality care delivery.

The traditional way of viewing health data and quality from a patient-centric focus is essential as a starting point for assessment of health information technology. However, the uninsured are a population that may place additional needs on the HIT system; the system must be able to recognize and respond to these needs. In addition, the Venn diagram of health care delivery needs to expand beyond the individual patient to embrace the communities and populations that reflect that patient's life (see diagrams). The system that provides care to the uninsured must pay attention to the elements beyond the traditional domains as well as ensuring that care at the time of a clinical visit is appropriate, affordable, and integrated into the larger health care safety net within the *community*.

The current medical model results in ongoing health inequities and inadequate access to care for many; without changes to health IT systems, providers will continue to deliver care that cannot impact the health disparities that result from these factors. We must move to the next level both clinically and technologically, using patient- and population-centric knowledge to determine what is important to uninsured patients and their communities. This work must be accompanied by a change in the care delivery model – a change that recognizes the needs of this special population, as exquisitely defined by this one attribute.

As the nation continues to emphasize and develop health IT, a unique opportunity exists to develop information systems that can help improve health status for individuals as well as a population health level. HIT solutions for the uninsured population can provide benefit to the larger US community.

Box 1 Regional Health Information Organizations (RHIOs): Community Approaches

As we know, the implementation of electronic medical and health records has the potential to help healthcare providers improve the safety and quality of their patient care. In addition, the possibility is present to also decrease costs and improve efficiency in caring for the uninsured who present for care at differing locations as well as sometimes, sporadically. However, despite these apparent benefits the cost of electronic health records remains the key barrier for community health centers and community providers who serve the uninsured and low income in our country. When costs are identified as the number one barrier to electronic records, it is not just the hardware and software costs, it is also the cost of having dedicated staff to plan, implement, train, troubleshoot, support, and continually evaluate the process of implementing electronic health records. Most local community providers and those caring for the

(continued)

Box 1 (continued)

uninsured do not have the human resources to manage this extensive transition process. Therefore, it is not surprising that less than 10% of safety-net providers have adopted electronic records, compared to 52% using electronic health records in the large medical groups (California Healthcare Foundation 2008). As the benefits are strongly touted to healthcare providers, healthcare administrators, and payers for the regional health information organizations, the funding is complex and requires a well-developed business plan. During the start-up phase, RHIOS rely mostly on grant funding, but as they reach the transition and production phases, their funding sources shift to member fees, transaction fees, and other earned income from utilization, cost and outcome data trending and reports. For those healthcare providers who are exclusively safety-net providers, their membership and access to RHIOS will need to be supported by other funding sources in order to truly provide quality and timely care for the uninsured as well as limit the costs of duplicative and unneeded services (Table 1).

Table 1 RHIO revenue streams

	Start-up phase	Transition phase	Production phase
Gifts/grants	84%	56%	34%
Member fees	7%	12%	28%
Transaction fees	0%	4%	8%
Other earned income	3%	4%	24%
All other	6%	24%	6%

Source: Healthcare IT Transition Group's 2007 Survey, "Sustainable RHIO Funding and the Emerging Business Model."

The development of Health Information Exchange Systems provides many benefits that include:

- Access to health information from hospitals, medical practices, laboratories, pharmacies, community health centers that improves quality and saves money
- Timely and effective care provided with quick data retrieval to address patient needs
- Savings of health care dollars – an estimated 31 cents of every dollar does for administrative costs currently (HIeHR Utility Project 2008) which health information exchange systems could work toward minimizing
- Up to $500 billion per year is spent on duplicative or unneeded care which access to timely patient information could avoid (HIeHR Utility Project 2008)

For safety-net providers, a collaborative community- or regional-based network for electronic medical/health record development seems the most cost effective and quality methodology to consider. Federal and state agencies along with other funding sources are seeing the benefits to be had by investing in this collaborative network. Some of the quite probable benefits of a network include focus on quality improvement, technical and operational support, and support of the mission for care of the uninsured, as well as sustainability and dependability. For healthcare systems caring for the uninsured, these are very critical factors. Some of the following initiatives are underway:

- California Electronic Health Record Network for Electronic Health Record Adoption is a collaborative funded by multiple sources that has developed a network for safety-net providers in California with the mission of ensuring access to affordable, quality health care for all Californians (http://www.chcf.org).
- Southern Arizona RHIO Coalition-Formed in the fall of 2004 with the immediate focus of dealing with the uninsured in Southern Arizona. However, within months, the recognition that a Regional Health Information Organization would benefit all providers and payers, not just the uninsured and those caring for them, changed the planning process. Today, the group's new name is the Southern Arizona Health Information Exchange and is midway in business development of a system that will share health information across all providers and ensure sustainability.
- HIeHR Utility Project-A state-based initiative funded by a Federal Medicaid Transformation Grant which focuses on developing and implementing a statewide, secure, online Health Information Exchange and Electronic Health Record system. A secure web portal will give authorized Medicaid providers quick access to needed care information. HIeHR Utility Project is also assisting healthcare providers in identifying the needs, plan, and potential resources to achieve the benefits of electronic health records, while working to mobilize resources and funding sources. (http://www.azahcccs.gov/eHealth)

Box 2 Government Initiatives Around Health Information Technology

Currently, the Department of Health and Human Services is providing guidance for the creation of standards for Health Information Technology Systems that will improve the efficiency and quality of patient care and health care systems. Various member agencies of the Department of Health and Human Services are working on funding, building, testing, and developing standards around HIT use. These include:

(continued)

Box 2 (continued)

- *American Health Information Community (AHIC)* which is a federal advisory board created in 2005 to make recommendations on how to develop and implement HIT. They represent and advocate for the health care consumer and help to build a broad and quality HIT system.
- *Office of the National Coordinator for Health Information Technology (ONC)* is working on creating a national seamless and secure information exchange for data and records. The ONC also advises the Secretary of Health and Human Services on HIT policies and initiatives and is leading the goal of making an electronic record available for most Americans by the year 2014.
- *Federal Health Architecture (FHA)* was established as an eGov Line of Business to increase efficiency and effectiveness in government operations. The FHA is responsible to support federal activities to enable federal agencies to exchange health data between and among themselves, with state, local, and tribal governments, along with private healthcare organizations.
- *Agency for Healthcare Research and Quality (AHRQ)* is funding research and development with over $166 million available for grants and contracts. This funding is to stimulate investment in HIT especially for the rural uninsured and underserved areas. AHRQ also provides technical assistance and shares knowledge and findings to speed progress along with electronic health systems.
- *Health Resources and Services Administration (HRSA)* promotes the use of health information technology and telehealth for the uninsured and underserved and/or have special needs. HRSA also works to assure that their policies are in concert with those of other governmental organizations regarding HIT development and adoption.
- *Indian Health Services (IHS)* IHS has been a leader in health information technology utilization. They capture both clinical and public health data using the resource and patient management system (RPMS). The RPMS electronic health record is available for all providers.
- *National Institutes of Health (NIH)* The NIH through the Nation Library of Medicine hosts an online medical database for consumers and healthcare professionals. MedlinePlus is free of charge and provides information about medications, an illustrated medical encyclopedia, interactive tutorials, and the most recent health and research reports.
- *Centers of Medicaid and Medicare Services (CMS)* CMS has a new electronic health record demonstration project to show that medical errors will decrease and quality of care will increase with the use of HIT. The project provides financial incentives for over five years to physician practices that utilize certified EHR systems to improve clinical measures. The more aspects of EHR utilized, the more bonuses available for physicians. CMS is encouraging other health care payers to also offer financial incentives for physicians to adopt electronic health records.

References

Agency for Healthcare Quality and Research (2008) Available at http://www.ahrq.gov. Accessed 13 Apr 2008

California Healthcare Foundation (2008) Creating HER networks in the safety net. Available at http://www.chcf.org. Accessed 13 Mar 2008

Dolan PL (2007) RHIOS hit financial stumbling blocks on path to national network. American Medical News, pp 22–24

Gibbons M (ed) (2008) eHealth: solutions for healthcare disparities. Springer Science, New York

Health Systems and Research Administration (2008) Available at http://www.hrsa.gov. Accessed 15 Apr 2008

HIeHR Utility Project (2008) Physicians and health information exchange. Available at http://www.azahccs.gov/eHealth. Accessed 18 Mar 2008

Immunization Information systems (2008) Available at http://www.cdc.gov/vaccines/programs/iis/default.htm.(2008). Accessed 13 April 2008

Landon B, Hicks L, O'Malley J (2007) Improving the management of chronic diseases at community health centers. N Engl J Med 9(356):921–934

McDonald C, Overhage J, Barnes M, Schadow G, Blevins L, Dexter PR, Mamlin B, and the INPC Management Committee (2005) The Indian network for patient care: A working local health information infrastructure. Health Aff 24(5):1214–1220

Rubenstein S (2009) Obama's Health IT Pick Pointed to Challenges for Doctors. The Wall Street Journal Digital Network. Available at: http://blogs.wsj.com/health/2009/03/20/obamas-health-it-pick-pointed-to-challenges-for-solo-doctors/. Accessed April 11, 2009.

U.S. Census Data. Available at: http://www.census.gov/prod/2005pubs/p23-208.pdf. Accessed 8 Apr 2008

Additional Resources

http://www.hhs.gov/healthit/onc/mission/ Office of the National Coordinator for Health Information Technology

http://www.hhs.gov/healthit/ Office of the National Coordinator for Health Information Technology Health IT initiatives

http://www.hhs.gov/healthit/healthnetwork/background Nationwide Health Information Network

http://www.cdc.gov/PHIN Public Health Information Network/ Center for Disease Control

http://www.myhealth.va.gov/ my health eVet at the Veterans Health administration

Agency for Healthcare Quality and Research http://www.ahrq.gov

Health Systems and Research Administration http://www.hrsa.gov

The Role of Government in Providing Health Care to the Uninsured

James E. Dalen

Nearly every developed country takes responsibility for critical public health matters such as sanitation and control of infectious diseases. In addition, most western countries also assume responsibility for ensuring that all its residents have access to health care. Unfortunately, the United States is not one of the nations that ensures access to health care to all its citizens.

There are two basic methods for a nation to ensure access to health care. The government may establish a national health service (NHS) to directly provide health services as in the United Kingdom, Spain, and Scandinavian countries. The other method is to ensure that all its citizens have health insurance by either providing health insurance, as in Canada, or requiring all its citizens to obtain health insurance, as in Germany, France, Switzerland, Taiwan and other countries.

The National Health Service Model

The United Kingdom (UK) is the prototype of the NHS model. In 1948, the government took over all hospitals in the UK, and all hospital-based health professionals including medical specialists and nurses became employees of the NHS. General practitioners (GPs) remained office based and became independent contractors to the NHS. Although GPs are not NHS employees, all their income is derived from the NHS in the form of capitation and bonuses.

In this system, health insurance is not required. Primary care and hospital care are available to all residents without charge. Prescription drugs are free for children, those aged 60 and older, and pregnant women. Others pay $15 per prescription. In some countries with an NHS, these services are free; in others there are copays which are usually waived for the retired and the poor.

This system is financed from general tax revenues, and therefore it must compete with other government services and programs each year. Unfortunately, this

J.E. Dalen
Professor Emeritus of Medicine and Public Health, University of Arizona, Tucson, AZ, USA

N.J. Johnson and L.P. Johnson (eds.), *The Care of the Uninsured in America*,
DOI 10.1007/978-0-387-78309-3_19, © Springer Science+Business Media, LLC 2010

Table 1 Health care statistics, 2003

Country	HCE/GDP	HCE/CAP	MD/100	% Insured
United Kingdom	7.7%	$2,231	2.2	100
Canada	9.9%	$3,001	2.1	100
Germany	11.1%	$2,996	3.4	100
Taiwan	6.0%[a]		1.3	100
US	15.0%	$5,635	2.3	84
China	5.5%	$ 55	1.6	22
OECD avg	8.8%	$2,394	3.1	NA

[a]2000

Source: OECD indicators: health at a glance (OECD 2005)

has led to chronic underfunding of the NHS in the UK. As shown in Table 1, the UK spent gross domestic product for health care compared to 8.8% for the 30 countries in the Organization for Economic Co-operation and Development (OECD 2005). This underfunding has caused a shortage of physicians and other health care workers and a shortage of modern health care facilities. The number of physicians per 1,000 citizens in the UK in 2003 was 2.2, compared to 3.1 for the 30 nations in the OECD (2005). There is a significant shortage of specialists in the UK. This shortage of health personnel has caused waiting lists for elective surgery and certain diagnostic tests such as CT scans and MRIs. In 1998 there were 1.3 million people on waiting lists (Klein 2006) and 30,000 of these patients had been on waiting lists for more than 1 year (Klein 2004). In order to circumvent waiting lists, many UK citizens purchase private health insurance. Since NHS specialists are allowed to practice part time outside the NHS, patients with private insurance can have diagnostic tests and elective surgery outside the NHS without a long wait.

In 2000, the UK initiated an NHS plan to decrease waiting lists (Klein 2001). Taxes were increased in order to increase funding for the NHS. Additional physicians and other health care workers were recruited. Diagnostic and Treatment centers were established, often staffed by physicians from other countries. These treatment centers perform orthopedic procedures, cataract surgery, and diagnostic tests such as MRIs and CT scans. This has greatly shortened the waiting lists (Klein 2004).

Under this system, all citizens have access to health care with minimal out-of-pocket expense. Patients have free choice of their general practitioner, but may not have free choice of specialists and hospitals. Those without private health insurance may have long waits for high-technology diagnostic tests and elective surgery. In some of the other countries with an NHS the option of private insurance is not available, and all citizens are equally exposed to waiting lists.

The NHS has been successful in two areas where the US has failed. It provides access to health care to all its citizens and it has controlled its expenditures for health care.

The Social Insurance Model

This model had its origins in Germany in the nineteenth century. Low-income workers and their employers were required to pay for social insurance which could be used for medical expenses. The insurance was administered by a number of "sickness funds" corresponding to a variety of occupations. By 1990, 90% of Germans had social insurance, and 10% of the population, certain government employees, self-employed, and very high-income citizens, were covered by private insurance (Brown and Amelung 1999). Germany was the first country to achieve universal health insurance coverage. This insurance is portable and permanent, and covers primary and secondary care and prescription drugs. Most services have copays which are waived for the retired, indigent, and chronically ill. Copays cannot exceed 2% of annual income.

Patients obtain their insurance by paying a premium of approximately 14% of their income to 1 of 420 "sickness funds" based on their occupation. The premium is shared with the employer. There is no extra charge for dependents. The premium for the unemployed is paid by unemployment insurance. Even though this payroll tax is mandatory, social insurance via "sickness funds" is seen as distinct from taxes and has greater support than taxes (Cuellar and Weiner 2000).

Health care is provided by the private sector rather than the government. Physician fees are negotiated nationally. Physician fees and hospital charges are paid by the sickness funds. Patients have free choice of GPs, specialists, and hospitals. Germany has more physicians per 1,000 population in 2003, 3.4, than the OECD average; 3.1 (OECD 2005) There is no rationing of health care, and, as in most countries with this model, there are minimal waiting lists. Germany spends 11.1% of GDP on health care compared to the OECD average of 8.8% (OECD 2005).

The role of the Federal government is to provide national standards and provide oversight of health care.

The Canadian Model

The Canadian model is a hybrid. The government provides health insurance, termed Medicare, to all its residents, but health care is delivered by the private sector rather than the government. All legal residents have access to physician care and hospital care without copays. Prescription drugs require copays. Drug costs are less than half the price in the US because the government controls drug prices. Patients have free choice of GPs, specialists, and hospitals. Health care is administered by the provinces with oversight from the Federal government. Administrative costs are 17% of all health care expenditures in Canada as compared to 31% in the US (Woolhandler et al. 2003).

More than half of all Canadian physicians are GPs. They see more patients per week than US physicians and they earn less.

As in the UK, health care is funded by general taxation, and as a result it is vulnerable to changes in the economy. The expenses are shared by the Federal government and the ten provinces and three territories. Originally, in the 1970s, the Federal share was 50%. By 2002 the government share had decreased to 16%. In 2003 the Federal share was guaranteed to be at least 25% of total health care expenses (Iglehart 2000). In the late 1980s and early 1990s, there were serious deficits in the national budget. As a result, in the 1990s major cuts were made in the health care budget. Hospital beds were reduced, some hospitals were closed, the number of medical students and medical residents and nursing students was reduced, and purchase of medical equipment was restricted. The percentage of GDP spent on health care decreased from 10.2% in 1992 to 9.3% in 1998. (Iglehart 2000) The predictable end result of these measures was a shortage of medical personnel and facilities which has led to waiting lists for elective surgery and certain diagnostic tests. The percentage of Canadians who were satisfied with their health care decreased from 61% in 1991 to 24% in 1999 (Iglehart 2000).

Unlike the UK, private insurance to cover physician or hospital care is not allowed in Canada. However, because of the recent waiting lists, private for-profit diagnostic and treatment centers are being established in some provinces even though they are illegal. This had led to fears that Canada may evolve into a two-tier system of health care: private clinics for the affluent and Medicare for the remainder of the population. (Steinbrook 2006) A major increase in health care expenditures in 2004 is expected to decrease waiting times by increasing the number of physicians and other health professionals.

Canada spends less on health care (9.9% of GDP) than the US (15.0%) (OECD 2005), yet all Canadians have access to health care without charge. Multiple studies have demonstrated that the quality of care in the US and in Canada is comparable (Lasser et al. 2006; Guyatt et al. 2007).

The US Model: Employment-Based Health Insurance

The majority of Americans have employment-based insurance which had its origins in World War II when wages were frozen by the Federal government. In order to compete for workers employers began to offer health insurance as part of a fringe benefit package. This soon became the dominant source of health insurance in the US. As shown in Table 2, in 2005, more than 60% of Americans younger than 65

Table 2 Source of health insurance in US, age <65, 2005

Employment based	63%
Private insurance	5%
Medicaid/SCHIP	11%
Military (CHAMPUS)	2%
None	18%

Source: Kaiser Commission on Medicaid and the Uninsured. October 2006

had employment-based health insurance (Kaiser Commission on Medicaid and the Uninsured 2006a, b). On the average, the employer pays 50–75% of the premium, and the employee pays 25–50%. Unlike social insurance in Europe, this health insurance is not portable and it is not permanent.

Not all employers provide health insurance. Some workers are afraid to leave their current job because the next employer may not provide health insurance. Nearly all employers who have more than a thousand employees provide insurers, whereas many small employers do not. The price of employer-provided insurance has increased more rapidly than the cost of living. From 2000 to 2006, the cost of employer-based health insurance increased by 87%, while inflation increased 18% (Kaiser Family Foundation Employer Health 2006). The constantly increasing price of health insurance makes it difficult for US businesses to compete with industries based on countries that have lower health care costs. As the costs of health insurance have escalated, employers have responded by increasing the employee's share of the premium, increasing deductibles, and/or increasing copays. The net result is increased out of pocket medical expenses for the employee. Some employees discontinue health insurance when the cost is increased. Some employers have stopped providing health insurance. The number of businesses offering health insurance decreased from 66% in 2001 to 61% in 2006 (Kaiser Commission on Medicaid and the Uninsured 2006a, b).

Since employment-based insurance is the primary source of health insurance in the US, as some employers stop providing health insurance, the number of uninsured Americans has steadily progressed. By 2005, 46 million, 15% of all Americans, were uninsured, and an additional 16% were underinsured (Kaiser Commission on Medicaid and the Uninsured 2006a, b). The majority of the uninsured are employed or the dependents of those employed.

In the absence of employment-based insurance, Americans have three options. They can purchase individual health insurance, or they may qualify for government-provided insurance or health care, or they can go without insurance.

Health insurance when purchased by an individual is even more expensive than when purchased by an employer. The average cost of family coverage in 2005 was $11,480 (Kaiser Family Foundation Employer Health 2006). It would be very difficult for a family with the US median family income to afford family coverage. The cost of private health insurance is even higher, or it may be impossible to obtain insurance, if any of the family members are old or if anyone has a chronic medical condition. Less than 10% of Americans have individually purchased health insurance (Kaiser Commission on Medicaid and the Uninsured 2006a, b). One reason for the high cost of US health insurance is that on average, one-third of the premium pays for billing and administration and profit to the insurance company. Only two-third of the premium is spent on health care (Kahn et al. 2005).

Prior to the passage of Medicaid and Medicare in 1966 there were few federal programs to provide health care for the elderly or the uninsured. City and county hospitals provided hospital care and outpatient care in some areas. The availability and the quality of care in these hospitals and clinics varied extensively across the nation.

Attempts to introduce universal health care in the US date back to 1912, when Theodore Roosevelt advocated national social insurance, to include health insurance. In 1935 Franklin Roosevelt wanted national health insurance (NHI) to be part of the social security act. He had to drop health insurance from the package in order to ensure passage of the Social Security Act. Harry Truman was a strong advocate of NHI in 1945 but was opposed by many forces including the American Medical Association. In 1951 it was suggested that NHI be limited to those eligible for social security benefits. In 1962, John Kennedy proposed that health insurance be added to the benefits of those eligible for Social Security. Finally, the strong arm of Lyndon Johnson secured passage of Medicare in 1965. President Johnson presented the first Medicare card to Harry Truman, and Medicare became effective in 1966.

The US Model: Medicare

All those eligible for Social Security or Railroad retirement benefits are eligible for Medicare when they reach age 65. In later legislation, patients with end-stage renal disease and the permanently disabled were also made eligible.

Medicare Part A covers inpatient hospital care, skilled nursing facility care, and home health care. It is funded by a payroll tax of 2.9% of all income. Employers and employees each pay 50%. This tax goes to the Medicare trust Fund and can only be spent for Medicare.

Medicare Part B covers physician services and outpatient care including X-rays and lab tests, and is financed by beneficiary premiums (25%) and the Federal government (75%). As more services are performed in the outpatient setting the cost of Medicare B is growing faster than Medicare A. Medicare Parts A and B have deductibles and copays that can be paid by optional supplemental ("Gap") insurance.

Coverage for prescription drugs, Medicare part D, became effective in 2006. Unlike Parts A and B, Medicare D is not administered by Medicare. Medicare D is administered by hundreds of private insurers. Two provisions of Medicare D have faced criticism (Dalen and Hartz 2005). Medicare is not allowed to negotiate drug prices with drug manufacturers as is done in nearly every other country. In addition, there is a gap (termed the "hole in the doughnut") in coverage once drug expenses exceed $2,250 (Iglehart 2004).

Initially, Medicare paid hospitals and physicians their usual charges or the prevailing charges. Hospitals are now paid by disease-related groups (DRGs). There is a set payment for hospitalization for various specific conditions (DRGs). The payment from Medicare does not vary with the length of hospitalization or the number of procedures performed. This has led to decreases in the length of stay in hospitals. Physicians are paid by a system called Relative Value Units (RVUs). Each procedure is assigned an RVU. For example a follow-up office visit for an established patient may be assigned an RVU of 1.0, and the performance of a coronary artery bypass graft may be assigned an RVU of 30. Payment to the physician is equal to the product of the RVU of that procedure times a dollar amount that is determined by Medicare annually.

After 40 years of experience Medicare has been very successful in providing care to 42 million enrollees (2005). More than 600,000 physicians and 5,000 US hospitals participate. The average spending per enrollee is $6,883, considerably less than the cost of private health insurance for younger, healthier patients. The administrative costs of this government-run program are less than 2% (Center for Medicare and Medicaid Services 2007a, b): less than the overhead of private US health insurers: 11–12% (Iglehart 2000).

The US Model: Medicaid

When Medicaid was enacted along with Medicare in 1966, it attracted little attention. Its original intent was to provide health care to those who are eligible for welfare and have children, and for those with low income who are blind or otherwise disabled. In the 1980s coverage was expanded to cover single women with children, children younger than six, and low-income Medicare patients. In 1997 the State Children's Health Insurance program (SCHIP) was established to expand Medicaid eligibility to uninsured children (Iglehart 2003). By 2006, 6 million children and 600,000 adults who did not qualify for other public programs were enrolled (Center for Medicare and Medicaid Services 2007a, b). It is estimated that between 7.5 and 10 million children remain uninsured.

By 2005, Medicaid covered more than 60 million Americans and expenditures of more than $300 billion exceeded those of Medicare (Iglehart 2007). Of the 60 million people receiving Medicaid, 72% are children and their parents. The remaining 23% are disabled adults and 7 million low-income Medicare patients ("dual-eligibles") (Iglehart 2007). However, children and their parents account for only 30% of Medicaid expenses. The disabled and the low-income Medicare patients, many of whom are in nursing homes, account for 70% of Medicaid expenses (Iglehart 2007). The administrative costs of Medicaid are 5.9% (Center for Medicare and Medicaid Services 2007b), higher than Medicare (<2%) but much less than private insurers (11–12%).

Medicaid is jointly funded by the Federal Government and the individual states. The federal government provides funds to states that operate approved medical assistance plans. Federal funds for Medicaid represent 40% of all federal funds received by states. Each state's share depends upon the state's per capita income. The federal share varies from a minimum of 50% to wealthy states to a maximum of 77% to the poorest state (Center for Medicare and Medicaid Services 2007b). As in Canada, where healthcare expenses are shared by the Federal and provincial governments, there are constant battles between Congress and the states as to the appropriate Federal share.

In order to qualify for Medicaid, the state must provide certain basic benefits to all those eligible for Medicaid as show in Table 3. A state may elect to provide the

Table 3 US medicaid benefits

Basic benefits	Optional benefits
In patient hospital care	Prescription drugs
Outpatient hospital care	Dental care
Physician services	Podiatry care
Lab and X-ray	Optical care
Prenatal care	
Vaccines	
Family planning services	
Home health care	

Table 4 What US medicaid pays for:

48% of nursing home care
40% of HIV/AIDS expenses
37% of all births
25% of children's health care
19% of all US prescription drugs

additional benefits shown in Table 3. If the state elects to provide additional benefits, the Federal government will share the expenses. Since most states do provide additional benefits Medicaid benefits are more extensive than Medicare or private insurance. There are minimal copays.

Each state administers its Medicaid program and determines the eligibility requirements. The eligibility rules have been described as being "legendary in their complexity." Eligibility is based on the individual or family income. These eligibility requirements vary widely among the 50 states. In some states those with a family income of less than three times the federal poverty level are eligible. In other states, only families with incomes less than the federal poverty level are eligible.

Each state also determines how much they will pay hospitals, physicians, and other health care providers. The per capita expenses per year per enrollee vary widely among the states. Medicaid reimbursement is much lower than private insurance and less than Medicare. As a result of low reimbursement 30% of US physicians did not participate in Medicaid in 2002 (Iglehart 2003). Medicaid patients in some areas are unable to find a primary care provider and therefore use expensive emergency room care.

There has been a progressive increase in the number of states that enroll Medicaid patients in HMOs. In 1992, 4 million were in HMOs; by 2002, 58% of all Medicaid patients, mostly mothers and children, were enrolled in HMOs (Iglehart 2003).

Medicaid, with total expenditures of $312 Billion in 2005, plays a critical role in financing US health care system as shown in Table 4. As Medicaid expenses have increased there has been increasing pressure from the federal government and the states to control costs. These pressures resulted in passage of the Deficit Reduction Act of 2005, which has a goal of cutting $26 Billion from Medicaid from 2006 to 2015 (Iglehart 2007). The cuts in expenses will come from copays and premiums and decreased benefits.

A major disadvantage of Medicaid as compared to Medicare is that it is funded by general tax revenues, rather than a designated payroll tax which pays for Medicare A. This makes the Medicaid budget more vulnerable to cuts in funding than Medicare. Since Medicaid is means-tested it is seen by many as "welfare" whereas Medicare is seen as a "right." The vulnerability of Medicaid funding is further increased because Medicaid recipients have much less political clout than the Medicare population.

Health Care in the Two Chinas: Taiwan

In 1949, Chiang Kai-shek and the Chinese Nationalist party fled from Mao Tse-Tung and the Chinese Communist Party on mainland China and settled on the island of Formosa, 124 miles from the mainland. They established a new nation Taiwan, the Republic of China. Mainland China became the People's Republic of China.

The new nation of 23 million on Taiwan established social insurance, similar to the German model. By 1980, 20% of the population was covered by social insurance; by 1995, 60% were insured. Most of the uninsured were the poor and children (Cheng 2003).

In 1995, they established Taiwan NHI. NHI is mandatory, and is financed through premiums and taxes. The NHI premiums are 4.6% of income and are shared by employees and employers. The average monthly premium for a family of four is $42 US. Employees pay 30% of the premium, the poor and the unemployed do not pay a premium. The nonpoor, self-employed pay 100% of the premium. The administrative overhead of the NHI was 2.2%, similar to US Medicare (Cheng 2003)

NHI covers in patient care, ambulatory care, lab tests, and prescription drugs. It also covers most preventive care and some home health care. There are modest copays which are capped at 10% of the national average income.

Health care is delivered by the private sector. There is free choice of physicians and hospitals. Referrals for specialty care are not required. There is no rationing, and no waiting lists. The number of physicians per 1,000 in 1999 was only 1.3, compared to 2.7 in the US (Cheng 2003). Taiwan physicians see more patients per week than in the US. Forty percent of physicians are in private practice in clinics and are paid fee for service. Fees are established by the NHI (Cheng 2003). Sixty percent are specialists practicing in hospitals and are paid salaries plus bonuses.

The majority of hospitals are nonprofit, and there are more beds per 1,000 (5.7) than in the US (3.6) (Cheng 2003). The NHI pays hospitals through a global budget.

The entire population has access to health care, and the percentage satisfied with their care in 2002 was 70% (Lu and Hsiao 2003). This has been accomplished with total health expenditures of only 6% of the Gross Domestic Product in 2000 (Lu and Hsiao 2003).

Provision of health care in Mainland China, the largest country in the world, with a population of 1.3 billion, is a formidable task. Although there are many huge cities, 70% of the population live in rural areas and are extremely poor.

Health care Under Mao Tse-tung from 1949 to 1976 has been well described by Blumenthal and Hsiao (2005). The communist government opened medical schools and schools for nurses and pharmacists. They built hospitals; by 1965 every county had a modern hospital. They blended traditional Chinese medicine with western medicine and stressed public health and prevention. The government controlled all hospitals and employed all doctors and health care workers. They established free urban and rural clinics. In addition to health care, the government provided wages, housing, education, and pensions.

Eighty percent of the population lived in communes in rural areas and worked on collective farms. They had access to a three-tier health care system (Blumenthal and Hsiao 2005). Village medical centers were the first tier. These village centers were staffed by 1.2 million "barefoot doctors" who were grade school educated and then had 2–6 months training in their village. They provided preventive care, vaccination, and could deliver babies and provide contraception advice. The emphasis of the village health centers was prevention, sanitation, and primary care.

The second tier for those in rural areas was township health centers: outpatient clinics with 10–30 beds. These served 10–30,000 and were manned by better trained assistant doctors. County hospitals staffed by medical school graduates that served 200–300,000 people were the third tier.

The twenty percent living in cities worked in state-owned collective enterprises also had access to a three-tier system of health care. The first tier was factory and neighborhood clinics manned by paramedical personnel. Tier two facilities were district hospitals, and tier three were municipal hospitals with medical school graduates.

The three-tier health care system established by Mao was very successful. Strong government public health programs focused on sanitation, immunization, and control of infectious diseases (Hesketh and Zhu 1997). Life expectancy increased from 38 to 68 years, and there was a marked decrease in infant mortality (Liu 2004a).

In the early 1980s there was dramatic shift in the Chinese economy to a profit-oriented capitalistic economy. Communes and collective farms were dismantled; agriculture was privatized. Money-losing government-run factories were closed. Government control and government funding to rural areas was markedly reduced (Liu 2004b).

The public health system was underfunded and dismantled. Public health and the provision of health care were delegated to the local authorities who lacked funding. The central government's share of health care expenditures decreased from 32% in 1978 to 15% in 1999 (Blumenthal and Hsiao 2005).

By 1998, only 9.5% of those in rural areas and 42 percent in urban areas had health insurance (Liu 2004a). Health care is paid out of pocket. Patients have to pay for immunizations. Many can't afford to pay, so are not immunized.

Hospitals have become privatized with minimal state support. They are not regulated by the government. Urban areas have modern hospitals for those who can pay. Patients without insurance must pay before they can be admitted to hospitals; when patients run out of funds they are discharged (Liu 2004a). Hospitals grossly overcharge for diagnostic tests and for prescription drugs which are overprescribed (Blumenthal and Hsiao 2005).

The average physician's salary is about the same as a taxi driver. The salary of physicians in rural areas is even less, so many have left rural areas. Physicians also increase their income by overprescribing and overcharging for prescription drugs and expensive diagnostic test. Physicians are not regulated; there are many poorly trained physicians and former barefoot doctors who provide services that they were not trained to do.

The government devotes only 5.5% of GDP to health care: $55 per capita per year (Blumenthal and Hsiao 2005). The number of physicians per 1,000 (1.6) and the number of hospital beds per 1,000 population (2.4) are much less than OECD averages (3.1, 4.3) (OECD 2005).

The current economy of China is one of the fastest growing in the world. Unfortunately health care in China is proceeding downhill at an equally rapid rate.

References

Blumenthal D, Hsiao W (2005) Privatization and its discontents – the evolving Chinese health care system. N Engl J Med 353:1165–1170

Brown LD, Amelung VE (1999) Mangled competition: market reforms in German health care. Health Aff 118:76–91

Center for Medicare and Medicaid Services (2007a) Available at: http://www.cms.hhs.gov/CapM. Accessed 27 Jun 2007

Center for Medicare and Medicaid Services (2007b) Available at: http://www.cms.hhs.gov/CFOR. Accessed 27 Jun 2007

Cheng TM (2003) Taiwan's new national health insurance program: genesis and experience so far. Health Aff 22:61–76

Cuellar AE, Weiner JM (2000) Can social insurance for long-term care work? The experience of Germany. Health Aff 19:8–25

Dalen JE, Hartz DJ (2005) Medicare prescription coverage: a very long wait for a very modest benefit. Am J Med 118:325–329

Guyatt G, Devereaux PJ, Lexchin J, Stone SB, Yalnizyan A, Himmelstein D, Woolhandler S, Zhou Q, Goldsmith LJ, Cook DJ, Haines T, Lacchetti C, Lavis JN, Sullivan T, Mills E, Kraus A, Bhatnagar N (2007) A systematic review of studies comparing health outcomes in Canada and the United States. Open Med 1:27–36

Hesketh T, Zhu WX (1997) Health in China: from Mao to market reform. BMJ 314:1543–1548

Iglehart JK (2000) Revisiting the Canadian health care system. N Engl J Med 342:2007–2012

Iglehart JK (2003) The dilemma of Medicaid. N Engl J Med 348:2140–2148

Iglehart JK (2004) The new Medicare prescription-drug benefit – a pure power play. N Engl J Med 350:826–833

Iglehart JK (2007) Medicaid revisited – skirmishes over a vast public enterprise. N Engl J Med 356:734–740

Kahn JG, Kronick R, Kreger M, Gans DM (2005) The cost of health insurance administration in California: estimates for insurers, physicians, and hospitals. Health Aff 24:1629–1639

Kaiser Commission on Medicaid and the Uninsured (2006a) Available at: http://www.kff.org/uninsured/7571.cfm. Accessed 28 Jun 2007

Kaiser commission on Medicaid and the Uninsured (2006b) Available at: http://www.kff.org/uninsured/7570.cfm. Accessed 27 Jun 2007

Kaiser Family Foundation Employer Health Benefits (2006) Available at: http://www.kff.org/insurance/7527/upload/7528. Accessed 27 Jun 2007

Klein R (2001) What's happening to Britain's national health service? N Engl J Med 345:305–308

Klein R (2004) Britain's national health service revisited. N Engl J Med 350:937–942

Klein R (2006) The troubled transformation of Britain's national health service. N Engl J Med; 355:409–414

Lasser KE, Himmelstein DU, Woolhandler S (2006) Access to care, health disparities in The United States and Canada: results of a cross-national population-based survey. Am J Public Health 96:1300–1307

Liu Y (2004a) China's public health-care system: facing the challenges. Bull World Health Organ 82:532–538

Liu Y (2004b) Development of the rural health insurance system in China. Health Policy Plan 19:159–165

Lu JFR, Hsiao WC (2003) Does universal health insurance make health care unaffordable? Lessons from Taiwan. Health Aff 22:77–88

OECD (2005) Health at a Glance OECD indicators. Available at: http://www.oecd.org/document/11/0,3343. Accessed 28 Jun 2007

Steinbrook R (2006) Private health care in Canada. N Engl J Med 354:1661–1664

Woolhandler S, Campbell T, Himmelstein DU (2003) Costs of health care administration in the United States and Canada. N Engl J Med 349:768–775

Think Nationally, Act Locally

Lane P. Johnson

Our favorite description of the United State Health Care system was one given by Dr. Terry Cullen in a lecture to a class of medical students in a Masters of Public Health (MPH) Program. Dr. Cullen described the US Health Care system as *a patchwork quilt with a lot of big holes in it* (Cullen 2008).

Approaching the question of what can be done to provide quality, lower cost, and accessible health care to the entire US population, the patchwork quilt is an apt metaphor. There are pieces of the quilt that are of excellent quality, pieces that do the job more than adequately, other pieces that are old and falling apart, and gaping holes that leave large sections of the bed uncovered. So what can one do with an old quilt? Commit to re-covering the entire structure? Patch the holes as best as one can? Throw it away and start again? Such is the dilemma that confronts the remodeling of the American Health Care System. What is not lacking is a wide spectrum of strong opinions about how it should be done.

It is not likely that the health care system will be made anew. An essay by Atul Gawande in the New Yorker (2009) does a wonderful job in outlining how most countries, when they have implemented national health care systems, have designed the system based upon the history, politics, policies, and institutions that were already in existence in that country. This is one reason why there is such a diversity of national health systems in countries across the world: government-run, employer-funded, private insurance based, separate national taxes for health care, etc.; each country's system reflects the political environment of that country at the time of the implementation of their national health care system.

The conservative political approach to the problem of health care coverage continues to consider market forces and managed competition as the driver of lower health costs. Consumers purchase a high-deductible and/or catastrophic health insurance plan, and have a health savings account with which they can purchase health care services by making choices among health service providers. Supplemental

L.P. Johnson
Arizona Health Sciences Center,
Tucson, AZ, USA
e-mail: lpj@email.arizona.edu

N.J. Johnson and L.P. Johnson (eds.), *The Care of the Uninsured in America*,
DOI 10.1007/978-0-387-78309-3_20, © Springer Science+Business Media, LLC 2010

insurance can be provided by employers or purchased on the open market (D'Angelo and Moffit 2006).

Contrary to the conservative approach is the HR 676, the United States National Health Insurance Act, introduced in 2007, which proposes a National Health Insurance Program to provide free health care including primary care and prevention, prescription drugs, emergency care, and mental health services for all individuals residing in the United States and in US territories. The bill currently has over 60 cosponsors (Govtrack.us 2007). Congressman Raul Grijalva (Dem-Arizona), a cosponsor, has stated that, while the bill is not popular with the current administration, or likely to pass in its present form, it is important in that it continues to press the issue of universal coverage that would otherwise not be on the table (Grijalva 2009).

The current administration's proposal tries to take the middle ground by suggesting that affordable, accessible health care for all Americans can be implemented using the existing system (The White House 2009). Provisions include:

- Require insurance companies to cover pre-existing conditions so all Americans regardless of their health status or history can get comprehensive benefits at fair and stable premiums.
- Create a new Small Business Health Tax Credit to help small businesses provide affordable health insurance to their employees.
- Lower costs for businesses by covering a portion of the catastrophic health costs they pay in return for lower premiums for employees.
- Prevent insurers from overcharging doctors for their malpractice insurance and invest in proven strategies to reduce preventable medical errors.
- Make employer contributions more fair by requiring large employers that do not offer coverage or make a meaningful contribution to the cost of quality health coverage for their employees to contribute a percentage of payroll toward the costs of their employees' health care.
- Establish a National Health Insurance Exchange with a range of private insurance options as well as a new public plan based on benefits available to members of Congress that will allow individuals and small businesses to buy affordable health coverage.
- Ensure everyone who needs it will receive a tax credit for their premiums.

Details as of this writing (April, 2009) are sparse, but some of the first specific suggestions by the administration include $634 billion for a reserve fund for health care reform, drug company discounts to Medicaid programs, cutting Medicare payments to health insurance companies providing comprehensive Medicare programs, cutting Medicare payments to hospitals for patients readmitted within 30 days of discharge, and decreasing payment to home health agencies (Pear 2009). While the details of these and many other policies remain to be revealed and fought over, the stage is certainly being set for some significant ideological and political battles.

As Dr. Dalen discussed in chapter "The Role of Government in Providing Health Care to the Uninsured," the United States has made at least five major efforts at implementing universal health care, most recently, in the early 1990s under the

Clinton administration. A critique of that effort has suggested that the process may have failed in part, at least, because of the following issues:

- There was insufficient congressional input to the plan's development despite public input prior to the proposal.
- The plan proposed the creation of a National Health Board in charge of regulating health care.
- Required standardized minimal benefits for each Insurance plan.
- Mandatory Employer Sponsored Health Coverage up to 80% of the full cost of the premium.
- The plan underestimated the polarity of the health care debate and the strength on both sides of the political spectrum coming together in opposition to the plan (Montgomery 2006).

Further, the Clinton reform effort did little to take on the established corporate and institutional stakeholders in the process, and also underestimated their power in opposing change (Oberlander 2007).

While the current administration is doing much to acknowledge and distance itself from the health reform failures of the past, there is much that hasn't changed in the national political arena. We believed this does not bode well for the prospects of national health reform in the short run.

What is the likelihood of a national health insurance program to cover the almost 50 million residents of the United States who do not have medical insurance being implemented at this time? From a historical perspective our belief is, not much. The longer answer begs a larger perspective of the political landscape of the national health system.

In order to begin to consider what the options for a national medical insurance program might look like, one must first consider the question: for whom is the current American Health Care system designed?

Certainly it is not designed for the patient. Complex, constantly changing, Byzantine regulations make it virtually impossible for even college-educated patients to figure out how to maneuver through the system.

Certainly it is not designed for the providers. Many experienced physicians, by and large, are looking for less complex ways of making a living. One of the fastest growing models of "primary care" is the "Concierge Medicine"; exclusive care of patients who have the means to pay directly for their medical service. Specialists spend more time doing procedures for which they can be reimbursed, and significantly less time actually taking care of patients. This is not a model that bodes well for the populace as a whole.

An even cursory look at the American Health Care System as it operates today reveals that it is designed to provide the highest return to the health insurance companies, pharmaceutical companies, and other medical vendors, and trial lawyers. It is no accident these three groups represent many of the largest contributors to both political parties on a national level. Look at Part D of Medicare. Look at tort reform. Look at any health insurance document. Look at the editorial page of the *Wall Street Journal*. They are all reflective of the power of the large stakeholders. This is why we believe it is unlikely that any national legislation will be successful in fundamentally changing the health care system in the United States in the near future.

The United States spends almost twice as much per capita as any other developed country. There is no question that there should be sufficient funding to provide basic health care for all US citizens and residents, if the political will existed to make the necessary changes. Sadly, that political will does not and is not likely to exist in the near future, given current special interests and the financial and political power they are able to wield.

Looking to the States

Interestingly, a number of states have not waited for the federal government to move forward on medical insurance coverage issues, but are finding their own methods to try to cover more, if not all, of their state residents. In most cases they are seeking ways to leverage funding that also includes federal support. The variety of approaches and successes will likely ultimately serve as a model for a national health program. There is, in addition, a variety of proposed federal legislation to help support these state efforts (Imas 2007).

The advantages of state programs for coverage include that a state legislature may be more accessible and have a greater potential for change in the short term than the federal government. Even in a relatively conservative state such as Arizona, initiative ballots have been successful in improving the eligibility requirements for the State Medicaid Program (Arizona Health Care Cost Containment System, or AHCCCS program). Vested interests may have less of a stranglehold on the state legislative process, and greater experimentation and variability are possible, taking into consideration state interests, priorities, institutions, and stakeholders. Countering these issues are the fact that most states likely cannot afford universal coverage programs without Federal assistance, and economic downturns are far more likely to affect eligibility in a state-level program. Most of these statewide efforts are reviewed in greater detail in chapter "Care of Underserved People with Mental Illness."

Hawaii is the grandfather of near-universal coverage for state residents. Established in 1975, the Prepaid Health Care Act required nearly all employers to provide health coverage for employees who work 20 h or more a week. This is the only state that has enacted an employer mandate, though some employers (government services, insurance agents and real estate sales persons on commission, approved seasonal employees, and sole proprietors with no employees) are exempted from the act. Employees must also contribute to the program. Under this act the medically uninsured rate fell from 30 % to 5%, though it has since risen to 10% (National Conference of State Legislatures 2008; Gauthier 2006).

Some of the boldest reforms seek to provide comprehensive, near universal, coverage. Maine, Massachusetts, and Vermont have proposed to use Medicaid to partly fund subsidized medical coverage, combined with other reforms that reflect local priorities (Burton et al. 2007).

The Dirigo Health Reform Act in Maine provides for small businesses, the self-employed, and eligible individuals without access to employer-sponsored insurance, an "affordable option" with people earning less than 300% of poverty level eligible for a sliding scale subsidy(National Conference of State Legislatures 2008; Kaiser Commission on Medicaid and the Uninsured 2008). However, there is at least some preliminary evaluation that suggests the program may not have substantially reduced the number of medically underinsured in Maine, and may be under-enrolled and underfunded (Sylvester 2009; Belluck 2007).

The Massachusetts Universal Health Care Package requires all residents to obtain health insurance (similar to automobile insurance) or pay a penalty, through a market-based system; combining federal funding through Medicaid, and a "fair and reasonable" contribution from employers. The Commonwealth Health Insurance Connector has been developed as a critical piece of the program to help businesses and individuals find affordable health insurance (Burton et al. 2007; Fahrenthold 2006; National Conference of State Legislatures, 2008; Kaiser Commission on Medicaid and the Uninsured, 2008). As of early 2009, evaluation showed that slightly more than 50% of previously medically uninsured are now insured, but that the program is much more expensive than was anticipated, forcing cuts to safety net providers, and forcing some insured patients to have to pay out-of-pocket for expenses they did not previously have to pay (Nardin et al. 2009; Sack 2009). Among the other unintended consequences of the Massachusetts Universal Health Care Package was the discovery that, given universal coverage, there are far too few primary care providers to take care of the number of patients who became eligible (Sack 2008).

Vermont's Catamount Health Plan, passed in 2006, has set a goal to assuring insurance coverage for 96% of state residents by 2010, through a subsidized private insurance "product" for families with incomes up to 300% of poverty levels, along with employer contributions. Vermont's program emphasizes management of chronic care, and includes funding from several sources, including an increased tobacco tax (Burton et al. 2007; Imas 2007; National Conference of State Legislatures 2008; Kaiser Commission on Medicaid and the Uninsured 2008). Evaluation of the program in 2008 suggests that this program is also suffering from increased costs, decreased funding from the state and federal sources, and is having more difficulty enrolling members than originally anticipated (Sidortsova 2008).

There are a number of other state efforts working to increase the number of state residents with medical insurance coverage. Illinois passed an act making insurance coverage available to all uninsured children; Pennsylvania has proposed a similar action. New Jersey has proposed raising the age of dependent status for health insurance to age 30, making 200,000 young adults (who are among the most likely not to have insurance) eligible for coverage. Other states in the process of proposing universal health coverage programs include California, Colorado, Connecticut, Kansas, Minnesota, New Mexico, New York, Oregon, Wisconsin, and Washington (Burton et al. 2007; Imas 2007; National Conference of State Legislatures 2008; Kaiser Commission on Medicaid and the Uninsured 2008). It should also be noted that at least one municipality, San Francisco, is working locally to reform medical insurance coverage for the uninsured by redirecting existing city funds, implementing a federal grant for expanding access, soliciting patient contributions, and legislating a requirement that business with more than 20 workers contribute a set amount to health care.(Sack 2007).

Gauthier (2006) suggests that the strategies that States should use in their efforts to expand coverage should include:

1. Design shared responsibility strategy to include state, employers, and individuals:

   - Expand public programs
   - Provide financial assistance to low income workers and employers to afford coverage
   - Require employers to offer benefit plans
   - Mandate individuals to purchase coverage
   - Require employers to offer and employees to take up insurance

2. Require insurers to raise age limit for dependents.
3. Pool purchasing power and promote new benefit designs to make coverage more affordable.
4. Develop reinsurance programs to make coverage more affordable in the small group and individual markets.

Moving Forward

It is tempting to look on the reform of medical insurance in the United States as an issue on par with the civil rights movement, with national reform being the logical outcome of demonstrations against unfair and unjust national priorities and policies. The sad fact remains, however, that the stalemate on the national level serves to support vested financial and political interests (of both parties) and is, in our opinion, unlikely to change soon.

We believe statewide efforts currently provide the best opportunity for reform over the short term, as it appears more likely stakeholders can be brought together, issues can be addressed, compromise can be achieved, programs can be hammered out, administered, evaluated, and improved on a state-by-state basis.

This is not to say it will be easy. But while it is frustrating to think of having to battle for health care reform in each and every state, state-centered efforts serve as a more realistic platform for individual, and local advocacy, and for the development of a set of programs that really must reflect more local conditions.

In this book, we have hopefully demonstrated how the differences among medically uninsured populations are equally as significant as the similarities. Solutions may best be developed on a patient by patient, clinic by clinic, community by community, county by county, and state-by-state basis, in collaboration with others. Similarly, statewide programs, policies, and financial issues need to look locally and then draw support nationally to continue to improve access for the medically disenfranchised. We believe it will be from these individual, local, and statewide efforts, ultimately, that a national program can finally be put into place. Then it will be time to celebrate.

Until then, it is time to get back to work.

References

Burton A, Friedenzohn I, Martinez-Vidal E (2007) State strategies to expand health insurance coverage: trends and lessons for policymakers, in State of the States 2007; Building hope, raising expectations, Robert Wood Johnson Foundation's State Coverage Initiatives Program. Available at http://www.commonwealthfund.org/publications/publications_show.htm?doc_id=461903. Accessed 10 May 2008

Belluck P (2007) As health plan falters, main explores changes. New York Times. April 30, 2007. Available at http://www.nytimes.com/2007/04/30/us/30maine.html?pagewanted=1&_r=1. Accessed 10 May 2008

Cullen T (2008) Class lecture on indigent Care, Issues and Trends in Public Health, MD-MPH Dual Degree Program, Tucson, AZ, October

D'Angelo G, Moffit RE (2006) Building on the successes of health savings accounts. The Heritage Foundation, October 20. Available at http://www.heritage.org/research/healthcare/wm1239.cfm. Accessed 5 Apr 2009

Fahrenthold D (2006) Mass. Bill requires health coverage, Washington Post, April 5, 2006. Available at http://www.gbio.org/maint/washington_post_4-5-06.pdf. Accessed 10 May 2008

Gauthier A (2006) Why not the best? A high performance health system in Hawaii. Hawaii Uninsured Project Fall Forum, October 2006. Available at http://www.healthcoveragehawaii.org/2006healthpolicyforum/Gauthier.Common wealth.10.23.06.ppt. Accessed 10 May 2008

Gawande A (2009) Getting there from here. The New Yorker. January 26, 2009. Available at http://www.newyorker.com/reporting/2009/01/26/090126fa_fact_gawande. Accessed 5 Apr 2009

Govtrack.us. (2007) United States National Health Insurance Act (or the Expanded and Improved Medicare for All Act), GovTrack.us (database of federal legislation) Available at http://www.govtrack.us/congress/bill.xpd?bill=h110-676&tab=summary. Accessed 5 Apr 2009

Grijalva R (2009) Healthcare Change Forum; February 14, 2009, Tucson, AZ

Imas K (2007) Under the microscope; states serve as laboratories for Universal Health Care Programs. State News; the council of state governments. February. Available at http://www.csg.org/pubs/Documents/sn0702UndertheMicroscope.pdf. Accessed 10 May 2008

Kaiser Commission on Medicaid and the Uninsured (2008) States moving towards comprehensive health care reform. Available at http://www.kff.org/uninsured/kcmu_statehealthreform.cfm. Accessed May 10, 2008

Montgomery K (2006) What was the Clinton Health Plan Proposal about, and why did it fail? Health Insurance; About.com. Retrieved 5 Apr 2009 from http://healthinsurance.about.com/od/faqs/f/clinton.htm

Nardin R, Himmelstein D, Woolhandler S (2009) Massachusetts' Plan: a failed model for health reform. Physicians for a National Health Program. February 18, 2009. Retrieved 5 Apr 2009 from http://pnhp.org/mass_report/mass_report_Final.pdf

National Conference of State Legislatures (2008) Comprehensive reforms; state examples, May 10, 2008, http://www.ncsl.org/programs/health/dhmaine.htm. Accessed 10 May 2008

Oberlander J (2007) Learning from failure in health care reform. NEJM 357(17):1677–1679

Pear R (2009) Obama offers broad plan to revamp health care. New York Times, 26 February 2009. Available at http://www.nytimes.com/2009/02/27/washington/27web-health.html. Accessed 5 Apr 2009

Sack K (2007) San Francisco to offer care for uninsured adults. New York Times, September 14, 2007. Available at http://www.nytimes.com/2007/09/14/us/14health.html. Accessed 11 May 2008

Sack K (2008) In Massachusetts, Universal coverage strains care. New York Times, April 5, 2008. Available at http://www.nytimes.com/2008/04/05/us/05doctors.html?scp=1&sq=%22strains%20care%22&st=cse. Accessed 5 Apr 2009

Sack K (2009) Massachusetts faces costs of big health care plan. New York Times, March 15, 2009. Available at http://www.nytimes.com/2009/03/16/health/policy/16mass.html?ref=policy. Accessed 5 Apr 2009

Sidortsova S (2008) Scoring catamount health. Vermont Public Interest Research and Education Fund. August, 2008. Available at http://www.vpirg.org/documents/CatamountScorecardIIFINAL.pdf. Accessed 5 April 2009

Sylvester B (2009) Health Experts Debate Baldacci's health plan. The Maine Campus, October 5, 2006.   Available   at   http://media.www.mainecampus.com/media/storage/paper322/ news/2006/10/05/   News/Health.Experts.Debate.Baldaccis.Health.Plan-2334104.shtml. Accessed 5 April, 2009
The White House (2009) Health Care. Available at http://www.whitehouse.gov/agenda/health_ care/. Accessed 5 April 2009

Resources

Ascension Health, Healthcare that leaves no one behind. http://www.ascensionhealth.org/ht_ leaves/main.asp

Cover the Uninsured, A Project of the Robert Wood Johnson Foundation. http://covertheunin-sured.org/

National Association of Community Health Centers, Access for All America Plan. http://www. nachc.com/access-for-america.cfm

National Conference of State Legislatures, Access to Healthcare and the Uninsured. http://www. ncsl.org/programs/health/h-primary.htm

St Luke's Health Initiative, A Catalyst for Community Health. http://www.slhi.org/

The Commonwealth Fund, Health Insurance. http://www.commonwealthfund.org/topics/topics_ list.htm?attrib_id=15 309

The Kaiser Family Foundation, Health Coverage and the Uninsured. http://www.kff.org/unin-sured/index.cfm http://www.nachc.com/access-for- america.cfm

Index